Cockburn Library, Yorkhill

T05532

616
047292
DOB
2013

Practical Treatment Options
for Chronic Pain in Children
and Adolescents

Library
Queen Elizabeth University
Hospital
Teaching & Learning Centre
0141 451 1216
library.qeuhc@ggc.scot.nhs.uk

15 JUL 2014

T   or before
                                     ow

Foreword I

This manual is a masterful, compelling, and satisfying read for all professionals in children's pain management. Going beyond the biomedical model, it provides a comprehensive appreciation of the physiology, psychology, pharmacology and familial/social aspects of common paediatric chronic pain syndromes. It emphasizes the broad impact of pain on the lives of children and teens, as well as the complicated process of recovery. Drs. Dobe and Zernikow achieve this by bringing us into the functioning of their inpatient treatment unit in Germany for children and teens with chronic pain. They share their intake procedures, assessment process and instruments, their well-developed decision-making processes, the nuances of their therapeutic program, interdisciplinary team's functioning and their research outcome – a tour de force!

What makes this chronic pain treatment program stand apart is the tight integration of clinical practice with their research program, based firmly within a biopsychosocial framework in the child-family systems context. In fact, they are consistently systems- oriented. A continuous flow-through of research findings informs the clinic's intake and treatment parameters, which in turn feeds their ongoing research. They give considerable attention to the patient's social, emotional, familial and physical systems. You'll note the well-integrated system of trained professionals – nurses, psychotherapists, physicians, psychologists and physiotherapists, and the different forms of psycho-biological treatment regimens to address and relieve pain that the children receive, either as outpatients or inpatients for 6 weeks in their 'Lighthouse' treatment unit.

With a 10-year history of treating some of the most distressed and pain-compromised children and teens in Germany (their patients aged 7–17 years have suffered chronic pain for an average of 3.5 years before starting treatment), the authors discuss their philosophy of care and treatment regimen in considerable detail. Their philosophy is based on principles that we've come to appreciate as critical for the effective treatment of children and teens. This includes principles of transparency, collaboration, requiring the child's commitment to treatment, incorporation of parents at pivotal decision and treatment points, challenging the patient's self-limiting behaviors, providing a well-organized treatment program that requires intensive work on the part of the child, and supporting the child's follow-through with engaging therapeutic relationships and active support to complete the program.

There is clinical brilliance and ingenuity in this intensive treatment program, particularly in the lively, sometimes challenging and strategic nature of their psychotherapy interventions, such as the 'Three Letters' in Chap. 6. There are aspects that some North American practitioners may find usual. The authors carefully explain their rationale and care in implementing these practices, their experience and research outcomes. One of these is that a child who does not take on all aspects of the program can be asked to leave. Under certain circumstances they can be invited to re-apply when they deem themselves ready. As part of that application they are required to write a convincing letter about what has changed and how they are now ready to fully engage with the 3-week treatment program.

Other novel practices are the 'Stress Day', an individually tailored challenge day, and 'Pain provocation' – an established cognitive behavioral strategy which ultimately provides the child with a greater sense of control over his or her pain. All of these techniques are described in sufficient detail for a clear appreciation of their therapeutic benefit. These are not boot camp techniques. They are implemented within empathic relationships and supportive and negotiable contexts, and consistently reflect their treatment approach of encouraging self-management.

Providing psycho-education on pain and ensuring that the children and teens understand it well enough to write about how pain is processed, is emphasized throughout this manual. With humor and transparency Drs. Dobe and Zernikow convey the idea that the doctor "isn't in charge of your body" and from the outset they change the relationship dynamic by asserting that it is the child who defines what is "the correct" pain perception, not the parents, psychotherapist or physician. A further declaration made early to the child and family is that sustained pain reduction cannot be achieved unless the child engages in learning and using active pain coping strategies. The authors provide detailed case examples of their multi-modal intake and treatment procedures, which makes their treatment system come to life. The child and family are required to make a commitment to this system, and it is evident that this is more than matched by a commitment by skilled personnel at every step along the trajectory towards pain relief.

Contrary to common practices, their treatment process is one that relies heavily and successfully on humor and playfulness as a therapeutic attitude for treating chronic pain. This is summed up by one of the teens in Chap. 4 who asks, "Why did you become a therapist, when you like to laugh so much?" This positive hope-giving attitude is supported by a therapeutic focus on enhancing the child's resources and problem- solving capacity – irrespective of the severity of the pain or symptoms of anxiety, depression or trauma.

Families of children with chronic pain suffer themselves. How to work with these families can sometimes present a particular challenge to the chronic pain team. Drs. Dobe and Zernikow address this from the very start and provide practical recommendations, case examples with dialogue, and strategies that help lay the groundwork for successful family teamwork. The parents, too, are part of the treatment process – and their learning and change provide for a better long-term outcome, once the child is discharged.

The hard truth of treating children and teens with chronic and complex pain is that there is no quick fix. I was heartened to read this statement by Dr. Boris Zernikow: "In a time of limited human resources and a shift to technical medicine the inpatient pain therapy program of the German Paediatric Pain Centre with its personnel-intensive multimodal approach focusing on the child and his/her family may seem to be a relic from the past. However, it is exactly that human approach that makes the program so successful."

Key, catchy phrases remind families and children of essential concepts in understanding pain, and these are reiterated throughout the treatment process. For example, Drs. Dobe, Kriszio and Zernikow discuss in Chap. 4 the "Three Thought Traps": 1."Everything is of pure psychological origin"; 2."Everything is of pure physical origin"; and 3."The pain must vanish at all costs". Debunking these commonly held myths as part of the initial psycho-education builds a solid foundation for the wide range of interventions that are explicated in this groundbreaking manual.

Chapter 6 is the heart of this manual on the treatment of paediatric chronic pain. This chapter alone is worth the price of the book. You'll be glued, as I was, to the discussion of how to assess and treat children who present with concomitant depression or trauma concurrent with their chronic pain. This is a unique contribution. In the paediatric pain literature to date, there is little research and discussion on children who have experienced trauma and present with chronic pain. We know clinically that their pain will not be successfully resolved without the skillful and sensitive concurrent treatment of the trauma and/or depression. Dr. Michael Dobe is masterful in his systematic exposition on how to engage the traumatized child. He discusses what images and therapeutic strategies are conducive to building psychological flexibility, adaptive cognitions and trust, while not re-traumatizing the child. Imaginative techniques, such as "The Safe Place", used to provide emotional stability and training in how to self-assess tension levels and use relaxation techniques, are but a few of the cognitive behavioral strategies that are well-described in this chapter.

Drs. Dobe and Zernikow have included in this manual contributions from their team members Drs. Wager, Kriszio, and Hechler. They explain in Chap. 3 the necessity of a comprehensive assessment and the use of standardized multi-modal instruments in determining the full scope of the emotional impact, cognitive, physical, social and familial impact/burden of chronic pain. Drs. Hechler, Dobe and Zernikow conclude the book with a well-written response to the question "Is it all worthwhile? – Effectiveness of intensive interdisciplinary pain treatment" by providing convincing evidence for the effectiveness of intensive interdisciplinary pain programs.

The authors generously provide a list of their questions, materials and in the appendix supply 19 worksheets to explore patients' resources and their stress factors. These worksheets are very useful and include descriptions with standardized instructions regarding the most important therapeutic interventions. They invite us to take these materials and worksheets with their detailed information and apply them in our own settings, whether in an outpatient or inpatient pain program. We should do so, as there is enough rich material, research, clinical cases and depth of understanding, whatever one's profession, for this substantial manual to remain a primary resource for pain practitioners for many years to come. It provides an excellent standard of care in the complex treatment of paediatric chronic pain in the second decade of the twenty-first century.

I congratulate Michael and Boris and their team on this superb contribution to the field of paediatric pain, and applaud their generosity in sharing their research, considerable clinical and teaching experience, and their assessment and treatment materials, which all add to the progress in treating chronic pain – one of the most exasperating of all pains.

Vancouver, BC, Canada   Leora Kuttner, PhD, Reg. Psych.

Foreword II

There are a number of textbooks in print on paediatric pain, but very few of them warrant inclusion of the word "Practical" in the title. Michael Dobe's and Boris Zernikow's *Practical Treatment Options for Chronic Pain in Children and Adolescents* provides an approach that is above all practical and useful for clinicians caring for children with chronic pain.

The presentation follows a logical progression, through epidemiology, mechanisms, assessment and measurement, therapeutic approaches, and development of a roadmap for clinical decisions about which patients require more routine versus more intensive treatment settings. The authors support many of their recommendations with a superb blend of case discussions, theoretical considerations, and outcome data. The tone throughout is child and family centered. The authors emphasize wellness and fostering a child's capacity to heal himself or herself.

Those of us who specialize in treatment of chronic pain in children are a relatively small club. There are stylistic differences among our treatment centers that reflect differences in theoretical models, in local expertise and training, in the cultural backgrounds of our patients and families, and in the type of health care system and larger society that surrounds us. Sometimes, a manual or textbook written in one language may translate poorly into another for linguistic reasons or for cultural reasons. As an English-speaking physician in the U.S., I find that Dobe and Zernikow's book translates very well linguistically, and it also translates well culturally. Among the predominantly English speaking countries, there are widely divergent health care delivery models and very different cultures, and these local factors may lead to modifications of some specific recommendations. Nevertheless, the core themes of the approach outlined in this book are immensely applicable across cultures and languages. I think that clinicians in a wide range of Anglophone countries, including the U.S., Canada, the UK, Australia, and New Zealand, will find the English edition of this book to be among the best "roadmaps" available for guiding treatment of chronic pain in children. In my opinion, this book will be extremely useful for a broad audience, including primary paediatricians, paediatric subspecialists, paediatric psychologists, physical and occupational therapists, child life specialists, nurses and many others worldwide. I salute Dr. Dobe and Prof. Zernikow for their superb and truly practical book.

Boston, MA, USA   Charles Berde, MD, PhD

Introduction

Anouk, a 13-year-old girl, presents at our paediatric outpatient pain clinic accompanied by her mother, after having undergone an extensive diagnostic investigation of her abdominal pain which yielded no pathological findings. Anouk has been suffering from chronic abdominal pain for about 4 years; the pain has been constant over the last 2.5 years. She has undergone various outpatient and inpatient diagnostic procedures, including esophagogastroduodenoscopy with biopsy, laparoscopy, appendectomy, and NMR with angiography, all yielding no clinically relevant findings, histology of the appendix included. During a laparoscopy 1 year ago, adhesions were successfully removed from her lower right abdomen, but she experienced only minimal improvement for a short while; during the last 6 months, the pain has been increasing again. For the last 3 months, Anouk has been unable to attend school due to abdominal pain; 2 months ago, Anouk stayed 4 days at a paediatric clinic for further diagnostic medical investigations. Since then, the intensity of the constant pain has actually increased, now scoring 7–9 on a numeric rating pain scale from 0 to 10 (0 = no pain, 10 = worst pain). Most of the time, Anouk slacks off and doesn't participate in any family activities, causing her parents to worry. Anouk told us that she was burdened and exhausted and was not able to concentrate anymore. According to her mother, the family burden due to these pain episodes was extraordinary, even impacting close relatives. Consequently, Anouk has feelings of guilt.

Anouk's case illustrates the fact that pain may be so strong and extensive that it severely affects the patient's and his/her family's lives. Pain is a universal experience. Mostly, pain is a sign of muscular tension or of minor injury (e.g., contusion) and will vanish quickly. This is typical of acute pain. But, if pain is present for a longer period of time (6 months in adults, 3 months in children) for at least 15 days/month, it is called chronic pain. Three to 5 % of all children and adolescents report severe chronic pain, also affecting different aspects of their lives (Huguet and Miro 2008).

Some of the children and adolescents (referred to as "children" from now on) will get sufficient help in primary care. But a substantial number of severely affected children remain who are strongly impaired in their daily lives. Most of these children might be effectively treated in an outpatient setting. Unfortunately, suitable paediatric outpatient clinics for children with chronic pain or equivalent treatment options are rare. Thus, it often proves impossible to arrange the indicated measures for children with chronic pain in an outpatient setting. Reasons for the paucity of outpatient treatment centers might be that only recently has attention been brought to the problem of diagnosing and treating chronic pain and recognizing it as an independent disease. It is only during the last few years that various medical and psychological university faculties and therapeutic medical schools/institutions have specialized in chronic pain and pain disorders in adults and children. As a consequence, a physician unaware of the pain disorder won't offer adequate treatment.

The lack of knowledge of many physicians, paediatricians, and therapists is also reflected in the fact that many children with chronic pain have a wrong diagnosis and receive insufficient treatment. We would like to emphasize that "simple" chronic pain is already of substantial negative impact for the patient's mental and psychosocial development. These children tend to miss school because of their pain. They attend fewer social activities than their healthy peers, and they more frequently show signs of depression (Palermo et al. 2009; Eccleston et al. 2004). Each month of insufficient treatment makes it more probable that the symptom of pain will become independent of physical input and lead to a chronic pain disorder. As seen in the case of Anouk, many patients and their families report a medical odyssey but have never been educated about chronic pain.

As mentioned before, untreated chronic pain frequently leads to pain-related absenteeism from school combined with a high emotional burden for the child and his/her family. Children like Anouk suffer pain disorders, diseases where pain has become an independent disease in such a way that it has a strong impact on thoughts, feelings, behavior, family life, or social activities. If the pain is not too severe, outpatient pain (psycho) therapy may be sufficient. But if the child is severely affected in his/her everyday activities and at school, outpatient pain treatment will in most cases not be effective, and participation in a multimodal inpatient pain therapy program is indicated (Hechler et al. 2009).

How should children with a chronic pain disorder be treated? Only since the end of the 1980s has the medical community engaged in the understanding and treatment of chronic pain disorders. Thus, it is not surprising that a treatment manual or even instruction for clinical practice for the treatment of paediatric chronic pain disorders is not yet available. Another point is the paucity of scientific data on paediatric inpatient pain therapy. So far, the inpatient pain therapy program of the German Paediatric Pain Centre (GPPC) is one of the few scientifically evaluated prospective and randomized inpatient treatment programs for children with chronic pain, irrespective of pain location, underlying cause, or duration of the pain disorder.

With this manual, we intend to integrate the latest scientific knowledge with our longstanding clinical experience in the treatment of children with chronic pain disorders and their families. Along with the explanation and detailed description of our clinical experience, we have included its theoretical background. Following our detailed manual, an experienced psychotherapist should be able to successfully treat children with a chronic pain disorder.

This manual should guide the psychotherapist or the medical doctor through the therapeutic process of treating children with chronic pain. The expert knowledge and therapeutic attitude imparted focus on clinical application and are suitable also in an outpatient setting, as are most of the methods illustrated in Chaps. 4, 6, and 7. Moreover, this manual should allow other inpatient institutions to offer effective inpatient pain therapy to children with a chronic pain disorder. Described in detail are the setting, inpatient routines, daily routines, as well as therapeutic work, interventions of the nursing and educational team (NET), and the therapeutic approach of including other professions based on the patient's needs. This will also allow minor modifications according to preexisting institutional or therapeutic concepts. We feel that the comprehensive description of the latest scientific knowledge, therapeutic attitude, education, treatment methods preferred by our team, and the institutional structure of the GPPC will help other institutions to successfully establish their own inpatient concept for the treatment of chronic pain in children.

Chapter 1 gives an overview of the latest epidemiological data. Chapter 2 summarizes the scientific state of the art with respect to the background and understanding of paediatric chronic pain. Chapter 3 describes the instruments useful in exploring chronic pain, while in Chap. 4 the necessary basic therapeutic knowledge is outlined in detail. Chapter 5 discusses the criteria for allocating patients to either the outpatient or the inpatient therapeutic setting. Chapter 6 delivers a comprehensive description of the inpatient paediatric pain management concept at the GPPC, not only listing the different tasks of the various professions but also giving practical hints for therapeutic interventions, illustrated by the presentation of sample clinical cases. An extra focus is set on imparting knowledge on working with the patient's family and the implementation of treatment approaches for children with chronic pain disorders concomitantly suffering, for example, psychotrauma or depression. Chapter 7 covers more general aspects of the therapeutic work with children suffering comorbid mental, psychosocial, or physical symptoms. Chapter 8 summarizes results from the latest effectiveness studies especially on inpatient pain treatment.

Chapter 9 includes some material for the clinical work. You will find various worksheets which help to explore patients' resources and psychological stress factors and some sheets just for getting acquainted with the patient. We also include descriptions of the most important therapeutic interventions, with standardized instructions.

We hope that the manual will reflect our enthusiasm for working with children with chronic pain and their families, and we wish the reader success in implementing the therapeutic program.

Datteln, Germany   Michael Dobe
Datteln, Germany   Boris Zernikow

References

Eccleston C, Crombez G, Scotford A, Clinch J, Connell H (2004) Adolescent chronic pain: patterns and predictors of emotional distress in adolescents with chronic pain and their parents. Pain 108(3):221–229

Hechler T, Dobe M, Kosfelder J, Damschen U, Hübner B, Blankenburg M, Sauer C, Zernikow B (2009) Effectiveness of a three-week multimodal inpatient pain treatment for adolescents suffering from chronic pain: statistical and clinical significance. Clin J Pain 25(2):156–166

Huguet A, Miró J (2008) The severity of chronic pediatric pain: an epidemiological study. J Pain 9(3):226–236

Palermo TM (2009) Assessment of chronic pain in children: current status and emerging topics. Pain Res Manag 14(1):21–26. Pain 108(3):221–229

Acknowledgement

Special thanks to Erik Michel and Leora Kuttner, who both made many suggestions for the improvement of this manual that, clearly, raised the quality of this work. We are grateful to Walter Magerl for his comments in Chap. 2 and all colleagues who enabled us to write this manual, especially the coauthors (Julia Wager, Rebecca Hartmann, Holger Kriszio, Tanja Hechler, and Jürgen Behlert) and the medical, therapeutic, and nursing team of the German Paediatric Pain Center, who gave the authors the necessary time to work on the manual by taking over some of their appointments and commitments.

Many, many thanks to my wife Stefanie for her constant emotional support, and to our children Jan, Marlon, and Noah, I'm so grateful for your presence!

Datteln, Germany   Michael Dobe

Contents

Abbreviations

ACC	Anterior Cingulate Cortex
APPT	Adolescent Paediatric Pain Tool
ARCS	Adult Responses to Children's Symptoms
AT	Autogenic Training
CASI	Childhood Anxiety Sensitivity Index
CBT	Cognitive-Behavioral Therapy
CGRP	Calcitonin Gene-Related Peptide
CNS	Central Nervous System
COX	Cyclooxygenases
CPM	Conditioned Pain Modulation
CRPS	Complex Regional Pain Syndrome
EEG	Electroencephalography
EMDR	Eye Movement Desensitization Reprocessing
FOPQ-C	Fear of Pain Questionnaire for Children
GPPC	German Paediatric Pain Centre
IASP	International Association for the Study of Pain
IHS	International Headache Society
IQ	Intelligence Quotient
JFMS	Juvenile Fibromyalgia Syndrome
JIA	Juvenile Idiopathic Arthritis
LTD	Long-Term Depression
LTP	Long-Term Potentiation
MB	Migration Background
MRI	Magnetic Resonance Imaging
NET	Nursing and Educational Team
NMDA	N-Methyl-D-Aspartate
NMR	Nuclear Magnetic Resonance
NO	Nitrous Oxide
NRS	Numeric Rating Scale
NSAID	Nonsteroidal Anti-inflammatory Drug
PCS-P	Pain Catastrophizing Scale for Parents
PMR	Progressive Muscle Relaxation according to Jacobson
PPC	Paediatric Pain Questionnaire
PPCI	Paediatric Pain Coping Inventory

PPCI-R	Paediatric Pain Coping Inventory-Revised
P-PDI	Paediatric Pain Disability Index
PPT	Pain Provocation Technique
PQCA	Pain Questionnaire for Children and Adolescents
PTSD	Post Traumatic Stress Disorder
QST	Quantitative Sensory Testing
RAP	Recurrent Abdominal Pain
RCT	Randomized Controlled Trial
SNRI	Serotonin Re-uptake Inhibitor
TENS	Transcutaneous Electrical Nerve Stimulation
TRPV1	Transient Receptor Potential Vanilloid Subtype 1
TTH	Tension-Type Headache
WDR-Neuron	Wide-Dynamic-Range Neuron

Epidemiology of Chronic Pain in Children and Adolescents

Michael Dobe and Boris Zernikow

"And I thought I was alone." – Jessica (15 years), chronic pain disorder with abdominal pain

Content

Abstract

Chronic pain is common in children and adolescents, affecting 20–25 % of this population. A total of 3 % of all children suffer severe chronic pain. In more than a half of those patients (1.7 %), the criteria for a chronic or somatoform pain disorder are met.

Children suffering from chronic pain are often surprised to learn that there are a great number of other children who also suffer chronic pain. Most patients feel alone with their pain in school or in their social environment. They feel misunderstood and excluded (Forgeron et al. 2011). On their first day on the pain ward, patients meet other children with chronic pain, who are well able to understand their

M. Dobe (✉)
German Paediatric Pain Centre (GPPC), Children's and Adolescents' Hospital,
Witten/Herdecke University, Dr.-Friedrich-Steiner Street 5,
Datteln 45711, Germany
e-mail: m.dobe@kinderklinik-datteln.de

B. Zernikow
German Paediatric Pain Centre (GPPC), Children's and Adolescents' Hospital,
Witten/Herdecke University, Dr.-Friedrich-Steiner Street 5,
Datteln 45711, Germany

Chair Children's Pain Therapy and Paediatric Palliative Care,
Witten/Herdecke University, School of Medicine,
Datteln 45711, Germany
e-mail: b.zernikow@deutsches-kinderschmerzzentrum.de

M. Dobe, B. Zernikow (eds.),
Practical Treatment Options for Chronic Pain in Children and Adolescents,
DOI 10.1007/978-3-642-37816-4_1, © Springer-Verlag Berlin Heidelberg 2013

symptoms. This usually relieves the affected children. Chronic pain in children and adolescents is quite common; the prevalence estimates reach 25 % (Perquin et al. 2000). However, most of those children are only mildly affected by their chronic pain. Representative samples indicate that about 5 % of all children suffer severe chronic pain, affecting their daily life to a moderate or high degree (Huguet and Miró 2008). This means that their school attendance, leisure activities, contact with family and peers, as well as their emotional health are negatively impacted (Palermo 2009; Huguet and Miró 2008). These children typically show distinct pain-specific emotions like fear of pain (Vlaeyen and Linton 2000; Simons et al. 2011) accompanied by a substantial tendency to catastrophize regarding existing or feared pain (Hermann et al. 2008).

Since this manual specifically deals with therapy for children with a pain disorder, the question is: how many children are affected by a pain disorder defined as a medical diagnosis (ICD-10 or DSM-IV)? In a representative survey in Germany comprising 3,021 adolescents and young adults (aged 14–24 years), Lieb et al. (1998 – only available in German language) discovered by means of semistructured interviews lasting 2 h that 1.7 % of the population meet the definition of pain disorder.

Studies on the prevalence of pain disorders in children aged 8–13 years are missing. Lieb et al., however, showed – based on symptom-focused anamnestic data – a significant increase in the prevalence of pain disorders starting at 11 years (some even starting at 4 or 5 years). At about 17 years, the prevalence decreases again. In accordance with the data of Lieb et al., Kröner-Herwig et al. (2007) report chronic headache with severe impairment of daily life in 3 % of all children aged 7–8 years. Patients on our pain ward (7–17 years) have already suffered chronic pain for an average of 3.5 years before starting this treatment (Dobe et al. 2011). All in all, there are indications that about 1.7 % of all children aged 8–17 years suffer from a pain disorder.

References

Dobe M, Hechler T, Behlert J, Kosfelder J, Zernikow B (2011) Pain therapy with children and adolescents severely disabled due to chronic pain: long-term outcome after inpatient pain therapy. Schmerz 25(4):411–422

Forgeron PA, McGrath P, Stevens B, Evans J, Dick B, Finley GA, Carlson T (2011) Social information processing in adolescents with chronic pain: my friends don't really understand me. Pain 152(12):2773–2780

Hermann C, Zohsel K, Hohmeister J, Flor H (2008) Dimensions of pain-related parent behavior: development and psychometric evaluation of a new measure for children and their parents. Pain 137(3):689–699

Huguet A, Miró J (2008) The severity of chronic Pediatric pain: an epidemiological study. J Pain 9(3):226–236

Kröner-Herwig B, Heinrich M, Morris L (2007) Headache in German children and adolescents: a population-based epidemiological study. Cephalalgia 27(6):519–527

Lieb R, Mastaler M, Wittchen HU (1998) Are there somatoform disorders in adolescents and young adults? First epidemiological findings based on a representative population sample. Verhaltenstherapie 8:81–93

Palermo TM (2009) Assessment of chronic pain in children: current status and emerging topics. Pain Res Manag 14(1):21–26

Perquin CW, Hazebroek-Kampschreur AAJM, Hunfeld JAM et al (2000) Pain in children and adolescents: a common experience. Pain 87(1):51–58

Simons LE, Sieberg CB, Kaczynski KJ (2011) Measuring parent beliefs about child acceptance of pain: a preliminary validation of the Chronic Pain Acceptance Questionnaire, parent report. Pain 152(10):2294–3000

Vlaeyen JW, Linton SJ (2000) Fear-avoidance and its consequences in chronic musculoskeletal pain: a state of the art. Pain 85(3):317–332

Pain Disorder: A Biopsychosocial Disease

2

Holger Kriszio, Julia Wager, Michael Dobe, Tanja Hechler, and Boris Zernikow

Contents

H. Kriszio • J. Wager • M. Dobe (✉) • T. Hechler
German Paediatric Pain Centre (GPPC), Children's and Adolescents' Hospital,
Witten/Herdecke University, Dr.-Friedrich-Steiner Street 5,
Datteln 45711, Germany
e-mail: m.dobe@kinderklinik-datteln.de

B. Zernikow
German Paediatric Pain Centre (GPPC), Children's and Adolescents' Hospital,
Witten/Herdecke University, Dr.-Friedrich-Steiner Street 5,
Datteln 45711, Germany

Chair Children's Pain Therapy and Paediatric Palliative Care,
Witten/Herdecke University, School of Medicine,
Datteln 45711, Germany
e-mail: b.zernikow@deutsches-kinderschmerzzentrum.de

M. Dobe, B. Zernikow (eds.),
Practical Treatment Options for Chronic Pain in Children and Adolescents,
DOI 10.1007/978-3-642-37816-4_2, © Springer-Verlag Berlin Heidelberg 2013

5

Abstract

Pain is an individual and purely subjective experience. Pain processing depends on both somatosensory and emotional brain areas (e.g., the limbic system). Therefore, pain is never a purely sensory perception, but always includes emotional determinants. Finally, the family and other social contexts of the child are important determinants of pain perception. Hence, in order to better understand the origin and perpetuation of pain disorders, biological and psychological factors as well as the social environment have to be taken into account. In this chapter, we describe biological, emotional, cognitive, and social factors that play a role in the origin, perpetuation, and amplification of pain disorders.

Pain is an individual and exclusively personal experience (Coghill et al. 2003; Turk and Okifuji 1999). Numerous areas of the central nervous system (CNS) take part in pain processing, i.e., somatosensory areas as well as emotional areas (e.g., the limbic system) (Melzack 2005). The International Association for the Study of Pain (IASP) also highlights the different dimensions in their definition of pain (IASP 1994) as "an unpleasant sensory and emotional experience associated with actual or potential tissue damage, or described in terms of such damage." Individual perception of pain with all its sensory and affective components makes a comprehensive assessment of the multidimensional pain experience indispensable (Schroeder et al. 2010). Pain experience is mostly operationalized by the description of individual pain perception (Schroeder et al. 2010).

The assessment of pain perception has a scientific basis, especially in adults. Typically, the components of pain intensity and pain quality (pain perception in a closer definition) are assessed separately (Geissner 1995). Sensory pain quality is, for example, characterized by the rhythm of the perceived pain or by its thermic characteristics. The affective component of pain is described in terms such as "tiring" or "horrible," delivering hints as to the weight of the individual psychological burden and the concurrent suffering (Geissner 1995; Nagel et al. 2002).

Finally, the patient's social environment is an important determinant of pain perception (McCracken et al. 2007; Eccleston et al. 2004). Compared to adults, in children, the social context is thought to be of much greater impact (Goubert et al. 2008). While the social context (e.g., parents) has an impact on the child's pain chronicity, the child's disorder also has an impact on his/her environment (e.g., burden on his/her parents).

The following sections will describe in detail the biological factors involved in the origin and perpetuation of pain disorders. Later sections give an overview of emotional, cognitive, and behavior-related processes contributing to the origin, perpetuation, or even amplification of pain disorders in children. For didactic purposes, it is not until Chap. 6 that we give an in-depth presentation of the important psychological or social determinants of pain disorders and a description of possible therapeutic interventions aiming to change those determinants.

2.1 Biological Determinants of Acute or Chronic Pain

2.1.1 Nociception

Nociception is purely biochemical/biophysical and results from neuronal changes as a response to actual or potentially damaging stimuli. Those changes and the processing of pain clearly show interindividual variability (Binder et al. 2011). Nociception comprises the subprocesses of transduction, transmission, modulation, and perception.

2.1.1.1 Transduction in Nociceptors

Transduction is the transfer of a biochemical/biophysical response caused by tissue damage into a neuronal answer. Tissue damage due to injury or inflammation induces local cellular release of various substances like K+ ions, H+ ions, ATP, and autacoids like histamine, serotonin, or bradykinin. For instance, in human beings, histamine is released particularly from mast cells, while serotonin originates nearly exclusively from thrombocytes. An important role is played by lipid mediators, like prostaglandins, leukotrienes, or other inflammatory mediators of the arachidonic acid cascade. The mediators of the arachidonic acid cascade are generated by enzymes called cyclooxygenases (COX) or lipoxygenase (LOX). The activity of the cyclooxygenases may be modulated by substances like acetylsalicylic acid, indomethacin, or ibuprofen. In addition, nociceptors have a secretory efferent function releasing vasoactive neuropeptides like substance P and calcitonin gene-related peptide (CGRP), which contribute to the local inflammatory response (neurogenic inflammation) and are important mediators in the neuro-immune interaction mediating chemotaxis, arteriolar smooth muscle relaxation, capillary vasodilation, and increased venolar permeability (leakage) allowing for extravasation of soluble and cellular components of the immune system into the extravascular space.

During the last several years, the investigation of pain focused on the relevance of the neuropeptide substance P, which is released by the endings of the unmyelinized nociceptive nerve fibers themselves. Substance P originates from the dorsal root ganglion cells and is released into the CNS as well as into the peripheral nerve. The nervous system is able to store substance P. The main effect of substance P seems to be a vasodilative effect, inducing microdilation and changes in the permeability of blood vessels. The resulting local edema may lower the threshold for neighboring nociceptive fibers. A new treatment modality is the deactivation of substance P. To this end, the alkaloid capsaicin is locally applied, inducing the release of substance P in peripheral neural endings, thus emptying its stores. Capsaicin acts as an agonist at the TRPV1 (transient receptor potential vanilloid subtype 1) receptor which is a nonselective cation channel that is also activated by means of heat and protons. Initially, capsaicin leads to increased local circulation, pruritus, and a burning sensation. Applied repeatedly, it may induce a sustained desensitization to external stimuli by initiating temporary retraction of the TRPV1-bearing endings from the exposed tissue. Neuropeptides are largely depleted from nociceptive neurons for several weeks by this excitotoxic treatment.

It is not yet clarified in every detail how these substances transform tissue injury into a pain signal, though a multifactorial reaction using direct and indirect signal transmission is favored. Local substances (H+ or K+ ions) are able to directly activate the nociceptive neurons, while prostaglandins indirectly sensitize the nervous system to physical as well as chemical stimuli.

2.1.1.2 Transmission

Nociceptors

Injury or inflammation activates several types of peripheral nerve fibers that process the nociceptive signal and transmit it to the CNS, where it is eventually transformed into the conscious experience of pain. Those nerve fibers are named nociceptors, and they make up the vast majority of afferents (up to 90 %) in almost all tissue. Some tissues, e.g., cornea, tympanic membrane, or dental pulp, are almost exclusively innervated by nociceptors. There are two types of nociceptors, visceral and peripheral (C-fibers; Aδ-fibers), with two subgroups each, appearing anatomically as free endings of nerve fibers. C-fibers are nonmyelinated nerve fibers that may be activated by mechanical, thermal (heat and/or cold), and a variety of chemical stimuli. They have conduction velocities of around 1 m/s. Aδ-fibers are thinly myelinated, allowing for much higher conduction velocities (10–25 times that of C-fibers), and they are also activated by mechanical, thermal, or chemical stimuli. Beyond this crude classification, nociceptors are a very complex system of afferents subdivided into many highly differentiated groups of sensors with diverse functions ranging from simple to polymodal sensors.

There are many C- as well as Aδ-fibers in the skin, muscles, and joints. In contrast, visceral structures exhibit many C-fibers, but just a few Aδ-fibers. C-fibers are generally more sensitive in almost any sensory modality than Aδ-fibers, making them prime candidates for detection of noxious events. Thresholds of Aδ-fibers are significantly higher than those of C-fibers. Their faster signal conduction enables the organism to withdraw quickly from a damaging stimulus, limiting stimulus impact at higher intensities in order to avoid permanent or at least further damage. Thus, for instance, after thermal injury, permanent tissue impairment (burning) may be limited or even avoided. The main feature of C- and Aδ-fibers is their ability to continue with signal transmission for a long time after acute tissue injury in order to signal to the organism that it should rest the respective body part or make it undergo treatment. Hence, healing is supported.

Sensitization

In Aβ fibers that transmit sensory information from non-noxious stimulus modalities (touch, proprioception), continuous or repeated stimuli lead to exhaustion, expressed as an increased threshold to the stimuli. In this respect, nociceptors are a unique type of sensor responding to repeated stimuli with increased sensitivity, lowered threshold, and a longer-lasting response beyond the actual stimulus impact (after discharge). In case of repeated or very severe painful stimuli, we find peripheral as well as central sensitization.

Peripheral sensitization is triggered by the release of locally acting substances from surrounding tissue and associated intracellular responses (e.g., increase of Ca^{2+} concentration in the peripheral nociceptor terminal) conjointly leading to a decrease of nociceptor threshold and an increase in suprathreshold stimuli. Additionally, insensitive (silent) terminals or branches may become sensitized, leading to an increase of receptive field size.

Triggered by long-lasting or repeated painful stimuli, the CNS and especially the dorsal horn respond with functional and structural changes (corresponding to histomorphologic changes) similar to cellular changes that parallel learning in other CNS areas, like the hippocampus. These neuroplastic changes are part of nociceptive central sensitization. Hyperalgesia, allodynia, or spontaneous pain with a concomitant increase in the painful body area is characteristic of central sensitization.

Chronic Pain

Chronic pain may also result from, or be amplified by, pathological changes of signal processing in the nervous system. As a consequence of insufficiently treated pain, there may arise changes in the CNS that increase the sensitivity to painful stimuli and that substantiate as hyperalgesia. There is much evidence that strong painful stimuli chronically amplify the synaptic transmission of pain information from peripheral to central. The induced synaptic changes at the spinal level (synaptic long-term potentiation, LTP) are similar to those that were initially identified in the hippocampus as components of cellular learning and of the creation of cognitive memory.

2.1.1.3 Modulation

Incoming pain information is modulated in the CNS. Afferent neurons of both the spinal nerves and the cranial nerves with their cell bodies in the dorsal roots ganglia or cranial nerve counterparts (e.g., the Gasserian ganglion of the trigeminal nerve) transmit nociceptive or sensory stimuli to the spinal dorsal horn. For a long time, it was believed that this level is a "hub," switching the incoming signal to the second neuron of the pain tract, but nowadays, we know that the processes in the dorsal horn are more complex. Even at that level of signal transmission, various synaptic or biochemical interactions result in summation effects or selection. Neuronal signals coming from primary afferents converge in the dorsal horn. There, by means of local inhibitory interneurons, they may be inhibited by segmental or descending control even before reaching a higher spinal level or the cerebrum.

According to the *Control Gate Theory* published in "Science" by Melzack and Wall in 1965, non-nociceptive stimuli are conducted to the dorsal horn via both large myelinated fibers and small nociceptive Aδ- and C-fibers (Melzack and Wall 1965). Since several peripheral neurons converge to one spinal neuron, this type of convergent neuron was named wide dynamic-range neuron (WDR neuron). The fact that different types of fibers converge to one neuron may be one of the several reasons why counterirritation, i.e., rubbing of the affected area after injury, sometimes alleviates the pain (other mechanisms are the activation of long-term depression (Treede 2008)).

The human organism inherited a very effective and highly preserved evolutionary endogenous pain-inhibiting system, the principal layout of which is found in even very primitive organisms, like snails or insects. According to requirements, this endogenous pain control is more or less active, depending on emotions. Based on that model, Melzack and Wall succeeded in explaining how after even the most severe injuries (i.e., accident) or under extreme emotional stress, some people – at least transiently – will not perceive pain from their injuries, even including a total lack of pain perception. Mediated by the monoaminergic neurotransmitters noradrenaline or serotonin, descending tracts of the brain stem are able to reduce the excitability of spinal nociceptive neurons directly or indirectly by stimulating inhibitory interneurons within the spinal gray substance. Some of these inhibitory neurons may release endogenous opioid peptides (i.e., endorphins) that stimulate opioid receptors, which may inhibit signal transduction to the WDR neuron by initiating opioid receptor-coupled potassium currents.

2.1.1.4 Perception

After having undergone modulation by interneurons, the second neuron of the nociceptive projection pathway is intraspinal. Its dendrites cross the midline of the spinal cord into the contralateral anterolateral funiculus (see Fig. 2.1).

The ascending nociceptive spinal tracts comprise several different parallel projecting tracts, namely, the spinothalamic, spinomesencephalic, spinoreticular, and spinoparabrachial tracts. The spinothalamic tracts can be further subdivided into the more lateral part (neospinothalamic tract) and a more medial part (paleospinothalamic tract). Pain signal conduction from neck or head areas follows a similar anatomical and physiological assignment via the trigeminal nerve with a first synaptic relay in the medullary dorsal horn, from which the second neuron projects into the neotrigeminothalamic and a paleotrigeminothalamic part, both crossing the midline running parallel with the spinothalamic tracts.

The neospinothalamic tract consists of large myelinated fibers that lead centrally and are switched to the third neuron of the pain tract in the ventral, posterior, and lateral parts of the thalamus. The third neuron projects parallel to the primary and secondary somatosensory cortices and nociceptive parts of the insula and operculum (in aggregate: the parasylvian cortex), which are all somatotopically organized. On its way, the neospinothalamic tract exhibits only a few synapses, and in humans and monkeys, it is more prominent than other nonprimate species.

The paleospinothalamic tract is composed of both short and long fibers and is less myelinated than the neospinothalamic tract. Many synapses help to transmit the signal into deeper brain structures like periaqueductal gray, cingulate cortex, hypothalamus, or the medial thalamic parts. From there, the signal pathway is more diffuse – and less somatotopically organized – into the limbic system and the frontal cortex.

Anatomical organization of both systems with their different numbers of synapses and their different grade of myelinization suggests that the neospinothalamic tract (exhibiting fewer synapses and faster signal conduction into the somatosensory cortex) is responsible for the signaling of acute pain. Its localization, and the scoring of its severity, allows the organism to quickly protect itself from the acutely

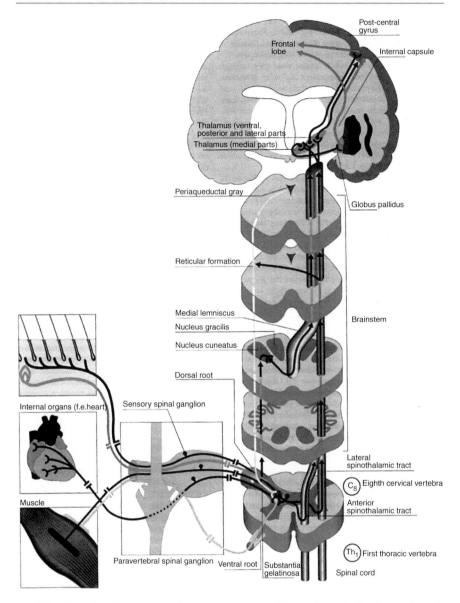

Fig. 2.1 The nociceptive system: nociceptors, ascending and descending spinal pathways, thalamic relay nuclei, subcortical and cortical projection areas (According to Brune et al. 2001, modified)

damaging stimulus or to stay away from the painful stimulus. The paleospinothalamic tract with its slower responses and its connections to, for example, the limbic system is thought to be primarily responsible for emotion and memory. This makes the paleospinothalamic tract the ideal candidate to be responsible for an arousal reaction or for reactions aimed at avoidance of further injury, i.e., behavioral changes, like avoidance behavior.

Obviously, conscious experience of pain goes far beyond the transmission of a signal from the peripheral nervous system to the CNS, which we term nociceptive processing. Pain is a multidimensional process including former experiences, emotions, cultural imprinting, and familial and social relationships. It is well known that the hypothalamus, the limbic system, and the medial parts of the thalamus are involved in motivational or emotional experiences and that they are connected to the paleospinothalamic tract. These systems are connected to other cerebral structures as well, i.e., the frontal cortex. Under pain, those phylogenetically old cortical areas, like the anterior cingulate cortex (ACC), are known to trigger autonomic reflexes like an increase in blood pressure, heart rate, or respiratory frequency (collectively termed pseudoaffective reflexes). The motivational and emotional state is of crucial influence in the spinal modulation of pain processing via descending tracts.

2.1.2 Pain Disorders

2.1.2.1 Migraine

Etymologically, migraine originally is described as typical hemicranial severe headache (Greek – hēmíkraira=half the head). Women suffer from migraine about three times as often as men. A similar gender distribution is found in adolescents.

So far, two migraine genes have been identified which are responsible for the rare familial hemiplegic migraine. There are many hints that genetic factors and hormonal factors – e.g. during the female cycle –are jointly responsible for triggering a migraine attack. In adolescent girls, starting with the menarche, and women, migraine without aura is frequently associated with menstruation. Therefore, the International Headache Society (IHS) included both menstrual migraine and menstrually related migraine in the IHS classification.

Unfortunately, the term "migraine" has developed in common language into a term for any type of severe headache. On closer examination, a headache termed "migraine" often does not comply with the criteria of the IHS. According to the IHS, migraine is defined as a sudden periodic headache, usually with a throbbing quality. This may be accompanied by symptoms such as nausea, vomiting, or increased sensitivity to light (photophobia) or auditory stimuli (phonophobia). Very often, symptoms increase in severity with physical activity. The patient withdraws, avoiding physical activity. Especially in younger children who are not able to verbally describe their photophobia or phonophobia due to their developmental age, their behavior delivers important diagnostic clues. If the migraine attack leads to transient neurological deficits preceding the pain, this is called an "aura." Manifestations of an aura may be visual or sensory disturbances of perception or motoric disturbances like paresis or expressive speech disturbances. The most common type of migraine is without aura, which has a higher attack frequency than migraine with aura. The diagnosis of migraine as a primary headache should not be given unless other neurological diseases can be excluded. The IHS defines the following diagnostic criteria for migraine (http://ihs-classification. org/en/):

A. At least 5 attacks fulfilling criteria B–D
B. Headache attacks lasting 4–72 h (untreated or unsuccessfully treated)[a, b]
C. Headache has at least two of the following characteristics:
  1. Unilateral location[c, d]
  2. Pulsating quality
  3. Moderate or severe pain intensity
  4. Aggravation by or causing avoidance of routine physical activity (e.g., walking or climbing stairs)
D. During headache, at least one of the following:
  1. Nausea and/or vomiting
  2. Photophobia and phonophobia[e]
E. Not attributed to another disorder

Sometimes, it is quite difficult to differentiate between migraine without aura and episodic tension-type headache (see below). In order to help children, parents, and professionals to differentiate tension-type headache from migraine in childhood, Table 2.1 lists the typical symptoms pinpointing the differences.

In case the patient falls asleep during a migraine attack and wakes up free of pain, the duration of the attack is calculated from the time of the first symptom until symptom-free awakening. Please note that especially in younger children, migraine headache is often described as double sided. The typical adult-type one-sided headache develops in adolescence or in young adulthood. Most migraine headache is localized frontotemporal. Especially in children, occipital pain (single or double sided) is seldom reported. Doing diagnostics in such cases, one should be careful not to miss space-occupying cerebral processes or structural lesions. During the migraine attack, cerebral blood flow does not show primary changes that would be characteristic of cortical spreading depression moving across the cortex in waves. However, perfusional changes in the brain stem may well exist as may secondary cortical changes as a consequence of pain activation. In contrast, in migraine with aura, there is a pathognomonic decreased perfusion underlying the neurological deficits. Thus, the "spreading depression" in migraine without aura is seen as pathophysiologically irrelevant. With certainty, the vasodilating substances nitrous oxide (NO) and calcitonin gene-related peptide (CGRP) are part of this process. For a long time, the vascular changes and the consecutive changes in perfusion were held primarily responsible for migraine. More recently, the sensitization of

---

[a] When the patient falls asleep during migraine and wakes up without it, the duration of the attack is calculated until the time of awakening.

[b] In children, attacks may last 1–72 h (although the evidence for untreated durations of less than 2 h in children requires corroboration by prospective diary studies).

[c] Migraine headache is commonly bilateral in young children; an adult pattern of unilateral pain usually emerges in late adolescence or early adult life.

[d] Migraine headache is usually frontotemporal. Occipital headache in *children*, whether unilateral or bilateral, is rare and calls for diagnostic caution; many cases are attributable to structural lesions.

[e] In young children, photophobia and phonophobia may be inferred from their behavior.

Table 2.1 Typical symptoms of tension-type headache and migraine in childhood

	Tension-type headache	Migraine
Frequent symptoms and typical course	Duration of headache 30 min to 7 days	Duration of headache 1–72 h
	Mild to moderate pain	Moderate to severe pain
	Double-sided	Frequently single-sided
	Pressing or tightening pain	Frequently pulsating
	Physical activity does not aggravate pain (most important criterion)	*Physical activity does aggravate pain* (most important criterion)
	Nausea and/or vomiting missing; sometimes absence of appetite mild photophobia or phonophobia	Nausea and/or vomiting photophobia and/or phonophobia
Less frequent symptoms	Neck pain	Aura (visual acuity impaired; flashes; restricted area of focused sight; paresis; etc.) preceding migraine attack
	Teeth grinding	Frequent yawning, ravenous appetite, extreme fatigue before the attack
	Dizziness	Double-sided pain
		Pressing or drilling pain
		Very short pain attacks
		Smell disturbances
		Abdominal pain
		Travel sickness even in periods free of migraine attacks
		Neck pain
		Cutaneous hyperalgesia
		Dizziness
		Paleness

perivascular nerve endings is seen as a possible pain trigger. Therefore, the possibility of migraine attacks being generated within the CNS is being discussed.

Meanwhile, we know about the relationship between migraine pain and neurotransmission. Data being gathered since the implementation of triptans into therapy are of special importance in clarifying these interrelationships. Triptans turned out to be very effective in the treatment of an acute migraine attack. Nowadays, it is undisputed that migraine is a complex neurobiological disease and not just the result of primarily vascular changes.

In spite of the severity of migrainous pain, there is no underlying destructive cerebral process. The only risk with migraine is not to treat it the right way, i.e., using analgesics at the very beginning of an attack. Treated with delay (i.e., not taking the medication until the patient can't stand the pain anymore), insufficiently (i.e., using a low drug dose), or in the wrong way (taking a nap instead of taking medication, using relaxation techniques *during* a migraine attack) make children suffer severe headaches more frequently. As time goes by, it becomes more probable that pain accompanied by fear of the upcoming pain attack is *learned*, establishing a *pain memory* and chronic headache.

2.1.2.2 Tension-Type Headache (TTH)

Tension-type headache is said to be the most frequent primary headache. Although its etiology and pathomechanisms are still unknown, the IHS defines this type of headache as a disease entity assigned to the primary headaches. It might well be that TTH comprises several different types of headache of still unknown origin. Meanwhile, many studies suggest that at least TTH with a severe course has a neurobiological origin.

It is helpful to distinguish between chronic TTH and episodic TTH. Chronic TTH leads to an impaired quality of life and has the potential to severely affect daily routine. Episodic TTH comprises two subtypes: the sporadic subtype, exhibiting pain less than once per month, and the subtype with more frequent attacks. The impact of the sporadic subtype on the patient's life is mild, while the subtype with more frequent attacks may result in life impairment similar to chronic TTH, leading to frequent usage of analgesics and frequent contact with health-care professionals, which may become a true financial burden to the family. Not only are medical doctors contacted due to persistent or recurrent headache; alternative practitioners and other health professionals are also visited. Some of them release spinal blockages; others blame the teeth or their position for the pain.

The first release of the IHS classification arbitrarily discriminated between patients with and without increased pain sensitivity of the pericranial muscles, a discrimination which turned out to be beneficial. The result of palpation of the neck muscles was helpful for discrimination. As mentioned earlier, pathophysiology of TTH is still unknown. Peripheral mechanisms seem to be of importance in sporadic and frequent episodic TTH, while the central mechanism seems to play a role in chronic TTH.

Infrequent Episodic Tension-Type Headache

Infrequent episodic TTH shows rare episodes of headache lasting minutes to days. The pain is double-sided and of pressing, tightening quality. It is mild to moderate and is *not* amplified by routine physical activity. There is no accompanying nausea, but there may well be photophobia or phonophobia.

Diagnostic Criteria for Infrequent Episodic TTH

A. At least 10 episodes occurring on <1 day/month on average (<12 days/year) and fulfilling criteria B–D
B. Headache lasting from 30 min to 7 days
C. Headache has at least two of the following characteristics:
   1. Bilateral location
   2. Pressing/tightening (non-pulsating) quality
   3. Mild or moderate intensity
   4. Not aggravated by routine physical activity such as walking or climbing stairs
D. Both of the following:
   1. No nausea or vomiting (anorexia may occur)
   2. No more than one of photophobia or phonophobia
E. Not attributed to another disorder

Frequent Episodic Tension-Type Headache

This diagnosis is characterized by frequent episodes of headache lasting minutes to days. The pain is typically bilateral, pressing or tightening in quality, and of mild to moderate intensity. It does not worsen with routine physical activity. It is not accompanied by nausea, but photophobia or phonophobia may occur.

Diagnostic Criteria for Frequent Episodic TTH

A. At least 10 episodes occurring on ≥1 but <15 days/month for at least 3 months (≥12 and <180 days/year) and fulfilling criteria B–D
B. Headache lasting from 30 min to 7 days
C. Headache has at least two of the following characteristics:
   1. Bilateral location
   2. Pressing/tightening (non-pulsating) quality
   3. Mild or moderate intensity
   4. Not aggravated by routine physical activity such as walking or climbing stairs
D. Both of the following:
   1. No nausea or vomiting (anorexia may occur)
   2. No more than one of photophobia or phonophobia
E. Not attributed to another disorder

Patients suffering migraine without aura frequently also suffer episodic TTH. A headache diary (see Sect. 3.5.2) is the tool of choice to analyze the co-occurrence of TTH and migraine. Since treatment is essentially different in those two types of headache, it is very important to educate patients and parents in the differentiation of the two types of headache in order to enable them to choose the appropriate therapy. This will also prevent the development of medication overuse headache in the long run.

2.1.2.3 Rheumatic Disease

The term "rheumatic disease" has its origin in the French doctor Guillaume de Baillou (1538–1616) who comprehensively described complaints of the musculoskeletal system. While the underlying theory of humoral pathology is long outdated, common language still uses the term, subsuming diseases of most different etiologies into the rheumatic spectrum disorder. The more specific immunologically mediated rheumatoid diseases are as follows:

1. Juvenile idiopathic arthritis
2. Collagenoses
3. Psoriatic arthritis
4. Reactive arthritis
5. Rheumatoid arthritis (= chronic polyarthritis)
6. Ankylosing spondylitis (M. Bechterew)
7. Vasculitis of different origin

Many readers will miss the diagnosis of juvenile fibromyalgia syndrome (JFMS). According to the latest guidelines, that diagnosis is subsumed under "chronic pain disease with somatic and psychic factors." The relationship between the symptoms of JFMS and psychic disorders like depression or posttraumatic distress syndrome were too obvious, which is in accordance with our clinical impression.

In paediatrics, the most frequent rheumatic diseases are reactive arthritis of different origin, frequently due to a recent infection, and juvenile idiopathic arthritis (JIA). The etiology of the latter is still obscure. It may well be that JIA comprises different yet unknown diseases. It goes without saying that causal treatment of JIA is not yet available. An important prerequisite for successful therapy is the early diagnosis and transfer of the patient to physicians with experience in the treatment of JIA. Only by doing so can early and effective treatment of both the inflammatory reaction and the pain be given. Effective control of any underlying disease and – if necessary – induction of remission, avoidance of joint contractures, or destruction leading to persistent physical disabilities as well as avoidance of impaired growth resulting in axial malposition are the main goals of quality rheumatologic treatment. Next to drug therapy, it is of utmost importance that the patient keeps moving and under no circumstances submits to passive pain control. Otherwise there is a high risk that the acute pain will become chronic, developing further into chronic pain disorder with somatic and psychic elements (called *pain amplification syndrome* by rheumatologists; see also Sect. 3.1).

Successful therapy should allow children a somatic and psychic development free of major disturbances. On an eleven-point scale, JIA patients rate their disease-related quality of life worse than their general quality of life (Feldman et al. 2000). Paediatric JIA patients score their quality of life lower than their healthy peers (Manschwetus 2003). Based on several JIA studies and the JIA national guidelines of the German scientific medical societies (AWMF), early diagnosis (within 1–2 months) and the assessment of disease activity are essential to rheumatologic therapy. To this end, there are various validated scales (i.e., PED ACR) available. Drug therapy should comply with the latest version of national or international guidelines.

Of special importance is physiotherapy and ergotherapy given by experienced and specifically trained therapists with the aims of maintenance or recovery of normal joint mobility, avoidance of contractures, stretching and activation of muscles, strengthening of muscles, and facilitation of physiological movements in order to avoid the development of relieving postures or false posture. In case of good disease control, participation in sports at school and other sporting activities is allowed and should be encouraged(!), since graded physical exposure has a positive effect on development and coping with the illness, and the risk of social isolation is minimized. As soon as acute inflammation has receded, training should be resumed, but only after the type of sports and training intensity are individually determined, since in inflamed joints sports that stress the joints may provoke an acceleration of destructive processes and lead to irreversible cartilaginous defects.

2.1.2.4 Minor Trauma and Complex Regional Pan Syndrome (CRPS) Types I and II

Blunt joint trauma and bruises primarily provoke an inflammation response similar to that seen in other types of arthritis. Both the vasoactive substances released by tissue damage and pain lead to locally increased blood flow and local edema. An injured joint may accumulate an increased amount of fluid (effusion). Local cooling of the joint will depress pain, inflammatory response, and edema. Nonsteroidal antirheumatics will also depress the inflammation. Skeletal or ligamental injuries need to be diagnosed as soon as possible to allow for targeted therapy. Any necessary immobilization should be as short as possible. If impairment is observed under immobilization, one should critically reevaluate therapy. One should be aware of thrombosis as well as nerve compression. When the acute injury is healed, the aim is to mobilize the joint as soon as possible in order to avoid the development of relieving posture or inappropriate straining of a joint.

Case Report Lotte (Age 14 Years), CRPS
Lotte is the second child in her family, with an older sister. When getting up one morning, Lotte gets her index finger caught between the mattress and bed. She immediately feels severe pain in her whole hand. Clinical examination by a surgeon reveals a strain of the capsule of the metacarpal joint. Radiologically, a fracture can be excluded. Lotte gets a cast on her hand. A few days later, the pain is increasing and nearly unbearable. Whole-hand allodynia develops. The affected hand is swollen, the skin has changed to doughy and shiny, the finger joints are fixed in flexion and massively swollen. Ibuprofen, metamizole, tilidine, and tramadol all are ineffective. A complex regional pain syndrome (CRPS) is diagnosed. Lotte gets pregabalin and inpatient multimodal pain therapy. During the course of treatment, the tropical changes decreased. Lotte is able to move her hand again. After discharge, she is able to write using her hand and to participate in school as usual.

CRPS may develop after all types of trauma to the distal parts of the extremities. By definition, symptoms do not follow the course of peripheral nerves or spinal roots. In extremely rare cases, the symptoms may spread to other extremities. The diagnosis is made according to the clinical picture since there are no other suitable diagnostic methods available. The diagnosis is by exclusion. Nuclear magnetic resonance (NMR) tomography, quantitative sensory testing (QST), or skeletal scintigraphy may be helpful. Complex regional pain syndrome develops with variable latency after injury of an extremity, i.e., trauma, or even diagnostic or therapeutic procedures, independent of type or grade of injury. Even a minor trauma may induce CRPS.

If the injury causes damage to a peripheral nerve and CRPS develops, the disease is named CPRS type II. If there is no nerve lesion present, it is CPRS type I. The International Association for the Study of Pain (IASP) defined sensitive and specific diagnostic criteria (Baron 2004; Harden et al. 2007).

Diagnostic Criteria IASP

1. The presence of an initiating noxious event or cause of immobilization.
2. Continuing pain, allodynia, or hyperalgesia with which the pain is disproportionate to any inciting event.

3. Evidence at some time of edema, changes in skin blood flow, or abnormal sudo-motor activity in the region of the pain.
4. This diagnosis is excluded by the existence of conditions that would otherwise account for the degree of pain and dysfunction.
   Note: Criteria 2–4 must be satisfied.

Generally, any findings assessed by a doctor are more important than the subjective symptoms as described by the patient. A sentinel characteristic of CRPS is that symptoms are not confined to the area of the injured nerve but tend to generalize, affecting the whole extremity.

The "Budapest" criteria of CRPS (Harden et al. 2007) are given below:

General definition of the syndrome:

CRPS describes an array of painful conditions that are characterized by a continuing (spontaneous and/or evoked) regional pain that is seemingly disproportionate in time or degree to the usual course of any known trauma or other lesion. The pain is regional (not in a specific nerve territory or dermatome) and usually has a distal predominance of abnormal sensory, motor, sudomotor, vasomotor, and/or trophic findings. The syndrome shows variable progression over time.

To make the clinical diagnosis, the following criteria must be met:

1. Continuing pain, which is disproportionate to any inciting event
2. Must report at least one symptom in *three of the four* following categories:
   (a) *Sensory*: Reports of hyperesthesia and/or allodynia
   (b) *Vasomotor*: Reports of temperature asymmetry and/or skin color changes and/or skin color asymmetry
   (c) *Sudomotor/edema*: Reports of edema and/or sweating changes and/or sweating asymmetry
   (d) *Motor/trophic*: Reports of decreased range of motion and/or motor dysfunction (weakness, tremor, dystonia) and/or trophic changes (hair, nail, skin)
3. Must display at least one sign *at time of evaluation* in *two or more* of the following categories:
   (a) *Sensory*: Evidence of hyperalgesia (to pinprick) and/or allodynia (to light touch and/or temperature sensation and/or deep somatic pressure and/or joint movement)
   (b) *Vasomotor*: Evidence of temperature asymmetry (>1 °C) and/or skin color changes and/or asymmetry
   (c) *Sudomotor/edema*: Evidence of edema and/or sweating changes and/or sweating asymmetry
   (d) *Motor/trophic*: Evidence of decreased range of motion and/or motor dysfunction (weakness, tremor, dystonia) and/or trophic changes (hair, nail, skin)
4. There is no other diagnosis that better explains the signs and symptoms

For research purposes, diagnosis should be applied when there is at least one symptom *in all four* symptom categories and at least one sign (observed at evaluation) in two or more sign categories.

Skin temperature is measured with suitable tools. All other symptoms are judged clinically. In order to answer point 4, especially the presence of diseases that can imitate CRPS must be excluded: rheumatic diseases, inflammation (i.e., infectious arthritis of any kind, postsurgical infections, polyneuritis, or radiculitis), thrombotic affections, compartment syndrome, or nerve compression syndrome. To this end, the patient should undergo biochemical investigations. It is *impossible* to diagnose CRPS exclusively by means of laboratory investigations like CRP or erythrocyte sedimentation rate.

Often it is difficult to discriminate CRPS from the results of a psychiatric disease. This is especially true with a dissociative disturbance with autoagressive components. Some of those diseases in fact are able to trigger CRPS, which complicates the situation. The course of disease should be documented using methods common in pain therapy, i.e., subjective (NRS) and semi-objective (QST) pain assessment, parameters of function (force/power, extent of mobility, circumference), and quantification of disturbances of the vegetative nervous system.

2.1.2.5 Insufficiently Treated Acute Pain

Insufficiently treated severe pain may lead to permanent sensitization of the CNS. Especially alterations at the spinal level are well investigated, and there is good reason to speculate that similar processes take place at the thalamus and cerebral level as well. Long-lasting changes lead to an increased sensitivity of spinal and thalamic nociceptive neurons to noxious stimuli. Clinically, this may manifest as pathologically increased algesia (hyperalgesia), even eliciting pain through non-nociceptive stimuli (i.e., by light touch or gentle cold stimuli, which manifest as dynamic mechanical or cold allodynia), or even as spontaneous pain. At the spinal level, the arising synaptic long-term potentiation (LTP) may be suppressed by local anesthetics and analgesics but not by general anesthesia. The pain-inhibiting tracts descending from the cerebrum to the spinal level are similarly effective. In humans, it is still difficult to erase pain memory by drug treatment (see below). Counterirritation measures like transcutaneous electric nerve stimulation (TENS) may however have the potential under special circumstances to actively bring the increased sensitivity of the nociceptive system back to normal. Recent work in animals and humans suggests that TENS may at least in part activate the mechanism of synaptic long-term depression (LTD) counteracting long-term potentiation (LTP).

2.1.3 Peripheral and Central Pain Sensitization and Inhibition

There are similarities between the processes at the cellular level resulting in use-dependent spinal "pain traces" and the hippocampal cellular processes that are regarded as the cellular basis of cognitive learning and memory. "Pain traces" in the nervous system often are called "pain memory"; however, they represent a nonconscious mechanism of use-dependent implicit learning and memory. In parallel to motor learning, where repeated stimuli (exercise) lead to specific and often highly automated sequences of motions (e.g., playing tennis, skiing, climbing), repeated pain experiences may "train" the brain with the result of a lower pain threshold and/or the feeling of pain even in the absence of pain triggers (e.g., chronic daily headache).

Imminent or already established tissue damage is recognized by nociceptors. Nociceptors are free endings of thin afferent Aδ- or C-type nerve fibers that exist in all organs except the CNS, ending in the spinal dorsal horn. On stimulation, they release the neurotransmitter glutamate. Binding of glutamate to AMPA receptors results in synaptic excitation of spinal dorsal horn neurons that themselves transmit the information either directly or indirectly via interneurons among other destinations via the thalamic nucleus to the cortex, thus potentially reaching consciousness. Finally, at the end of the signaling chain in the somatosensory cortex, the conscious perception of "pain" is generated.

The release of glutamate is proportional to the intensity of the painful stimulus. On strong painful stimuli, great amounts of glutamate are spinally released, resulting in both short-lived excitation of dorsal horn neurons and recruiting involving activation of NMDA glutamate receptors – precipitating sustained changes of spinal nociceptive neurons. The specific features of the NMDA receptor channel are of eminent clinical significance. This nonselective ligand-gated ion channel is permeable to Ca^{2+} ions, and calcium is an important messenger in the intracellular signaling chain that via numerous cell functions is partially held responsible for central sensitization. Importantly, NMDA receptors are partially blocked by magnesium ions and only become permeable to sodium and calcium ions after releasing magnesium from their binding sites in the channel pore by concomitant depolarization, which may occur, e.g., by depolarization of the neurons by glutamate acting at AMPA receptors. Full sensitivity also affords allosteric modulation of the NMDA receptor at the glycine binding site (usually by binding the amino acid D-serine, which is present in high concentrations in almost all areas of the CNS). Glutamate also acts in parallel at G-protein-coupled metabotropic glutamate receptors, which modulate the sensitivity of ionotropic NMDA receptors. Strong excitation with concomitant strong intracellular increase of calcium elicits nociceptive sensitization by endpoints of various intracellular signaling pathways, like phosphorylation of ionotropic glutamate receptors by various protein kinases, inactivation of protein phosphatases, changes in the ionotropic glutamate receptor subtypes by receptor translocation (e.g., replacing the GluR2 by GluR1 AMPA receptor subtype), altered gene expression by induction activation of transcription factors (immediate early genes), and eventually structural changes of the nociceptive neuron, like increase of size and numbers of synaptic spines. Cotransmission by nociceptive neuropeptides (substance P, CGRP, and others) further contributes to nociceptive sensitization of postsynaptic neurons. Collectively, these mechanisms may lead to permanent amplification of synaptic efficacy (i.e., long-term potentiation of synaptic transmission). Long-term potentiation (LTP) is thought to be the central cellular mechanisms of central sensitization to nociceptive stimuli and even cross talk of non-nociceptive inputs into nociceptive pathways. As a consequence of long-term potentiation in the nociceptive system, minor painful stimuli may already result in a distinct excitation of nociceptive dorsal horn neurons. Usually, this sensitization subsides with half-lives of several hours and may fully resolve within 1–3 days. However, recent studies in humans have shown that some subjects may be particularly prone to long-lasting central sensitization in such a way that even very short-lasting strong noxious stimuli may elicit experimentally induced long-term potentiation of pain sensitivity lasting many days or weeks, i.e., transforming decremental early nociceptive or pain LTP into sustained late LTP (Pfau et al. 2011). In case of repeated or ongoing painful stimuli, functional synaptic changes may persist until death. Hence, it is most important to avoid the onset of neural pain memory. Synaptic long-term potentiation and the concomitant central sensitization to pain are induced by calcium influx into nociceptive neurons of the dorsal horn and stimulation of glutamate receptors of the NMDA subtype.

Functional changes of the magnitude of synaptic transmission may spontaneously regress after some time (hours to years), while apoptosis or necrotic cell death are irreversible. The degree to which compensatory effects like an increase in receptor sensitivity to GABA might compensate for the loss of inhibiting neurons awaits further investigation.

This knowledge allows for preventive measures as follows:

1. Avoidance/attenuation of glutamate release from nociceptive Aδ- und C-fibers using peripheral nerve block techniques (infiltration, regional, or plexus anesthesia)
2. Inhibition of nonphysiological excitability of afferent nerve fibers in peripheral neuropathies or presynaptic inhibition of transmitter release (i.e., spinal anesthesia using opioids that bind to *pre*synaptic opioid receptors)
3. Blunting the glutamate effect at the NMDA receptor channel by means of pharmacologically blocking the NMDA receptor (for instance, by using ketamine, dextrometorphan, or other NMDA receptor blockers) or restricting the postsynaptic calcium response using blockers of voltage-gated calcium channels (e.g., gabapentin) or restricting the excitability of postsynaptic nociceptive dorsal horn neurons by opening potassium channels (by, e.g., opioids that bind to *post*synaptic opioid receptors)

Even a deep general anesthesia is unable to avoid the manifestation of cellular pain memory, and sedatives do not protect from sensitization because those drugs have insufficient impact at the spinal level.

Human being has a very potent intrinsic pain defense mechanism originating at the brain stem level. At the spinal level, nociceptive neurons are inhibited pre- or postsynaptically by long descending tracts by the release of endogenous opioids, monoamines, and inhibiting amino acids. These substances are able to prevent calcium influx via NMDA receptor channels and/or act directly on voltage-gated calcium channels (VGCC), thus protecting from central sensitization. The intrinsic pain control is always active and may be additionally activated by acute stress or painful stimuli.

If intrinsic pain control is insufficient, sensitivity to pain is increased and the manifestation of pain memory is potentially enhanced. Supposedly, inter- and intraindividual differences in efficacy of intrinsic pain control are one of the reasons for differences in pain chronicity under presumably similar underlying diseases and burdens of pain. Nowadays, the clinical value of preventive analgesia is judged very discordantly. The inconclusive scientific data may originate in the fact that some of the patients may be sufficiently protected by their intrinsic pain control, preventing the establishment of pain memory and central sensitization, rendering preventive analgesia unnecessary and of no additional effect due to lack of headroom (Yarnitsky 2012). In fact, it has been demonstrated recently that the SNRI duloxetine is inefficient in subjects with intact conditioned pain modulation (CPM, as experimentally tested by the cold pressor test), but acts readily as an analgesic in patients exhibiting a lack of CPM.

One may intervene in the path of signal transduction in order to reverse sensitization by using measures of counterirritation, therapeutically exciting sensible nerve fibers. This can be accomplished using transcutaneous electrical nerve stimulation (TENS) or physical modes of pain control, i.e., the application of heat or cold. Some counterirritative measures are able to inhibit pain for some hours, or even days, the effect lasting longer than the nerve stimulation itself. Recent in vivo and in vitro studies showed that the synaptic transmission between Aδ- or C-fibers and the spinal neurons is permanently inhibited provided the parameters of stimulation are chosen right (synaptic long-term inhibition). Even the long-term potentiation of spinal synaptic transmission may be reversed.

In order to do so, it is necessary to excite the Aδ-type nerve fibers. Unfortunately, the necessary stimuli intensities are often perceived as a bit painful. Hence, the stimulus is mostly applied with only low frequency (1–3 Hz), presumably activating paths of spinal neural transmission that at least partially reverse sensitization. If the intensity of the stimulus is such that only low-threshold Aβ-fibers are excited, sensed by the patient as non-painful paresthesia, there will be no lasting effect. Exciting all afferent nerve fibers, including the high-threshold C-fibers, would not only be very painful to the patient, but moreover, it may also be unnecessary for maximum effect or even be detrimental, overruling the specific ameliorating pain-depressing effect of Aδ-nociceptor stimulation. This is in accordance with clinical observation that long-term analgesia using TENS or acupuncture can be reached only if a painful stimulus is used.

2.1.4 Pain and Gender

Numerous studies have investigated the gender-specific differences in pain prevalence. A good example is the German Children's and Adolescent's Survey (KiGGS) of the Robert Koch Institute. There, more than two-thirds of the children aged 3–10 years and three-fourths of those aged 11–17 years reported on pain during the last 3 months. Overall, pain prevalence was the same in boys and girls. But, the 11–17 year old girls complained of significantly more headache, back pain, or abdominal pain during the last 3 months than the age-matched boys. These findings are in accordance with several similar studies.

Pain localization varies with age and gender. Pain intensity is higher in girls, reflecting the findings in chronic pain in an outpatient setting (Keogh and Eccleston 2006) and those of a study on inpatient children with pain (Hechler et al. 2010). LeResche et al. (2005) investigated the relationship between puberty development and pain sensitivity and found stage of puberty a better predictor for pain than age. It is still unclear if these findings reflect hormonal changes (as is speculated with the clustering of migraine in girls aged 12 years and up; see Sect. 2.1.2) or are better explained psychosocially in role finding or role expectation and their accompanying conflicts.

2.1.5 Genetic Determinants

There is good reason to assume that human pain sensitivity is partially genetically determined. The "fakir gene" has long been known. This is a gene mutation first seen in a Pakistani family whose members are unable to sense pain. This gene coding for a sodium channel has the effect that affected people are unable to respond adequately to impairing environmental stimuli. Pain development and processing, however, are not monogenetically determined. Pain processing is determined by the cooperation of various genetic factors, more and more influenced by learning processes with increasing age. A single mutation does not necessarily grant increased or blunted pain sensibility or various degrees of efficacy of analgesics in affected individuals.

Numerous methods are used to find candidate genes. Human geneticists are looking in large families for genomic markers that are present in affected family members, but not in unaffected ones. If a marker is located next to a relevant pain gene, it should be more frequently found in affected individuals than in healthy ones. Single nucleotide polymorphisms (SNPs) are especially frequent. In those, a single nucleotide of DNA is exchanged, possibly resulting in a changed protein relevant in signal transmission.

Is has long been known that pain runs in families and consequently an analysis of pain in index subjects predicted pain sensitivity in their families (Birklein et al. 2008). There are more than 40 genes identified that play a role in perception of pressure, pain with cold or heat, or pain processing. Examples are the COMT gene, the OPRM1 gene, and the TRPV1 gene. If the gene coding for the μ opioid receptor was affected and a substantial 11 % of the population are carriers of that polymorphism, pressure sensitivity was altered. A certain gene mutation coding for the capsaicin- and heat-sensitive vanilloid receptor TRPV1 found in 37 % of the population resulted in a blunted pain response to cold, but only homocygous allele carriers showed a markedly blunted response. Activation of TRPV1-bearing C-nociceptors is essential for central sensitization, and a snap of the TRPV1 receptor presumably resulting in a lack-of-function mutation of TRPV1 has recently been shown to prevent nociceptive sensitization in patients with neuropathic pain (Binder et al. 2011).

Several genes have been identified whose transcription and/or translation is triggered by pain, including genes from the IEG (immediate early genes) group; the gene products of these genes are detectable in dorsal horn neurons within minutes after a painful stimulus. So far, the significance of the post-pain changes in the phenotype of the nociceptive neurons has not been clarified in every detail. It may well be that they contribute to central sensitization, too. Or they are a meaningful adaptation to increased neuronal activity. A pronounced increase in the concentration of calcium ions in neurons is able to trigger programmed cell death (apoptosis) or necrotic cell death. Obviously, inhibiting (antinociceptive) spinal dorsal horn neurons are especially sensitive to triggered cell death, since after peripheral nerve lesions or trauma to peripheral tissue, the number of neurons using the inhibiting neurotransmitter GABA decreases. A loss of spinal GABA-ergic inhibition results in severe types of hyperalgesia, allodynia, or spontaneous pain.

Preventive analgesia is an option only in case of expected pain exposure, which opens an avenue for prevention of chronic pain development by combined pre- and postsurgical management using drugs with a potential antihyperalgesic profile of action. Unfortunately, patients often undergo treatment only when pain memory, and therefore chronic pain, is already established. This may pose substantial therapeutic difficulties, since none of the officially approved drugs (centrally acting opioids effective in prevention included) seems to have the potential to erase pain memory.

2.2   Psychological Determinants

Pain perception is subjective and thus an individual experience (Coghill et al. 2003). It comprises biological, psychological, and social (context) components (Flor and Diers 2007). This is true with acute as well as chronic pain. The multidimensionality of pain becomes evident when the numerous components of central pain processing with the involvement of different areas of the CNS are considered. Apart from somatosensory areas, other areas determine the pain experience, e.g., those responsible for emotions, like the limbic system (Melzack 2005).

The significance of psychological or social factors can be illustrated by many examples. If, for example, a child is hurt during play, he/she will typically not take notice of the pain at first. The more pain becomes chronic, irrespective of the biological component, the more the significance of psychological and psychosocial factors increases. This is also reflected by the diagnostic criteria of pain disorders which will be presented in detail in Chap. 3.

For a pain therapist, it is important to realize the connection between these different dimensions. If he/she focused on just one dimension, it would be impossible in most cases to successfully treat paediatric pain (see "The Three Thought Traps"; Sect. 4.1). In contrast, a multimodal approach allows for successful therapy. The effectiveness of the multidisciplinary concept presented in this manual has been proven in many studies (see Sect. 8.2).

2.2.1   Learning Pain

Learning theories assume that the development of chronic pain is favored by reinforcement. Reinforcement of pain-specific behavior may arise from avoiding pain or from parental reactions to the child's pain. If a child lies down because of a headache, this may decrease his/her pain. That pain reduction may have various causes. Whatever the cause, this behavior will become more frequent during headache due to the fact that the headache indeed initially decreased. This is a classic example of operant conditioning. Apart from this, there are less direct learning processes. We would like to give an example of fear of pain. Children with recurrent or chronic pain often experience an increased fear of pain. In consequence, that fear may cause the child to continuously avoid any kind of potentially painful activities. Reinforced avoidance behavior will consolidate that fear of pain (Vlaeyen and Linton 2000; Asmundson 2012), and a vicious cycle has started.

A child's pain behavior is also influenced by his/her parents' behavior. According to learning theory, receiving more attention from the parents when experiencing (and reporting) pain will lead to a positive reinforcement of pain. Such behavior is typical in parents of children with chronic pain and is triggered by worries, distress, or negative cognitions like catastrophizing thoughts (Jordan et al. 2007; Goubert et al. 2006; Maciver et al. 2010). At the same time, due to their affinity for catastrophizing, parents of children with chronic pain tend to react solicitous when their child shows pain behavior (Vervoort et al. 2011). However, in our experience, there are also parents who increasingly react dismissively or aversively to their child's pain. Unfortunately, research in this field is still rare (Goubert et al. 2005). Often, the child's disorder results in substantial disturbances of the parent–child interaction (reproach: "You don't believe me that I am in pain!"), and this further amplifies pain. Irrespective of the type of parental reaction, it is important to discuss during treatment the (mostly unintended) consequences of their behavior.

Parents or close attachment figures of children with chronic pain often suffer chronic pain themselves (Merlijn et al. 2003). This may hint at a process of model learning and is in accordance with our clinical experience. However, other mechanisms may also be at play (e.g., processes of empathy (Goubert et al. 2006)). This field is still open to debate.

2.2.2 The Role of Cognitions

Pain experience is influenced by the subjective appraisal of the situation and the possibilities of dealing with it. Appraisals have an impact on coping strategies, and coping strategies again have an impact on pain experience.

Coping with pain may be either behavioral or mental (Hechler et al. 2008). Coping oriented to solutions (problem-focused coping) aims to change the circumstances and in most cases results in active pain coping behavior. If the child is less engaged in problem-focused coping, he/she is prone to show a more passive pain coping behavior (Walker et al. 2007). Depending on the degree to which the coping aims at changing circumstances, pain may either become accepted or increasingly negative ideas will develop (Walker et al. 2007). Active pain coping and acceptance of the pain are strategies proven effective in pain therapy (Wicksell et al. 2007; Wicksell et al. 2009). This illustrates the most important relationship between pain-related cognitions and the coping strategy used (active versus passive). The close relationship of experience and behavior is illustrated in the "Fear-Avoidance Model" of chronic pain (Asmundson et al. 2012).

Typical pain-related cognitive coping strategies are positive self-instruction, cat-astrophizing thoughts or cognitive distraction. Especially catastrophizing correlates with increased pain scores and increased emotional burden (Hermann et al. 2007; Crombez et al. 2003). In the long run, this will lead to substantially increased perception of body signals, the so-called somatosensory amplification (Rief and Barsky 2005; Nakao and Barsky 2007). Section 6.4.6 elucidates the importance of somatosensory amplification in interoceptive conditioning. In contrast, mental dis-traction will reduce pain (Chambers et al. 2009). Importantly, cognitive strategies are not equally suitable for all children. Sometimes, acceptance-based interventions not aiming at mental distraction should be preferred over classical cognitive coping strategies, a fact repeatedly pointed out by Wicksell et al. (2007, 2009). Section 6.4.3 suggests in detail which strategies aiming at cognition and appraisal might match which patient.

Physical rest, avoidance, and seeking social support are typical pain-related cop-ing behaviors following dysfunctional cognitions. Coping behaviors following helpful cognitions are, for example, behavior-related distraction and search for information. Passive pain coping strategies are positively correlated with an increased pain score, shown in an outpatient study on paediatric abdominal pain (Walker et al. 2007) and in an inpatient sample during the course of disease (Dobe et al. 2011). Especially in girls, seeking social support is associated with an increased pain score (Hechler et al. 2008; Hechler et al. 2010). Both mental- and behavior-related distraction result in reduced pain scores (Reid et al. 1998). In Sects. 6.4.3 and 6.5.5, interventions on coping strategies aimed at changing dysfunctional cog-nitions are demonstrated by means of case reports.

2.2.3 The Role of Emotions

Apart from cognitions, emotions are relevant in the understanding of chronic pain, since each pain event – even in chronic pain – is associated with feelings of fear and threat. The degree of a child's impairment due to pain is individually variable. Individual cognitions and the individual coping strategies of the child and his/her parents have a huge impact on chronic pain. The presence of catastrophizing ideas and seeking social support are relevant predictors of emotional impairment in chronic pain (Eccleston et al. 2004). The correlation between chronic pain and emotions was studied, mainly focusing on depression, anxiety, critical life events, and posttraumatic stress disorder (PTSD) (for a detailed discussion, see Sects. 6.4.6 and 6.5.2).

In a recent outpatient study, nearly a quarter of the paediatric study population with severe chronic pain showed increased scores for depression and anxiety (Zernikow et al. 2012). In an inpatient study population, nearly 50 % of the patients reported increased scores in at least either anxiety or depression before therapy (Hechler et al. 2009). Burba et al. (2006) were able to show that more than half of the patients with chronic pain were unable to notice or describe their own feelings (alexithymia). This is partially compatible with our clinical experience. Many children are not or are only insufficiently able to assign their perceptions of physiological processes to the various emotional qualities. Whether this is a consequence of their pain disorder (according to their parents, many of these children were formerly well able to reflect on their thoughts and emotions) or a factor favoring the development of pain disorders is still under dispute. Sections 4.3, 6.4.3, and 6.6.3 will describe various interventions improving differential perception of feelings on an interactive level.

Depression and anxiety may arise from chronic pain or they may perpetuate or amplify the pain due to social withdrawal or to difficulties in falling asleep and/or remaining asleep. Numerous models try to explain the complex interactions (Fernandez and Boyle 2002). First results favor a multifactorial process with mutual negative interactions, which may differ interindividually.

General anxiety and school aversion play an important role in chronic pain (Zernikow et al. 2012). In the assessment of chronic pain, it is always advisable to account for any school problems. Testing for dyslexia may be indicated in order to exclude the possibility that continuous distress in school due to that disorder perpetuates chronic pain.

Fear specific to pain is of special importance in the "Fear-Avoidance Model" of chronic paediatric pain (Vlaeyen and Linton 2000; Asmundson et al. 2012).

This model – primarily developed for musculoskeletal pain but also transferable to other pain conditions – postulates that pain-related fear plays a central role in the maintenance and exacerbation of chronic pain. According to this model, dysfunctional appraisals about pain and its consequences, such as catastrophizing thoughts, increase pain-related fears. This leads to avoidance behavior in order to escape situations which may trigger pain. Avoidance behavior will result in a general decrease in activity and physical fitness but also an increase in mood disturbances (Vlaeyen and Linton 2000). Furthermore, people with an increased fear of pain pay more attention to possibly pain-related stimuli; therefore, their focus will be on pain-related stimuli and away from other tasks necessary for normal everyday functioning (Vlaeyen and Linton 2000). In children, increased fear of pain is associated with increased pain-related disability (Martin et al. 2007; Simons et al. 2011; Turk and Wilson 2010). Additionally, children with fear of pain also report more pain-related catastrophizing (Simons et al. 2011). Interventions to counteract pain-related fear avoidance are demonstrated in Sect. 6.4.5. Other research shows that fear of pain is also influenced by interoceptive conditioning functioning (Vlaeyen and Linton 2000). Studies with adult chronic pain patients show that they have a more precise perception of physical processes (Scholz et al. 2001; Katzer et al. 2012). An association between increased interoceptive perception and negative appraisals of those processes leads to maladaptive interoperception, i.e., (neutral) interoceptive stimuli are associated with fear of pain (De Peuter et al. 2011). Studies in children to support the assumption that they are more prone to maladaptive interoception do not yet exist. In Sect. 6.4.5, we will give details on this scientific background and any therapeutic interventions based thereon.

Adolescents with PTSD often experience somatoform disorders (Essau 2007). Even the experience of negative critical life events and permanent emotional distress contributes to the development of pain disorders (Asmundson et al. 1999; Essau 2007). A pilot study on chronic pain and critical life events was able to show that children and adolescents severely impaired by their pain report a high number of such events (Bauer et al. 2010 – only available in German language). Since comorbidity of children with pain disorders and adjustment disorder or PTSD is high, the respective scientific background and any interventions based thereon are an issue of Sect. 6.5.2.

2.3   Social Determinants

Discussing learning processes, coping strategies, and emotions, it became apparent that chronic pain in children and adolescents cannot be isolated from its context factors. The social environment of the child, especially his/her family, peer group, and school, plays a more or less important role in the origin of pain disorders.

The family's role in chronic pain and pain-related impairment was verified in a model (Palermo and Chambers 2005) focusing on the individual parental features (catastrophizing thoughts, worries). It is emphasized that these features must be seen as a dyadic relationship (i.e., quality of parent–child interaction) which is imprinted by the whole-family system. Social systems can only be understood in their full complexity.

So far, studies explicitly investigating the impact of the patient's peer group are scarce. A study by Merlijn and colleagues suggests that peers reward and amplify pain-free behavior (Merlijn et al. 2003). They were able to show that peers pay attention to their friends suffering chronic pain especially during episodes free of pain, but lower their attention during pain episodes. According to this, Forgeron et al. (2011) found that children with chronic pain often feel misunderstood by their peers since they desire increased attention and understanding especially when pain is increasing. The described peer behavior as contrasted with the patient's expectations could explain our clinical impression that many children experience social exclusion in the course of disease (and not the other way around).

Children with pain disorders tend to miss school (Eccleston and Malleson 2003; Dobe et al. 2011). Irregular attendance at school has numerous consequences for the child. Frequently, school achievement drops markedly, sometimes resulting in repeating a class and endangering the child's educational development. On the social level, these children become more and more distant from their classmates and lose contact with peers. Finally, absenteeism from school provokes reactions and attributions of teachers. It is more the rule than the exception that teachers interpret chronic pain in a dualistic way; they attribute the pain either to an organic or a psychological cause (Logan et al. 2007). Dependent on his/her interpretation, the teacher's understanding may vary from overwhelming empathy and understanding (organic cause) to lacking empathy and understanding (psychological cause).

There is a paucity of scientific literature with respect to the social determinants of the development and perpetuation of pain disorders in children. According to our clinical experience, social and psychosocial factors contribute to the development and perpetuation of many children's pain disorders. Studies evaluating the effectiveness of our multidisciplinary inpatient pain therapy do not allow us to draw any firm conclusions on the role of the numerous social factors or the effectiveness of certain systemic interventions, since many different social or psychosocial factors were taken into account. Hence, the various family therapeutic or systemic procedures as described in Sect. 6.6 and Chap. 7 are mainly based on our clinical experience.

References

Asmundson GJ (2012) Do attentional biases for pain depend on threat value of pain and competing motivation toward non-pain goals? Pain 153:1140–1141

Asmundson GJ, Norton PJ, Norton GR (1999) Beyond pain: the role of fear and avoidance in chronicity. Clin Psychol Rev 19(1):97–119

Asmundson GJ, Coons MJ, Taylor S, Katz J (2002) PTSD and the experience of pain: research and clinical implications of shared vulnerability and mutual maintenance models. Can J Psychiatry 47(10):930–937

Asmundson GJ, Noel M, Petter M, Parkerson HA (2012) Pediatric fear-avoidance model of chronic pain: foundation, application and future directions. Pain Res Manag 17:397–405

Baron R (2004) Mechanistic and clinical aspects of complex regional pain syndrome (CRPS). Novartis Found Symp 261:220–233; discussion 233–238, 256–261

Bauer K, Hechler T, Dobe M, Hamann M, Vocks S, Zernikow B (2010) Critical life events in adolescents with chronic pain. Effects on the outcome of pain therapy? Article published in German. Schmerz 24:138–139

Binder A, May D, Baron R, Maier C, Tölle TR, Treede RD et al (2011) Transient receptor potential channel polymorphisms are associated with the somatosensory function in neuropathic pain patients. PLoS One 6:e17387

Birklein F, Depmeier C, Rolke R, Hansen C, Rautenstrauss B, Prawitt D et al (2008) A family-based investigation of cold pain tolerance. Pain 138(1):111–118

Brune K, Beyer A, Schafer F (2001) Schmerz – pathophysiologie, pharmakologie, therapie. Springer, Heidelberg/New York/Tokio

Burba B, Oswald R, Grigaliunien V, Neverauskiene S, Jankuviene O, Chue P (2006) A controlled study of alexithymia in adolescent patients with persistent somatoform pain disorder. Can J Psychiatry 51(7):468–471

Chambers CT, Taddio A, Uman LS, McMurtry CM et al (2009) Psychological interventions for reducing pain and distress during routine childhood immunizations: a systematic review. Clin Ther 31(2):77–103

Coghill RC, McHaffie JG, Yen YF (2003) Neural correlates of interindividual differences in the subjective experience of pain. Proc Natl Acad Sci U S A 100(14):8538–8542

Crombez G, Bijttebier P, Eccleston C, Mascagni T, Mertens G, Goubert L et al (2003) The child version of the pain catastrophizing scale (PCS-C): a preliminary validation. Pain 104(3):639–646

De Peuter S, Van Diest I, Vansteenwegen D, Van den Bergh O, Vlaeyen JW (2011) Understanding fear of pain in chronic pain: interoceptive fear conditioning as a novel approach. Eur J Pain 15:889–894

Dobe M, Hechler T, Behlert J, Kosfelder J, Zernikow B (2011) Pain therapy with children and adolescents severely disabled due to chronic pain: long-term outcome after inpatient pain therapy. Schmerz 25(4):411–422

Eccleston C, Malleson P (2003) Managing chronic pain in children and adolescents. We need to address the embarrassing lack of data for this common problem. BMJ 326(7404):1408–1409

Eccleston C, Crombez G, Scotford A, Clinch J, Connell H (2004) Adolescent chronic pain: patterns and predictors of emotional distress in adolescents with chronic pain and their parents. Pain 108(3):221–229

Essau CA (2007) Course and outcome of somatoform disorders in non-referred adolescents. Psychosomatics 48(6):502–509

Feldman DS, Hedden DM, Wright JG (2000) The use of bone scan to investigate back pain in children and adolescents. J Pediatr Orthop 20(6):790–795

Fernandez E, Boyle GJ (2002) Affective and evaluative descriptors of pain in the McGill pain questionnaire: reduction and reorganization. J Pain 3(1):70–77

Flor H, Diers M (2007) Limitations of pharmacotherapy: behavioral approaches to chronic pain. Handb Exp Pharmacol 177:415–427

Forgeron PA, McGrath P, Stevens B, Evans J, Dick B, Finley GA et al (2011) Social information processing in adolescents with chronic pain: my friends don't really understand me. Pain 152(12):2773–2780

Geissner E (1995) The Pain Perception Scale – a differentiated and change-sensitive scale for assessing chronic and acute pain. Rehabilitation 34(4):XXXV–XLIII

Goubert L, Craig KD, Vervoort T, Morley S, Sullivan MJ, de C Williams AC et al (2005) Facing others in pain: the effects of empathy. Pain 118(3):285–288

Goubert L, Eccleston C, Vervoort T, Jordan A, Crombez G (2006) Parental catastrophizing about their child's pain. The parent version of the Pain Catastrophizing Scale (PCS-P): a preliminary validation. Pain 123(3):254–263

Goubert L, Vervoort T, Sullivan MJ, Verhoeven K, Crombez G (2008) Parental emotional responses to their child's pain: the role of dispositional empathy and catastrophizing about their child's pain. J Pain 9(3):272–279

Harden RN, Bruehl S, Stanton-Hicks M, Wilson PR (2007) Proposed new diagnostic criteria for complex regional pain syndrome. Pain Med 8(4):326–331

Hechler T, Dobe M, Kosfelder J, Damschen U, Hübner B, Blankenburg M, et al (2009) Effectiveness of a three-week multimodal inpatient pain treatment for adolescents suffering from chronic pain: statistical and clinical significance. Clin J Pain 25:156–166

Hechler T, Kosfelder J, Denecke H, Dobe M, Hübner B, Martin A et al (2008) Pain-related coping strategies in children and adolescents with chronic pain. Validation of a German version of the Paediatric Pain Coping Inventory (PPCI revised). Schmerz 22:442–457

Hechler T, Kosfelder J, Vocks S, Mönninger T, Blankenburg M, Dobe M et al (2010) Changes in pain-related coping strategies and their importance for treatment outcome following multimodal inpatient treatment: does sex matter? J Pain 11(5):472–483

Hermann C, Hohmeister J, Zohsel K, Ebinger F, Flor H (2007) The assessment of pain coping and pain-related cognitions in children and adolescents: current methods and further development. J Pain 8(10):802–813

IASP Task Force on Taxonomy (1994) Part III: pain terms, a current list with definitions and notes on usage. In: Merskey H, Bogduk N (eds) Classification of chronic pain, 2nd edn. IASP Press, Seattle, pp 209–214

Jordan AL, Eccleston C, Osborn M (2007) Being a parent of the adolescent with complex chronic pain: an interpretative phenomenological analysis. Eur J Pain 11(1):49–56

Katzer A, Oberfeld D, Hiller W, Gerlach AL, Witthöft M (2012) Tactile perceptual processes and their relationship to somatoform disorders. J Abnorm Psychol 121:530–543

Keogh E, Eccleston C (2006) Sex differences in adolescent chronic pain and pain-related coping. Pain 123(3):275–284

LeResche L, Mancl LA, Drangsholt MT, Saunders K, Korff MV (2005) Relationship of pain and symptoms to pubertal development in adolescents. Pain 118(1–2):201–209

Logan DE, Catanese SP, Coakley RM, Scharff L (2007) Chronic pain in the classroom: teachers' attributions about the causes of chronic pain. J Sch Health 77(5):248–256

Maciver D, Jones D, Nicol M (2010) Parents' experiences of caring for a child with chronic pain. Qual Health Res 20(9):1272–1282

Manschwetus H (2003) Quality standards and certification of patient education in rheumatology. Z Rheumatol 62(2):21–23

Martin AL, McGrath P, Brown SC, Katz J (2007) Anxiety and sensitivity, fear of pain and pain-related disability in children and adolescents with chronic pain. Pain Res Manag 12:267–272

McCracken LM, MacKichan F, Eccleston C (2007) Contextual cognitive-behavioral therapy for severely disabled chronic pain sufferers: effectiveness and clinically significant change. Eur J Pain 11(3):314–322

Melzack R (2005) Evolution of the neuromatrix theory of pain. The Prithvi Raj Lecture: presented at the third World Congress of World Institute of Pain, Barcelona 2004. Pain Pract 5(2):85–94

Melzack R, Wall PD (1965) Pain mechanisms: a new theory. Science 150(3699):971–979

Merlijn VP, Hunfeld JA, van der Wouden JC, Hazebroek-Kampschreur AA, Koes BW, Passchier J (2003) Psychosocial factors associated with chronic pain in adolescents. Pain 101(1–2):33–43

Nagel B, Gerbershagen HU, Lindena G, Pfingsten M (2002) Development and evaluation of the multidimensional German pain questionnaire. Schmerz 16(4):263–270

Nakao M, Barsky AJ (2007) Clinical application of somatosensory amplification in psychosomatic medicine. Biopsychosoc Med 9:1–17

Palermo TM, Chambers CT (2005) Parent and family factors in pediatric chronic pain and disability: an integrative approach. Pain 119(1–3):1–4

Pfau DB, Klein T, Putzer D, Pogatzki-Zahn EM, Treede RD, Magerl W (2011) Analysis of hyperalgesia time courses in humans after painful electrical high-frequency stimulation identifies a possible transition from early to late LTP-like pain plasticity. Pain 152(7):1532–1539

Reid GJ, Gilbert CA, McGrath PJ (1998) The Pain Coping Questionnaire: preliminary validation. Pain 76(1–2):83–96

Rief W, Barsky AJ (2005) Psychobiological perspectives on somatoform disorders. Psychoneuroendocrinology 30(10):996–1002

Scholz OB, Ott R, Sarnoch H (2001) Proprioception in somatoform disorders. Behav Res Ther 39:1429–1438

Schroeder S, Hechler T, Denecke H, Müller-Busch M, Martin A, Menke A et al (2010) German Pain Questionnaire for Children, Adolescents and Parents (DSF-KJ). A multimodal questionnaire for diagnosis and treatment of children and adolescents suffering from chronic pain. Schmerz 24(1):23–37

Simons LE, Sieberg CB, Carpino E, Logan D, Berde C (2011) The fear of pain questionnaire (FOPQ): assessment of pain-related fear among children and adolescents with chronic pain. J Pain 12:677–686

Treede RD (2008) Highly localized inhibition of pain via long-term depression (LTD). Clin Neurophysiol 119(8):1703–1704

Turk DC, Okifuji A (1999) Assessment of patients' reporting of pain: an integrated perspective. Lancet 353(9166):1784–1788

Vervoort T, Huguet A, Verhoeven K, Goubert L (2011) Mothers' and fathers' responses to their child's pain moderate the relationship between the child's pain catastrophizing and disability. Pain 152(4):786–793

Vlaeyen JW, Linton SJ (2000) Fear-avoidance and its consequences in chronic musculoskeletal pain: a state of the art. Pain 85(3):317–332

Walker LS, Smith CA, Garber J, Claar RL (2007) Appraisal and coping with daily stressors by pediatric patients with chronic abdominal pain. J Pediatr Psychol 32(2):206–216

Wicksell RK, Melin L, Olsson GL (2007) Exposure and acceptance in the rehabilitation of adolescents with idiopathic chronic pain – a pilot study. Eur J Pain 11(3):267–274

Wicksell RK, Melin L, Lekander M, Olsson GL (2009) Evaluating the effectiveness of exposure and acceptance strategies to improve functioning and quality of life in longstanding pediatric pain – a randomized controlled trial. Pain 141(3):248–257

Yarnitsky D, Granot M, Nahman-Averbuch H, Khamaisi M, Granovsky Y (2012) Conditioned pain modulation predicts duloxetine efficacy in painful diabetic neuropathy. Pain 153:1193–1198

Zernikow B, Wager J, Hechler T, Hasan C, Rohr U, Dobe M et al (2012) Characteristics of highly impaired children with severe chronic pain: a 5-year retrospective study on 2,249 pediatric pain patients. BMC Pediatr 12(1):54

Diagnostics of Chronic Pain in Children and Adolescents

Julia Wager, Holger Kriszio, Michael Dobe,
Tanja Hechler, and Boris Zernikow

> *"Wow, that's a lot!" – Markus (14 years), when answering the pain questionnaires*

Contents

J. Wager • H. Kriszio • M. Dobe (✉) • T. Hechler
German Paediatric Pain Centre (GPPC), Children's and Adolescents' Hospital,
Witten/Herdecke University,
Dr.-Friedrich-Steiner Street 5, Datteln 45711, Germany
e-mail: m.dobe@kinderklinik-datteln.de

B. Zernikow
German Paediatric Pain Centre (GPPC), Children's and Adolescents' Hospital,
Witten/Herdecke University,
Dr.-Friedrich-Steiner Street 5, Datteln 45711, Germany

Chair Children's Pain Therapy and Paediatric Palliative Care,
Witten/Herdecke University, School of Medicine,
Datteln 45711, Germany
e-mail: b.zernikow@deutsches-kinderschmerzzentrum.de

M. Dobe, B. Zernikow (eds.),
Practical Treatment Options for Chronic Pain in Children and Adolescents,
DOI 10.1007/978-3-642-37816-4_3, © Springer-Verlag Berlin Heidelberg 2013

Abstract

By definition, a pain disorder is a biopsychosocial phenomenon. Irrespective of their individual proportion, diagnostics in pain disorders must always assess biological, psychological, and social factors in order to get the full picture. Medical diagnostic procedures investigate injuries, physical diseases, or inflammation as possible causes, or contributors, to pain. Psychological diagnostic procedures assess the emotional burden of pain, emotional determinants, the appearance of dysfunctional cognitions or coping strategies, and the degree of pain-related impairment of the child's life. Diagnostics of social factors check for dysfunctional behavior within the family system or elsewhere, and the relationship between the pain disorder and dysfunctional behavior within the family, school, or peer group. Apart from the assessment of problematic influences, it is important to identify the child's and his/her family's specific resources. This chapter describes the procedures necessary for a comprehensive assessment.

Markus (see above) is not the only one making such a remark when filling out the battery of questionnaires. Many patients and parents react similarly, seeing our series of questionnaires for the first time. However, in most cases, the initial reaction that the questionnaires are too much work changes once they are completed. Often the patient and his/her family feel taken seriously and realize that some of the questions, covering details of the patient's medical history and pain experience, were never asked before. Completing the questionnaire gives them a chance to express their personal views and ideas on the pain.

Questionnaires are an important tool in the diagnostics of chronic pain. Generally, questionnaire-based diagnostics should be kept to a minimum in order not to overburden the patient and his/her parents. On the other hand, all important aspects of the pain condition should be covered. Furthermore, questionnaire assessment always needs to be supplemented by diagnostic interviews and medical examinations.

In this chapter, we will first discuss the diagnostic criteria of pain disorders. This will be followed by a description of recommended medical diagnostic procedures usually performed without questionnaires. Questionnaires, however, are the standard tool for the assessment of the psychological and social aspects of the disorders.

3.1   Definition of Pain Disorders

The DSM-IV has two diagnoses regarding pain disorders, both subsumed under somatoform disorders. The DSM-IV distinguishes between *pain disorder associated with psychological factors* (307.80) and *pain disorder associated with both psychological factors and a general medical condition* (307.89). The respective diagnostic criteria are given in Table 3.1.

In both disorders, a biopsychosocial view is important since there are both physical and psychosocial determinants of the disorder. The main differences between the two diagnoses are the factors triggering and maintaining the pain condition.

Table 3.1 DSM-IV criteria for pain disorder

General criteria: pain disorder

A. Pain in one or more anatomical sites is the predominant focus of the clinical presentation and is of sufficient severity to warrant clinical attention

B. The pain causes clinically significant distress or impairment in social, occupational, or other important areas of functioning

C. Psychological factors are judged to have an important role in the onset, severity, exacerbation, or maintenance of the pain

D. The symptom or deficit is not intentionally produced or feigned (as in factitious disorder or malingering)

E. The pain is not better accounted for by a mood, anxiety, or psychotic disorder and does not meet criteria for dyspareunia

Pain disorder associated with psychological factors (307.80)

Psychological factors are judged to have the major role in the onset, severity, exacerbation, or maintenance of the pain. (If a general medical condition is present, it does not have a major role in the onset, severity, exacerbation, or maintenance of the pain.) This type of pain disorder is not diagnosed if criteria are also met for Somatization disorder

Pain disorder associated with both psychological factors and a general medical condition (307.89)

Both psychological factors and a general medical condition are judged to have important roles in the onset, severity, exacerbation, or maintenance of the pain. The associated general medical condition or anatomical site of the pain is coded on Axis III

For the treatment of pain disorders, it is important to identify any underlying physical disease since repeatedly relapsing (inflammatory) processes may cause pain (typical examples thereof are migraine or juvenile arthritis). Those types of underlying diseases should be treated with analgesics (for details, see Sect. 6.7.2). Apart from that, the presence of any underlying chronic physical disease does not change the further therapeutic approach to the pain disorder (for a more detailed view, see Sect. 7.6).

The biopsychosocial criteria relevant to the diagnostics of pain disorders underscore the importance of a detailed pain history comprising medical as well as psychosocial factors. Apart from psychological diagnostic assessment, it is advisable to talk to the previously treating physician/therapist, e.g., the family doctor. For the evaluation of treatment, it has proved useful in our experience to repeatedly assess the various dimensions of the pain.

3.2 Medical Diagnostic Procedures

As in all areas of medicine, a detailed medical history is of utmost importance and may provide hints on which diagnostic steps should follow, apart from the obligatory thorough physical examination. In children and adolescents, physicians should try to apply the least burdening (also including radiation protection) and least invasive procedure. Certain procedures depend on the patient's cooperation. If for an MRI examination a sedative or anesthesia are necessary (e.g., with younger children), risks and benefit should be carefully weighed.

Invasive procedures should only be applied in order to clarify a *specific* hypothesis. Some diagnostic procedures may even traumatize the patient; this should be avoided at all costs. Pain caused by taking blood for "routine blood chemistry" is unnecessary and avoidable, especially if there is no sound reason to expect a gain in information. Any necessary procedure should be performed under local anesthesia, for instance, using EMLA®. One should refrain from performing procedures explicitly requested by the parents, but not medically indexed.

3.2.1 Exclusion of Secondary Headache

The physician should be aware of which cranial structures are sensitive to pain when trying to exclude secondary headaches. Pain-sensitive structures are the skin, periosteum, and aponeuroses. In the field of ENT, pain-sensitive structures are the nasal conchae, the various sinuses, and the ear. The eyes are pain sensitive as are the dura mater, arachnoidea, and the cerebral vessels, but not so the greater part of the brain itself, where nociceptors are missing. The posterior cranial fossa and its content are sensibly innervated by the upper ipsilateral cervical roots via the glossopharyngeal and the vagus nerve. The middle and the anterior cranial fossae are innervated by the ipsilateral trigeminal nerve. By experimental stimulation of the C1 root, pain sensation is provoked in the area of the ipsilateral eye, and frontally, which shows that those areas are obviously innervated by C1.

This knowledge allows for the pinpointing of the causes of pain. In most children with headache, there is no physical cerebral correlate. The goal is to identify those patients with secondary headache who will benefit from causal therapy.

One should take into account:
1. Preceding head injury
2. Inflammation of the sinus
3. Arterial hypertension
4. Increased pressure of cerebrospinal fluid (hydrocephalus; pseudotumor cerebri)
5. Any kind of space-occupying process
6. Vasculitis (arteriitis)
7. Meningitis
8. Aneurism of cerebral vessels
9. Hypoglycemia, especially in diabetics
10. Metabolic disorders like hypo- or hyperthyroidism
11. Any adverse effects of drugs

Apart from the neurological examination in headaches of so-far-unknown origin, an EEG and an ophthalmologic examination are often indicated, including testing visual acuity and papilledema in order to exclude the possibility of increased cerebral pressure. Adequate equipment and expertise allow for a sonography of the papilla and the eyeball. Medical imaging (computer tomography; MRI) helps detect anatomic anomalies, space-occupying processes, or inflammation and vascular diseases. The most appropriate procedure can best be chosen in discussion with the radiologist in order to avoid any unnecessary burden or diagnostics not leading to the results necessary for confirming hypotheses.

3.2.2 Exclusion of Secondary Abdominal Pain

Abdominal pain in children is in most cases benign. But abdominal pain as a sign of an acute abdomen may indicate life-threatening diseases and may lead to permanent complaints limiting everyday activity. Since the interrelationships are complex, a physical cause should be excluded in any case of acute or chronic abdominal pain. Patients with functional abdominal pain not caused by an underlying organic disease sometimes undergo unnecessary invasive diagnostic procedures and long-lasting inappropriate therapeutic trials or diets that are ineffective. This will make the child and his/her parents insecure; kindergarten or school is not attended regularly, and quality of life is diminished due to the pain but also due to the time spent at the doctor's or in hospital (for details, see Sect. 4.6.1).

Characteristics of abdominal pain differ. In most cases, the child will report unspecific periumbilical pain normally attributed to functional pain (Sect. 4.6.2). In any case of sustained pain, basic diagnostics are indicated. A detailed medical history is helpful in order to get an overview of investigations already performed and to rapidly start with necessary diagnostic measures not yet performed. The following questions have proved helpful for us in the assessment of abdominal pain:

1. Is there a circadian rhythm of complaints?
2. Is the pain associated with meals?
3. Is the pain associated with eating certain foods?
4. Is any food avoided due to intolerance?
5. How is the frequency of bowel movements and stool consistency? Any blood observed in the stool?
6. Is there any stool lubrication?
7. Is the pain constant or intermittent?
8. In girls, is there any correlation with menstruation?
9. Any unintended loss of weight?

Since the abdomen is mainly connected to C-fibers, the patient is usually unable to precisely localize the painful organ. Since this is not the place to discuss the differentials of an acute abdomen, we will focus on chronic abdominal pain. Medical history and supplemental examinations are necessary in the diagnostic process. The following diseases should be excluded:

1. Chronic inflammation of the bowel (Crohn's disease; ulcerative colitis)
2. Ulcus disease
3. Gastrointestinal tumor

4. Mesenteric ischemia
5. Meckel diverticulum
6. Endometriosis
7. Ovarian tumor
8. Stenosis of the small intestine (following radiation; adhesions)
9. Post-surgery functional disorder (adhesions)
10. Disaccharide deficiency (fructose malabsorption; lactose malabsorption)
11. Celiac disease
12. Metabolic disorder (diabetes mellitus; Fabry's disease)
13. Chronic hereditary pancreatitis.

The incidence of carbohydrate malabsorption has substantially increased during the last number of years. One should know that a pathologic H2-breathing test in the absence of adequate clinical signs under exercise *by no means* proves a fructose or lactose malabsorption. Be aware of all the therapeutic consequences following a false-positive diagnosis. Dietary restrictions will add to the emotional burden. Balancing the risks and benefits, a diet only makes sense in our view in severe cases of carbohydrate malabsorption. *By no means* should a diet be prescribed in the absence of pathological clinical signs (Sect. 4.6).

3.2.3   Exclusion of Secondary Muscle or Joint Disease

Musculoskeletal pain may originate from various causes. In children, it is advisable to reconstruct the medical history, questioning the parents and the child independently. The medical history should be extended to the weeks before the onset of disease. Especially in children, it is well known that various (minor) infections may trigger reactive arthritis. There are reports of joint complaints after the use of certain antibiotics or other drugs.

(Noninvasive) joint sonography may deliver first clues to the diagnosis. Changes in the cortical bone may indicate an osteomyelitis. In case of any findings, sonography should be supplemented with conventional x-ray or MRI. Nontraumatic pain of the musculoskeletal system may be due to aseptic osteonecrosis (i.e., Perthes disease) or chronic nonbacterial osteomyelitis. In most cases, radiological findings will lead to the correct diagnosis. The diagnosis of juvenile idiopathic arthritis requires testing the blood chemistry (CRP, erythrocyte sedimentation rate, quantitative immunoglobulin in serum, complement system).

Generally, with back pain that is unresponsive to active measures such as training the back muscles or omitting excessive sports activities (in adolescents!), excluding a secondary cause is recommended, for instance, by doing x-ray imaging, scintigraphy of the skeleton, MRI of the affected spinal part, or blood chemistry (leucocytes, erythrocytes, platelets, blood smear, inflammatory parameters).

The following diseases are of importance in secondary back pain (Table 3.2).

Table 3.2 Diagnoses with chronic back pain

Diseases of the back	Diseases beyond the back
Aneurysmatic bone cyst	Disorder of a parenchymal abdominal organ
Non-inflamed necrosis	Leukemia
Protrusion of an intervertebral disc	
Inflammation	
Functional – "blockade" of the vertebral joints	
Bone tumor (benign; malignant)	
Osteoporosis	
Post-accident (i.e. fracture)	
Rheumatism	
Scheuermann's disease	
Spondylolistesis	

3.3   Psychological Diagnostic Procedures

In Chap. 2, we discussed the role of psychological factors extensively, both in the development and the maintenance of chronic pain. It is important to examine these factors in the psychological assessment. Generally, questionnaires are a valuable basic psychological diagnostic tool. However, they should never act as a substitute for a clinical interview or in-person talk; instead they are meant for screening or for building hypotheses (Andrasik and Schwartz 2006).

3.3.1   Assessment of Pain-Related Cognition and Coping Strategies

Walker et al. (2005) demonstrated that passive coping strategies (e.g., catastrophizing, social withdrawal) are positively correlated with increased pain symptoms (e.g., pain intensity), high pain-related impairment, and increased depressive symptoms after 3 months. Adaptive strategies, such as acceptance or self-encouragement, are negatively correlated with depressive symptoms (Walker et al. 2005). A meta-analysis on cognitive-behavioral therapy (CBT) of chronic pain in childhood and adolescence found that education in active coping strategies plays a central role in CBT (Eccleston et al. 2002). This study also reports that coping strategies in childhood and adolescence are not stable over time (Gil et al. 1997). Therefore, any therapy should aim at the reduction of passive coping strategies and teach active coping strategies (Walker et al. 2005). Sections 6.4.7, 6.5.3, and 6.6.3 focus on the implementation of active coping strategies into everyday life, both on the ward and in the family. Hechler and colleagues (2010b) showed that 3 months after the inpatient therapy at the German Paediatric Pain Centre (GPPC), passive pain coping and the search for social support were reduced. Changes in coping behavior were associated with a decrease in pain intensity and pain-related disability in everyday life (Hechler et al. 2010b). Questionnaires for the assessment of pain-related cognition and coping strategies are the Waldron/Varni Paediatric Pain Coping Inventory (PPCI (Varni et al. 1996)), the Pain Response Inventory (PRI (Walker et al. 1997)), and the Pain Coping Questionnaire (PCQ (Reid et al. 1998)) presented in Table 3.3.

Table 3.3 Tools for the assessment of psychological parameters in chronic pain

Construct	Questionnaire	Author (s)	Appropriate age (years)
Cognition and behavior			
Cognitive self-instruction, seek social support, strive to rest, be alone, cognitive refocusing, problem-solving self-efficacy	Waldron/Varni Paediatric Pain Coping Inventory (PPCI)	Varni et al. (1996)	5–16
Three higher-order factors: active, passive, accommodative coping; 13 subscales	Pain Response Inventory (PRI)	Walker et al. (1997)	8–18
Three higher-order factors: approach, problem-focused avoidance, emotion-focused avoidance; 8 subscales	Pain Coping Questionnaire (PCQ)	Reid et al. (1998)	7–17
Emotions			
Affective and evaluative pain perception	Varni/Thompson Paediatric Pain Questionnaire (PPC)	Varni et al. (1987)	5–15
Affective and evaluative pain perception	Adolescent Paediatric Pain Tool (APPT)	Savedra et al. (1993)	8–17
Fear of pain	Fear of Pain Questionnaire for Children (FOPQ-C)	Simons et al. (2011a)	8–17
Fear sensitivity	Childhood Anxiety Sensitivity Index (CASI)	Silverman et al. (1991)	6–17
General anxiety	Revised Child Anxiety and Depression Scale-2 (RCMAS)	Reynolds and Richmond (2008)	6–19
Depression	Children's Depression Inventory (CDI)	Kovacs (1981)	7–17
	Revised Child Anxiety and Depression Scale (RCADS)	Chorpita et al. (2000)	8–18
Emotional functioning	Paediatric Quality of Life Inventory (PedsQL)	Varni and Bernstein (1991)	2–18
Psychological well-being	Kidscreen-27	Ravens-Sieberer (2006)	8–18

Note: This table lists a selection of tools for the assessment of significant psychological parameters in a patient with a pain disorder. However, other validated questionnaire measuring those constructs may be used

3.3.2 Assessment of Emotion

The assessment of emotion is also important in the diagnostics of chronic pain. We would like to distinguish between pain-related and general constructs.

Affective pain perception, which reflects emotional impairment due to pain, may be assessed using the Varni/Thompson Paediatric Pain Questionnaire (PPC (Varni et al. 1987)) which includes a list of adjectives describing the pain. The child is asked to pick the descriptions best matching his/her pain experience. Children describe their pain perception as "sad," "cruel," or "tiring." A further tool to assess the affective pain perception using an approach similar to the PPC is the Adolescent Paediatric Pain Tool (APPT (Savedra et al. 1993)).

A tool to assess pain-related fears and avoidance behavior is the Fear of Pain Questionnaire (FOPQ-C (Simons et al. 2011b); Table 3.3). That questionnaire is constructed to assess fear of pain as well as avoidance of activities. Knowledge of the degree of pain-related fear is important to numerous therapeutic interventions, since in active pain coping, the exposure with the patient's own fears is necessary. Our clinical impression is that many children with pain disorders suffer extensive pain-related fears.

Anxiety sensitivity is strongly correlated with the degree of fear of pain (Martin et al. 2007). With ongoing chronicity, the anxiety sensitivity increases, activating the fear system by a feedback loop. The Childhood Anxiety Sensitivity Index (CASI (Silverman et al. 1991)) is a suitable tool for the assessment of that variable. Sections 2.2.2 and 6.4.6 comment in more detail on the role of anxiety sensitivity in the origin and chronicity of pain disorders and in suitable therapeutic interventions.

Avoidance behavior based on pain-related fears leads among other things to impairment of everyday life and depression, again increasing pain-related fears (Lethem et al. 1983). Furthermore, depression and fears may amplify specific pain-related fears through passivity, avoidance behavior, and loss of initiative. Hence, especially in the field of chronic pain, one should also assess general emotional impairment, such as depression or general anxiety. The degree of emotional impairment is strongly correlated with the type of coping strategy used (Eccleston et al. 2004).

There are several tools for the assessment of general anxiety and depression; some are listed in Table 3.3. Psychological well-being as a subdimension of health-related quality of life may also be assessed.

3.3.3 Assessment of Resources and Projective Diagnostics

Often, an examination of abilities, resources, aims, and personal moments of happiness is omitted, though this information is as important for therapy planning as the assessment of current problems in the patient's life. In Chap. 9 are worksheets for projective diagnostics (#6 "Complement the sentences"), for the assessment of resources and to get to know each other (#1 "Everything I judge as good…"; #2 "Everything I judge as bad…"; #5 "'Wanted' Poster"), and for the assessment of special resources and stress factors (#3 "The 5 best events, the 5 worst events"; #4 "3 things that should change soon…").

The worksheets presented in Chap. 9 are an addition to the validated diagnostic tools described earlier. The worksheets are meant to allow the child to express his/her own personality, goals, stress factors, family interactions, wishes, hopes, and hobbies in a pleasant and discrete written way. In contrast to the other tools presented in this chapter, those worksheets are neither validated nor scientifically evaluated. Therefore, the worksheets are nothing but suggestions and may be extended or shortened at will. All patients receive those six worksheets on the first day of their inpatient stay. Their task is to complete them before their first therapeutic appointment on the next day and hand them over to the NET or to the therapist. According to the therapist's individual ideas, the worksheets can be used as a basis for talks to assess resources and stress factors (for detailed instructions with regard to the first two personal therapeutic appointments, see Sect. 6.3).

3.4   Assessment of the Social Environment

Together with psychological aspects, social components like pain-related family interactions or general family stress factors are important determinants of the perpetuation of pain disorders. In this respect, extreme caring/protective parental behavior or constantly talking about pain may focus the patient on his/her pain and may thus intensify the pain (Walker et al. 2006). Distracting parental behavior may reduce pain instead (Walker et al. 2006) (for more information on integrating the family into therapy, see Sect. 6.6). Nonfamily aspects may also be important in the manifestation and perpetuation of chronic pain. Distress, e.g., due to school problems or conflicts with peers, may favor the perpetuation of pain (Miro et al. 2007).

The assessment of both parental behavior and parental cognitions related to their child's painful episodes is mandatory in order to assess family factors. Another important aspect is the assessment of satisfaction with the family, school, and peer setting (Kidscreen-27) (see Table 3.3). One tool for the assessment of parental behavior is the Adult Responses to Children's Symptoms (ARCS (Van Slyke and Walker 2006)), which examines protective, minimizing, and encouraging/monitoring parental behavior towards the child's pain. Since increased pain-related devotion and attention may be an issue in the manifestation and maintenance of paediatric pain disorders, it is generally helpful if distracting behavior is increased within the family and attentive reactions are shown irrespective of the child's pain (Sect. 6.6.3). Apart from pain-related interactions, the whole family system is of importance. Behavior-related interactions in particular can best be assessed by direct observation, such as observing communication between the parents on the ward or an extended interview with the child, his/her family, or the child's therapist.

It is much easier to assess pain-related catastrophizing ideas by means of questionnaires than by behavior-related interactions. Parental cognitions are examined using the Parental Catastrophizing Scale (PCS-P (Goubert et al. 2006)). That tool determines the extent of catastrophizing manifested as feelings of helplessness, rumination, or magnification. To our knowledge, a validation study of this questionnaire has not yet been published in English.

3.4.1   Working with Genograms

In our experience, it is always helpful to construct a family genogram in addition to the results received from questionnaire assessment. This is not the right place to give detailed information on the theory, background, or construction of a genogram (for more information on the topic, see McGoldrick et al. (2008)). At the GPPC, the construction of a genogram, starting with information on the grandparents, is part of the admission interview with the child and his/her parents. The genogram is conducted together with the physician, the pain therapist, and a member of the NET (for technical details, see Sect. 6.6.1).

3.5   Multimodal Pain Assessment Tools

As already mentioned, to diagnose pain disorders, several dimensions of the pain experience should be examined. In clinical practice, the assessment of a multidimensional pain history is another important diagnostic approach, in addition to the previously described pain diagnostics, delivering lots of information about all three dimensions of pain within a short time (Nilges et al. 2007).

3.5.1   Pain Questionnaire for Children and Adolescents

The "*Pain Questionnaire for Children and Adolescents*" (PQCA (Schroeder et al. 2010)) is a multidimensional questionnaire. It was originally developed in Germany and is now translated into English (to receive a copy, e-mail B. Zernikow@Kinderklinik-Datteln.de). The PQCA allows the structured assessment of general medical and pain history; makes an estimate of pain-related impairment, appraisals, and attitudes; and assesses other pain-triggering and intensifying factors. In addition, it delivers preliminary information on factors of the social environment (family, kindergarten, school) possibly relevant to the pain (Sect. 3.4). There are predefined answers as well as open questions where the child may describe his/her pain and its consequences. Table 3.4 lists the main components of the PQCA.

Table 3.4 Components of the "Pain Questionnaire for Children and Adolescents" (PQCA (Schroeder et al. 2010))

1. Sociodemographic data and family history
2. Pain characteristics
3. Pain triggering and pain modulating factors
4. Previous examinations and previous therapies
5. Pain-related impairment
6. Cognitive-emotional and behavioral effects; subjective concept of the disorder

Apart from the numerous single items assigned to the diverse main components, the PQCA also includes two scales. Pain-related impairment in everyday life is rated by the *Paediatric Pain Disability Index* (P-PDI (Hübner et al. 2009)). This 12-item scale assesses the frequency of the child being kept from various everyday activities and scores from 12 to 60. A score of 36 or higher indicates an extremely high pain-related disability (Dobe et al. 2006, 2011). The questionnaire is validated in German for the self-assessment of children aged 11 years and up. In younger children, the parents' answers may be used. A validation of the English version has not yet been performed, but will be done in the near future.

Another scale that is part of the PQCA is the Pain Perception Scale for Adolescents (Wager et al. 2010). This scale assesses the affective pain perception as a measure of pain-related emotional impairment (Sect. 3.2) as well as sensory pain qualities such as "pressing," "pulsating," or "burning" which may be useful in the differential diagnostics of primary headaches. A validation study of the German version indicates that adolescents aged 11 years and up may rate their pain perceptions themselves. In younger children, parents' answers may be used. Again, this scale has so far not been validated in English, but a validation study will be undertaken in the near future.

Tools for assessing pain intensity vary according to the child's age. Adolescents aged 11 years or older score pain intensity on a numeric rating scale (0 = no pain at all, 10 = worst pain (von Baeyer et al. 2009)). Since in younger children that scale is less suitable (von Baeyer et al. 2009), the child version of the PQCA contains a faces pain scale (Faces Pain Scale Revised, FPS-R (Hicks et al. 2001)).

There are three different versions of the PQCA: (1) for children aged 4–10 years, (2) for adolescents aged 11–18 years, and (3) for parents or the main carer of the patient. The different versions were developed based on the patients' respective developmental level. Hence, the questionnaire for children comprises assessment modules different to those for adolescents and is much shorter. In children lacking the necessary ability to read or write, their parents are asked to read the questions aloud and record their child's answers. The parent version of the questionnaire allows for an extended collection of information as well as the assessment of parental perspectives with regard to their child's pain problem. The PQCA for the first contact is extensive; there are shorter versions for the application in the course of treatment in order to assess treatment effects. The latter may be used every three (or more) months.

The PQCA is especially suitable for preparing the first contact with a patient since apart from a great deal of medical, psychological, and social information, it also assesses the criteria necessary for recommending (or not) inpatient pain therapy (Chap. 5). E-mail B.Zernikow@kinderklinik-Datteln.de to receive the electronic version of the questionnaire free of charge.

3.5.2 Pain Diary

Especially in children with headache, a pain diary is a valuable tool for both diagnostics and the assessment of the effects of various therapeutic measures. With respect to treatment, it may be helpful to use a pain diary in order to distinguish between different headache diagnoses (e.g., migraine vs. tension-type headache). During the course of treatment, a pain diary may be applied in order to check the child's ability to distinguish between different kinds of headache, if therapeutic measures are effective, or if trigger factors can be identified.

Keeping a diary allows a continuous and prompt recording. Diaries are a reliable source of information in the diagnostics of headache (Phillip et al. 2007), and, in direct comparison, they allow the child to recognize changes in the course of treatment. Furthermore, they help strengthen self-controlled action (Hechler et al. 2010a). Diaries should record the main parameters of pain (intensity, frequency, and duration). Of further interest are trigger factors, consequences of pain, pain medication, emotional well-being, impairment, attendant symptoms as well as applied coping strategies (Hechler et al. 2009). If pain comes in attacks or is recurrent, the pain diary should be kept for an extended period of time (e.g., three months) (Kröner-Herwig et al. 1992). Much more problematic is the use of pain diaries in children with pain disorders, since the diary may contribute to an intensified pain perception by making the patient focus on his/her pain. It is an individual decision if keeping a pain diary makes sense – there should be a good balance between gaining information and pain amplification. In inpatient pain therapy at the GPPC, many children keep their diary just for the first few days of treatment. At days 4–7, we switch to the documentation of distraction where the patient doesn't record the instantaneous pain intensity anymore but instead the active distraction method he/she used with which type of headache, and how efficient this strategy was.

The authors developed a headache diary assessing some criteria of primary headache of the International Headache Society (IHS). Based on recorded pain intensity and accompanying symptoms, headache diaries are a good tool for diagnosing migraine at a glance. Since the time of drug application is exactly recorded, they also allow us to rate the effectiveness of medication. Furthermore, a week's documentation facilitates the recognition of any pattern of weekdays with pronounced pain or changes in the course of pain during a week (to receive a copy of the English version of the diary free of charge, e-mail B.Zernikow@kinderklinik-Datteln.de).

References

Andrasik F, Schwartz MS (2006) Behavioral assessment and treatment of pediatric headache. Behav Modif 30(1):93–113

Chorpita BF, Yim L, Moffitt C, Umemoto LA, Francis SE (2000) Assessment of symptoms of DSM-IV anxiety and depression in children: a revised child anxiety and depression scale. Behav Res Ther 38(8):835–855

Dobe M, Damschen U, Reiffer-Wiesel B, Sauer C, Zernikow B (2006) Multimodal inpatient pain treatment in children – results of a three-week program. Schmerz 20(1):51–60

Dobe M, Hechler T, Behlert J, Kosfelder J, Zernikow B (2011) Pain therapy with children and adolescents severely disabled due to chronic pain – long-term outcome after inpatient pain therapy. Schmerz 25(4):411–422

Eccleston C, Morley S, Williams AC, Yorke L, Mastroyannopoulou K (2002) Systematic review of randomised controlled trials of psychological therapy for chronic pain in children and adolescents, with a subset of meta-analysis of pain relief. Pain 99(1–2):157–165

Eccleston C, Crombez G, Scotford A, Clinch J, Connell H (2004) Adolescent chronic pain: patterns and predictors of emotional distress in adolescents with chronic pain and their parents. Pain 108(3):221–229

Gil KM, Wilson JJ, Edens JL (1997) The stability of pain coping strategies in young children, adolescents, and adults with sickle cell disease over an 18-month period. Clin J Pain 13(2):110–115

Goubert L, Eccleston C, Vervoort T, Jordan A, Crombez G (2006) Parental catastrophizing about their child's pain. The parent version of the Pain Catastrophizing Scale (PCS-C): a preliminary validation. Pain 123(3):254–263

Hechler T, Dobe M, Kosfelder J, Damschen U, Hübner B, Blankenburg M, Sauer C, Zernikow B (2009) Effectiveness of a three-week multimodal inpatient pain treatment for adolescents suffering from chronic pain: statistical and clinical significance. Clin J Pain 25(2):156–166

Hechler T, Blankenburg M, Dobe M, Kosfelder J, Hübner B, Zernikow B (2010a) Effectiveness of a multimodal inpatient treatment for pediatric chronic pain: a comparison between children and adolescents. Eur J Pain 14(1):97.e1–97.e9

Hechler T, Kosfelder J, Vocks S, Mönninger T, Blankenburg M, Dobe M, Gerlach AL, Denecke H, Zernikow B (2010b) Changes in pain-related coping strategies and their importance for treatment outcome following multimodal inpatient treatment: does sex matter? J Pain 11(5):472–483

Hicks CL, von Baeyer CL, Spafford PA, van Korlaar I, Goodenough B (2001) The faces pain scale-revised: toward a common metric in pediatric pain measurement. Pain 93(2):173–183

Hübner B, Hechler T, Dobe M, Damschen U, Kosfelder J, Denecke H, Schroeder S, Zernikow B (2009) Pain-related disability in adolescents suffering from chronic pain: preliminary examination of the pediatric Pain Disability Index (P-PDI). Schmerz 23(1):20–32

Kovacs M (1981) Rating scales to assess depression in school-aged children. Acta Paedopsychiatr 46(5–6):305–315

Kröner-Herwig B, Plump U, Pothmann R (1992) Progressive relaxation and EMG biofeedback in the treatment of chronic headache in children. Results of an explorative study. Schmerz 6(2):121–127

Lethem J, Slade PD, Troup JDG, Bentley G (1983) Outline of a Fear-Avoidance Model of exaggerated pain perception–I. Behav Res Ther 21(4):401–408

Martin AL, McGrath P, Brown SC, Katz J (2007) Anxiety and sensitivity, fear of pain and pain-related disability in children and adolescents with chronic pain. Pain Res Manag 12(4):267–272

McGoldrick M, Gerson R, Petry S (2008) Genograms: assessment and intervention. W.W. Norton & Company, New York\London

Miro J, Huguet A, Nieto R (2007) Predictive factors of chronic pediatric pain and disability: a Delphi Poll. J Pain 8(10):774–792

Nilges P, Köster B, Schmidt CO (2007) Pain acceptability – concept and verification of the German version of the Chronic Pain Acceptance Questionnaire. Schmerz 21(1):57–67

Phillip D, Lyngberg A, Jensen R (2007) Assessment of headache diagnosis. A comparative population study of a clinical interview with a diagnostic headache diary. Cephalalgia 27(1):1–8

Ravens-Sieberer U (2006) The KIDSCREEN questionnaires – quality of life questionnaires for children and adolescents – handbook. Pabst Science Publisher, Lengerich

Reid GJ, Gilbert CA, McGrath PA (1998) The Pain Coping Questionnaire: preliminary validation. Pain 76(1–2):83–96

Reynolds CR, Richmond BO (2008) Revised children's manifest anxiety scale-second edition manual. Western Psychological Services, Torrance

Savedra MC, Holzemer WL, Tesler MD, Wilkie DJ (1993) Assessment of postoperation pain in children and adolescents using the adolescent pediatric pain tool. Nurs Res 42(1):5–9

Schroeder S, Hechler T, Denecke H, Müller-Busch M, Martin A, Menke A, Zernikow B (2010) German Pain Questionnaire for Children, Adolescents and Parents (DSF-KJ) – a multimodal questionnaire for diagnosis and treatment of children and adolescents suffering from chronic pain. Schmerz 24(1):23–37

Silverman WK, Fleisig W, Rabian B, Peterson RA (1991) Childhood anxiety sensitivity index. J Clin Child Psychol 20(2):162–168

Simons LE, Sieberg CB, Carpino E, Logan D, Berde C (2011a) The Fear of Pain Questionnaire (FOPQ): assessment of pain-related fear among children and adolescents with chronic pain. J Pain 12(6):677–686

Simons LE, Sieberg CB, Kaczynski KJ (2011b) Measuring parent beliefs about child acceptance of pain: a preliminary validation of the Chronic Pain Acceptance Questionnaire, parent report. Pain 152(10):2294–2300

Van Slyke DA, Walker LS (2006) Mothers' responses to children's pain. Clin J Pain 22(4):387–391

Varni JW, Bernstein BH (1991) Evaluation and management of pain in children with rheumatic disease. Rheum Dis Clin North Am 17(4):985–1000

Varni JW, Thompson KL, Hanson V (1987) The Varni/Thompson Pediatric Pain Questionnaire: I. Chronic musculoskeletal pain in juvenile rheumatoid arthritis. Pain 28(1):27–38

Varni JW, Waldron SA, Gragg RA, Rapoff MA, Bernstein BH, Lindsley CB, Newcomb MD (1996) Development of the Waldron/Varni pediatric pain coping inventory. Pain 67(1):141–150

von Baeyer CL, Spagrud LJ, McCormick JC, Choo E, Neville K, Connelly MA (2009) Three new datasets supporting use of the numerical rating scale (NRS-11) for children's self-reports of pain intensity. Pain 143(3):223–227

Wager J, Tietze AL, Denecke H, Schroeder S, Vocks S, Kosfelder J, Zernikow B, Hechler T (2010) Pain perception of adolescents with chronic functional pain: adaptation and psychometric validation of the Pain Perception Scale (SES) by Geissner. Schmerz 24(3):236–250

Walker LS, Garber SJ, Van Slyke DA (1997) Development and validation of the Pain Response Inventory for children. Psychol Asses 9(4):392–405

Walker LS, Smith CA, Garber J, Claar RL (2005) Testing a model of pain appraisal and coping in children with chronic abdominal pain. Health Psychol 24(4):364–374

Walker LS, Williams SE, Smith CA, Garber J, Van Slyke DA, Lipani TA (2006) Parent attention versus distraction: impact on symptom complaints by children with and without chronic functional abdominal pain. Pain 122(1–2):43–52

The Basics of Treating Pain Disorders in Children and Adolescents

4

Michael Dobe, Holger Kriszio, and Boris Zernikow

Contents

M. Dobe (✉) • H. Kriszio
German Paediatric Pain Centre (GPPC), Children's and Adolescents' Hospital,
Witten/Herdecke University,
Dr.-Friedrich-Steiner Street 5, Datteln 45711, Germany
e-mail: m.dobe@kinderklinik-datteln.de

B. Zernikow
German Paediatric Pain Centre (GPPC), Children's and Adolescents' Hospital,
Witten/Herdecke University,
Dr.-Friedrich-Steiner Street 5, Datteln 45711, Germany

Chair Children's Pain Therapy and Paediatric Palliative Care,
Witten/Herdecke University, School of Medicine,
Datteln 45711, Germany
e-mail: b.zernikow@deutsches-kinderschmerzzentrum.de

M. Dobe, B. Zernikow (eds.),
Practical Treatment Options for Chronic Pain in Children and Adolescents,
DOI 10.1007/978-3-642-37816-4_4, © Springer-Verlag Berlin Heidelberg 2013

Abstract

This chapter presents the basics necessary for professionals to provide effective treatment of pain disorders in children and adolescents. These basics are independent of the actual therapeutic setting or the therapists' medical or therapeutic backgrounds. The reader will get to know the "Three Thought Traps" favoring the development of pain disorders. We then discuss the necessity of active pain coping strategies and of integrating the family into the therapy. We present important aspects of drug-based pain therapy and medical background information on the most important biological determinants of chronic headache, abdominal pain, or back pain in childhood and adolescence. Finally, we discuss therapeutic attitude and the functionality of pain.

In this chapter we present several principles which should be followed independent of the actual therapeutic setting or methodology in order to achieve the most beneficial treatment outcome in paediatric pain disorders. Any therapeutic interventions based on these principles are presented in Chap. 6. Some aspects (e.g., the "Three Thought Traps") are based on our own clinical experience. Other aspects arise from scientific knowledge (e.g., indication for and risk of analgesic usage). Certainly, the list of relevant aspects could be endless. But, from our experience, adhering to the basics discussed in this chapter suffices to build a sustainable therapeutic relationship with the child and his/her family which is the foundation stone of successful paediatric pain therapy.

4.1 "Three Thought Traps"

Working with children with chronic pain and their parents or the numerous therapists over the years, we learned about many attempts to explain the phenomenon of pain disorders. Generally, most of the different explanatory attempts differ due to individual cultural, biographical, or professional backgrounds and follow a dualistic world view. Those simple explanatory attempts seem to keep one grounded in times of helplessness, and by their straight relationship of cause and effect, they give hope ("Having found the cause I will eliminate it, and with it the unpleasant effect (the pain)"). Following such a problem-solving strategy is understandable from a patient's and his/her family's point of view. However, it is damaging if a professional helper system supports, or even amplifies, such thinking. Of course, it is tempting to seek a monocausal explanation for pain disorders in the specific areas the therapist is familiar with. But, scientific findings show that such an approach is wrong, and according to personal experience, it hinders the healing process. A monocausal explanatory attempt and its respective treatment make further chronicity of pain symptomatology even more probable (Flor and Diers 2007).

In spite of their obvious differences, the various monocausal explanatory attempts may be classified into three approaches. We call them the "Three Thought Traps."

The First Thought Trap: "Everything Is of Pure Psychological Origin"

Here chronic pain is seen as the result of a suspected or actual mental conflict while neglecting the influence of any biological factors. Normally, it is not the affected child but his/her parent(s) (in most cases just one of them) and/or the therapist being trapped in this thought. They make statements typical of this trap, such as "You are in pain because … (take one of the following: … you don't want to go to school; … you don't fight; … you have conflicts with your boyfriend/girlfriend; … you are under too much stress; …)."

Certainly, psychological conflicts may negatively influence the experience of pain mediated by concomitant physical stress and anxiety. But rarely would this alone cause chronic pain. Furthermore, this thought invalidates the child's own perception. His/her impairing pain experience is not taken seriously, or even worse, between the lines they are accused of exaggerating their pain in order to avoid unpleasant activities. Processes of sensitization and conditioning as well as clearly somatic influences, such as migraine or irritable bowel syndrome, remain unconsidered. And even worse, there is no good way out for those children. The more they try to show their environment how severe their pain is, the more they are perceived as being hysterical, or they are told they just imagine their pain. If they try, however, to stay active despite their pain, nobody will believe that they actually experience pain. In our experience, the First Thought Trap often leads to an impaired child-parent relationship and/or a dropout of therapy in a case where one of the parents or the therapist remains trapped in the First Thought Trap. In such a constellation, many children report feeling left alone and resign from therapy.

The Second Thought Trap: "Everything Is of Pure Physical Origin"

This Thought Trap is the most frequent approach to explain the suffering and the impairment caused by a pain disorder. The simple logic behind this Thought Trap is that something "feeling" so bad has to have a bad cause. This will lead to the paradoxical effect – well known to most physicians – that parents and their child aren't relieved at all if medical examinations don't reveal any pathologic result or at least no result exhibiting a causal relationship to the presented symptoms.

In consequence, the child will undergo more and more medical investigations all leading to the abovementioned effect. As time goes by, the child will lose faith that he/she will get help by someone since "no underlying cause" can be identified. The more investigations are performed, the higher the probability that a somewhat suspicious but clinically insignificant (random) result will arise. Furthermore, these investigations inherit a certain measurement error, and one should be aware that the human factor is present in conducting, analyzing, and evaluating the investigation. Normal values reflect only a part of the population. Genetic variants where a "suspicious" result is normal are often not taken into account. Not being aware of those statistical considerations, a suspicious finding may result in even more insecurity for the patient and in more or less amateurish and bizarre explanations (often based on self-performed Internet enquiry), and those findings may erroneously be set into a causal relation with the symptomatology.

At the same time, the child and his/her parents may be encouraged in their Thought Trap by their contact with the professional helper. Repeatedly, parents reported about therapists who assigned an abnormal occlusion, vertebral blockade, wrong nutrition, a special type of ametropia, or "inner imbalance" as the *only* cause of the child's chronic pain. (In this regard, we would like to emphasize that we consider especially a monocausal explanation model as problematic. The mentioned factors may well *contribute* to a pain disorder. However, it is very unlikely that they would be the only cause.)

The effect is especially drastic if therapeutic recommendations derived from a monocausal explanatory model result in a substantial financial burden for the family (e.g., treatment costs to be privately paid), a substantial restriction of quality of life (rigid change of nutritional habits), or physical endangering of the child (e.g., unnecessary surgical procedures or only minimally effective daily intake of analgesics for several months). Luckily, many parents intuitively decline such treatment recommendations or interrupt therapy if the hoped-for improvement doesn't materialize. Such decisions should not be considered a lack of compliance but a sign of healthy reflection.

Finally, with people following this Thought Trap, we face the risk of further deterioration of the situation. The search for and the fight against what is seen as the somatic "cause" results in frustration and hopelessness and consequently more passivity and resignation.

The Third Thought Trap: "The Pain Must Vanish at All Costs"

Simplified, this Thought Trap is the exaggeration of the First or Second Thought Trap (mostly the Second Thought Trap) combined with an additional very low acceptance of pain. The child, his/her parents, and often the previous therapists agreed that under no circumstances should pain be accepted but should be fought like an enemy.

It is our experience that especially for children stuck in the Third Thought Trap and suffering low pain tolerance, often other psychological factors play an important role; Furthermore, the Third Thought Trap induces exaggerated inherent focusing on the issue "pain"; this combined with low pain acceptance mostly results in a fast and pronounced increase in helplessness in the child and his/her parents.

In this Thought Trap, a combination of such unfavorable factors bears the risk of a treatment endangering quality of life and health. The lack of success in finding the "cause" leads to pronounced helplessness and puts a lot of pressure on the professional helper system to eventually "do something." Such a situation may result in a lack of objectivity and measures or therapies that are not indexed. A lack of objectivity may result in the prolonged prescription of not medically indexed analgesics (in case of headache or backache), or surgical procedures (appendectomy where conservative measures are ineffective). Restrictive diets (e.g., free of lactose or even fructose in clinically insignificant disaccharide deficiency and chronic abdominal pain not associated with nutrition), restriction of physical activity, or the drastic reduction of all kinds of stressors (e.g., home schooling instead of attending regular classes) are just as harmful.

To summarize, the Three Thought Traps are based on our clinical experience and are not necessarily a comprehensive description. In most cases there is an artificial focus on just one aspect of the pain disorder, and concomitantly the other two factors are ignored (Chap. 2). Sometimes the child and his/her parents switch between the different Thought Traps. It is interesting to see that there are very few children and families with a fixation on social factors as the cause, such as "Other people are to blame for my child suffering chronic pain." For the successful treatment of pain disorders, it is most relevant to acknowledge that a prerequisite is the resolution of the Thought Trap(s) in the child *and* his/her parents. Hence, the right education from the very beginning (starting with the first contact with the therapist) is crucial for the course of treatment. For an in-depth discussion of age-appropriate education adapted to the child's developmental stage, see Sect. 6.3.2.

4.2   Active vs. Passive Pain Coping Strategies

It is crucial for an effective therapy to take the pain coping style favored by the child and his/her family into account (Sects. 2.2 and 2.3.). Put simply, all attempts to cope with pain and its respective therapies may be classified into active or passive coping strategies. While both active and passive coping strategies have their place in everyday life and in acute pain, the rule of thumb for pain disorders is: the more passive the worse. Why is that? After all, the child and his/her parents (mostly) concomitantly report that avoidance of physical activity or passivity leads to a slight reduction of pain symptoms. However, the three main reasons for using active coping are as follows:

First, in pain disorders avoidance of physical activity or exaggerated passivity (lying down, resting) will – nearly inevitably – result in an increase in body awareness in the long run. In an environment nearly devoid of stimuli, the patient will focus more on any (endogenous) stimulus (in this case, specifically on pain), amplifying pain perception and finally leading to consolidation of pain memory (Sect. 2.2).

Second, in the course of the pain disorder, there is a secondary dysfunctional development that is not directly part of the pain symptomatology. We are all familiar with the experience of the first day back at work after a holiday or a leave due to illness. The restorative effect of the holiday only lasts a short time once we are again under the stress of work. This manual is not the right place to discuss the responsible complex regulatory loops of the sympathetic nervous system. Simplified, our ability to cope with everyday stressors depends on biological laws that become obvious in endurance training. After some weeks of running three times a week for an hour, one won't be out of breath anymore. But, after a longer interruption of the regular training schedule, part of the training effect has vanished and has to be reestablished. What does this have to do with pain symptoms? If for several weeks up to several months a child avoids physical activity, or is passive, his/her ability to cope with everyday stressors is diminished, and he/she will experience exhaustion, distress, or tension more quickly. Confronting a child with a pain disorder with a normal amount of everyday activity will provoke a moderate to pronounced increase in pain at the beginning. This will strengthen the child's and his/her family's belief that avoidance of physical activity or passivity is best for pain reduction, and confronting everyday duties is best done when the pain "is gone" or at least significantly reduced. Such an interpretation – as understandable as it may be – turns the cause-and-effect relationship upside down and will consolidate the chronicity of symptoms. In consequence, this often results in social withdrawal, fear of (non-)achievement, or fear of school.

Third, passivity and avoidance of physical activity reduce self-esteem in the long run since the experience of success is missing, and as time goes by self-doubts and fear of the future increase. In the end, all this causes an amplification of pain in a vicious cycle.

In our experience, especially at the beginning of pain therapy, interviews with the child and his/her family focus on the topic of activity and passivity. Many parents fear hurting their child trying to enforce active pain coping. The child's fear is that pain will become unbearable with more activity. The authors feel the best way to show that those fears are unfounded is to give a brief overview of the following scientific data:

In outpatient and inpatient pain therapy of both children *and* adults suffering chronic pain, *independent* of the cause of the physical pain (even after a slipped disk, accident, rheumatic disease, or any other inflammatory process), the implementation of an active pain coping strategy is a prerequisite for long-term success (Claar et al. 2008; Eccleston et al. 2004; Hermann et al. 2007; Hechler et al. 2010). Not to be misunderstood: in acute pain, e.g., immediately after an accident or a sports injury, physical rest is medically indicated for a short time but not for weeks or months. In Sects. 6.6.2 and 6.6.3, we present in detail a method for getting the parents and their child involved in active pain coping.

4.3 Integration of the Family System

"My mother's love doesn't help me." – Jan (12 years)

According to Sects. 4.1 and 4.2, the close integration of the family in the therapy is a prerequisite for successful paediatric pain treatment. But education with respect to the Three Thought Traps and the child's support in active pain coping strategies are not the only reasons to integrate the family system.

Often, parents have strong ties with their child and can intuitively judge the situation quite well. However, they are trapped in interdependencies with other important attachment figures and/or their perception is easily influenced by others. Well-meaning advice starts with "The child doesn't drink enough" and extends to "You were never able to exert your will with your child," "How could you send your child to school with so much pain?" or "If I were you, I would look after my child in need." Parents or their children report variants of these forms of advice and reproaches. In order for the parents to be able to withstand this pressure, it is important for us to strengthen them with helpful information (e.g., handing out the parents' guide "How to stop chronic pain in children: a practical guide" (Dobe and Zernikow 2013); Sect. 6.6.7); the same applies to handling teachers, physicians, or therapists not familiar with this matter. Strengthening the parents is also important in order to avert the jeopardy of ongoing medical investigations or placebo treatment instead of effective therapy.

And there are still some other reasons to integrate the family system, namely, the presence of various interactions within the family during or after pain therapy that perpetuate the pain.

1. There is evidence that decreased satisfaction in the parental relationship and specific concomitant interactions have a negative impact on paediatric headache (Quiring et al. 2007; see Logan et al. 2012, for an overview).

2. On the other hand, increased concerns and worries of the family may cause other conflicts to be pushed back while the child's pain becomes the main focus of family interaction (e.g., more frequent inquiry on pain, searching the Internet for new treatment modalities, disputes on the right approach or the truth about the diagnosis (especially in separated parents), or permissive parenting style due to feelings of guilt).

3. Intensified querying about the pain often results in a phenomenon we mischievously call "sentimental pap" (Sect. 6.6.3). All kinds of negative emotions may exaggerate the pain experience. The child, however, is asked about nothing else but the pain, thus putting nothing but the pain into focus. In this case, we observe that with ongoing chronic pain many children increasingly lose the ability to distinguish between their various negative emotions. This is especially harmful if the child has been insufficiently trained before to distinguish between various emotions.

4. If one or both of the parents also suffer from a pain disorder, this is very unfavorable for their child's pain symptomatology. Children with parents having a history of chronic pain are at an increased risk of developing pain disorders (Merlijn et al. 2003). And many children report being upset that the one family member suffering the most pain gets the most care and attention. This does not necessarily mean that the child will adopt this mostly disliked pattern of interaction. But, since it threatens the child's basic needs, it must be a part of education for the affected parent and has to be considered in pain therapy.

5. Affected parents may find it more difficult to encourage their child with active pain coping. Empathy is evoked via cerebral processes resulting in activation of mirrored processes in the observer (Loggia et al. 2008). Thus, in parents with chronic pain, perceiving their child's pain results in an increase in their own pain. Parental support for a child's active pain coping strategies is a significant success and should be reinforced by praise.

6. Finally, aspects of the family learning model play an important role in the manifestation or perpetuation of pain disorders (e.g., to what degree parents cope actively or passively with demands or emotional crises). Certainly, not every unfavorable interaction pattern should become a matter of discussion within the family. Normally, children are well able to decide what makes sense for them in the long run and what doesn't. If, however, during her emotional crises a mother

tends to lie weeping in her child's arms, in the long run the child will be overburdened by the situation, and alternative solutions have to be sought (e.g., psychotherapy for the mother).

While the logic underlying our approach (e.g., not asking about the pain) should be evident by now, it is not yet clear at first glance which type of family interaction is counterproductive for long-term success *after having completed* pain therapy. The two most important determinants are:

1. After some time (on average, children coming for inpatient pain therapy have been suffering chronic pain for 3–4 years already (Dobe et al. 2011)), the pain disorder usually has a moderate to strong impact on the development of the child's autonomy, which is a consequence of increasing passivity along with social withdrawal. The resulting proximity to the family system is experienced as being either pleasant or unpleasant depending on the individual child and his/her family. The normal development of autonomy is hereby often hampered. Successful pain therapy in a child with chronic pain results in catching up with the "missed" autonomy conflicts. In order to allow for a good long-term thera-peutic relationship with the whole family system, we highly suggest discussing this aspect of treatment well at the beginning of therapy and asking the parents for their "consent" for this type of "adverse effect" of successful pain therapy (for details of our approach, see Sect. 6.6).

2. Emotional exhaustion ("emptiness") or sometimes depression (mostly in moth-ers) is another aspect of family interaction frequently manifesting itself towards the end of effective pain therapy. This may happen once the threat (pain) to the well-being of the beloved child has been averted. The occurrence of such symp-toms in the parents depends on numerous biographic factors. No outsider can grasp the emotional burden on the parents when their child suffers chronic pain. Hence, we recommend treating the parents with respect and avoiding blaming them or making them feel causally responsible for their child's disorder. In Sect. 6.6 we will discuss therapeutic approaches to this conflict between child and parents, one that is not easy to resolve.

To put it plainly: For successful and lasting treatment of paediatric pain disor-ders, it is of the utmost importance that the whole family system be closely involved from the start.

4.4 Using Analgesics in Paediatric Pain Disorders

One should have a diagnosis before using analgesics in children, as is usual in drug therapy. As a next step, the physician has to decide if analgesic therapy is useful with this diagnosis. Pain medication has the potential for adverse effects. For instance, with ibuprofen, adverse gastrointestinal effects are frequent (an inhibited prostaglandin synthesis results in disturbance of the gastric mucous membrane). While analgesics are very helpful with many acute pain conditions, they are at the same time not proven with most chronic ones.

Using analgesics makes sense only if a sustained nociceptive stimulus is part of the chronic pain disease (e.g., neuropathic pain, arthritis, inflammation) or in case of recurring acute pain in addition to chronic pain (e.g., migraine). In such cases it is important to inform the child and his/her parents of the effects that can be expected from the analgesic (it won't eliminate the pain disorder) and how to use the analgesic properly (e.g., take the *full* dose *as soon as possible* during a migraine attack, and take an additional reduced dose "if pain becomes unbearable"). In chronic pain disorders, common analgesics have frequently proven not very effective in clinical trials; this is also our clinical experience (Sect. 8.1). Nevertheless, on a daily basis we see children at our outpatient clinic who have been taking analgesics for months or even years even though the desired effect has not been seen. They argue: "I fear my pain will become worse if I stop taking the medication." This fear of increased pain when stopping medication makes them accept the risk of severe adverse effects. Frequently, the children become physically addicted (e.g., with opioids). During opioid weaning an increase in pain is indeed observed. Section 4.5.4 deals especially with analgesics and their adverse effects in paediatric headache.

To summarize, neither scientific data nor our clinical experience prove that – except in acute pain – analgesics are beneficial in paediatric pain disorders. In fact, one could better think of the Third Thought Trap in a case of continual and substantial use of analgesics (Sect. 4.1). Many children and their parents are not properly informed about analgesics (they may not have been informed of the risks of analgesics abuse). They are shocked when learning about the possible adverse effects of daily drug consumption. Generally, we recommend limiting the usage of analgesics (e.g., if we are uncertain that there is an underlying rheumatic disease, or in acute backache) to a certain time period and communicate that decision to the child and his/her parents together with a warning of possible adverse effects. A reduction in pain after taking analgesics is *not* always due to the analgesics. To a great extent, seemingly successful drug therapy in pain disorders is a brief *placebo* effect *not* resulting in decreased pain-related restrictions of daily activities.

4.5   The Basics on Paediatric Headache

Section 2.1.2 discussed the biological background of the most important types of paediatric headache (migraine, tension headache) at length. Section 3.2.1 presented the medical diagnostic procedures necessary to exclude secondary paediatric headache. In this section we summarize the most important definitions and facts of primary paediatric headache.

4.5.1   Primary vs. Secondary Headache

Every fifth to sixth child reports headache with a frequency of at least once a weak (Perquin et al. 2000) which may be primary (headache not due to physical disease) or secondary (headache as a symptom of an underlying somatic disease). The International Headache Society classifies headache into more than 100 different types. Fortunately, paediatric chronic headache is usually of primary origin; paediatric secondary headache is a rarity. How to differentiate primary from secondary headache is discussed in Sect. 3.2.1.

4.5.2 Paediatric Migraine with or Without Aura

About 6 % of children and adolescents suffer migraine (Bigal et al. 2007). Even infants may show symptoms typical of migraine that respond well to standard medical treatment. Often, a migraine treated insufficiently, incorrectly, or not at all plays an important role in the development of pain disorders with the main pain localization in the head. Hence, for the planning and implementation of paediatric headache therapy, it is important to diagnose the migraine with/without aura with certainty and treat it sufficiently.

The biological background of migraine was discussed in Sect. 2.1.2. The patients and their parents, however, need a much shorter summary focusing on the practical aspects of the subject.

How to best educate a child and his/her parents on the complex biological interplay that happens during a migraine attack? In the following you will find an example educational explanation aimed at older children and their parents.

Example: Migraine Education

The disposition towards migraine is inherited. Simply speaking, a child inherits a "migraine generator" from his/her parent. A migraine generator is an area of the brain where cerebral cells seem to be very sensitive to any kind of pronounced "change." Those brain cells don't care about the nature of the change, be it psychological distress, a variation in hormone levels, daily schedule, sleep habit, or a change in the weather. In some children even certain smells or foods may stimulate those cells. Depending on the frequency and intensity of these changes, the migraine generator discharges in more or less regular intervals, in a similar way to a short-circuited battery. But how does this lead to pain or accompanying symptoms (nausea, vomiting, intolerance to noise or light, impaired vision) when the brain is devoid of nociceptors?

The migraine generator is cross-linked with numerous brain areas. Brain cells, the diameter of the blood vessels, and their sensitivity to stimuli are altered via the neural network or changes in the cerebral neurotransmitters in a manner in which even the blood pulsating through the vessels is perceived as pain ("pulsating" pain). Activation of the neural connections to the vomiting center provokes nausea. You can imagine how busy the brain is with the numerous stimuli during a migraine attack. Therefore, children appear different during a migraine attack; often they become very tired, irritable, or very excited.

The next step is to explain why it is important to take the analgesic as early as possible and in the right dose.

"The migraine attack leads to chaos in the brain. Once it starts, it is difficult to interrupt it – especially since enteral analgesics aren't readily absorbed. But if an analgesic – the most frequently used is ibuprofen – is taken at the very beginning of the migraine attack, there is enough time for the analgesic to be absorbed and transported into the brain. Luckily, that drug has the power to stop the migraine attack even before the attack reaches its peak. So, pain and the other symptoms of the attack are reduced and the child develops a feeling of control, resulting in less fear of the next attack, less distress, and therefore fewer migraine attacks in the long run. The child will use less medication by taking the analgesic on time because then he/she has to take them less often. Furthermore, the child will miss less school which will also lower the stress level and the number of migraine attacks."

People consistently say that a special diet is favorable in migraine. However, recent studies do not support this claim. The fact is that even before migraine-related headache is present, some parts of the brain are dysfunctional. For instance, some migraine patients primarily long for chocolate during a migraine attack and later develop a headache. They eat some chocolate, and when the attack is over, they think that the chocolate was the trigger, when in fact the appetite for chocolate was part of the attack. Consuming chocolate between migraine attacks (e.g., if prompted to do so) will not lead to an attack in those children. Children and adolescents rarely report always getting severe headache shortly after consuming a specific type of nut, or some specific chocolate. Those children mostly know about those relationships and thus avoid those foods. There is *no* necessity for a specific diet (e.g., diet free of lactose, fructose), and we don't recommend any specific diet in patients suffering headache. Generally, a diet will lead to reduced quality of life and indirectly to a deterioration of symptomatology. It is clear that a healthy and balanced diet is good for any child independent of the presence of migraine.

4.5.3 Paediatric Tension-Type Headache

In contrast to what is seen in adults, paediatric patients often report similar symptoms during both migraine and tension headache. For instance, paediatric migraine is often bilateral, while in adults it is almost invariably unilateral and easily distinguished from tension-type headache (http://ihs-classification.org/en/). This is probably to do with cerebral maturation during childhood and adolescence. At least 10 % of all children and adolescents suffer tension-type headache (Anttila 2006). In contrast to migraine-related headache, tension-type headache should *not* be treated with analgesics. Frequently taking analgesics in tension-type headache increases the probability of developing medication overuse headache (Piazza et al. 2012;

Sect. 4.5.4). Tension-type headache is especially easy to handle using simple behavioral measures (Sect. 6.4). In our experience it is sufficient for those patients to just have a few appointments for education, training some psychological technique, and educating the parents on how to react to their child's pain (Hechler et al. 2011). Now, here is an example of education for tension-type headache.

Case Report: Education for Tension Headache

"Normally, tension-type headache is double-sided, of light to moderate headache intensity with a more or less pressing quality. Often it starts shortly before, during, or after psychological stress (e.g. having to concentrate in school; experiencing boredom), or with lack of physical exercise or poor spinal posture (e.g. sitting crooked for hours in front of the computer playing games). Explained roughly, there is a cerebral dysregulation of neurotransmitters resulting in the perception of "too much" pain. Moving around or going for a walk will lead to recovery from the pain. Tension-type headache is one of the headaches most responsive to treatment, and it is completely harmless. (*Advice*: show the pain diary of the GPPC – available via http://www.deutsches-kinderschmerzzentrum.de/aerztetherapeuten/frageboegen-und-tagebuecher/schmerztagebuecher/ – to the child and his/her parents. For typical symptoms of paediatric tension headache, see Chap. 2, Table 2.1)."

4.5.4 Paediatric Headache and Medication Overuse Headache

In frequent headaches there is the great risk of augmented analgesics use. Continual or intermittent but daily headaches in fact can often be considered headaches whose frequency is increased by the augmented use of analgesics. Beware of medication overuse headache in any child taking analgesics for headache for a longer time (>10 day/month) (Piazza et al. 2012). In these children the frequent analgesic use may have induced cerebral changes resulting in increased pain perception (Zeeberg et al. 2009). The only way to get rid of the headache is to wean from the analgesics in a controlled manner; this usually cannot be managed in an outpatient setting. Our recommendation is to wean from medication under the supervision of a specialized therapist or to consult a specialized institution in order to provide adequate therapeutic support for the withdrawal.

4.5.4.1 Summary

In light of so much information on paediatric headache, we would like to summarize the essentials. All cases of paediatric headache should be medically investigated. Most cases are harmless and generally accessible to treatment. Using a pain diary for meticulous observation is a prerequisite for sustained treatment effect. In addition to psychological therapeutic measures, migraine also requires analgesic treatment during attacks. It is our experience that good migraine drug therapy will decrease attack frequency. There is *no* proven connection between diet and headache. Since headache occurs with changes in lifestyle, experience, physical processes of the sympathetic or parasympathetic nervous systems, or neurobiological processes, there is generally a close temporal relationship between headache and the presence of those psychological or social factors. This close temporal relationship will gradually disappear with increasing sensitization or chronicity until it has vanished as is the case in severe pain disorders with permanent headache.

4.6   The Basics on Paediatric Abdominal Pain

As in headache, we distinguish primary (benign, not originating from inflammation or other physical disease) from secondary abdominal pain (originating from physical disease). Chronic abdominal pain is frequent in children and adolescents and, like headache, mostly a primary symptom.

4.6.1   Primary vs. Secondary Abdominal Pain

For the differentiation of primary from secondary abdominal pain, the patient should undergo a detailed physical examination performed by a paediatrician experienced in gastroenterology who will decide on supplemental medical investigations according to the criteria from Sect. 3.2.2.

Functional abdominal pain is typically located around the navel (periumbilical). The pain originates from the intestines and can be tracked down to hypersensitivity of the intestinal muscular layer induced by psychological stress. This phenomenon is well known in popular lore as "having butterflies in one's stomach"; "having a fist in one's stomach out of rage," "the way to someone's heart is through the stomach," or "soiling one's pants out of fear" are some of the idioms that reflect the close relationship between emotion and intestinal reaction or bodily sensation. The reader will know the bad feeling in the stomach with concomitant nausea or loss of appetite just before a difficult exam.

Many children or parents are not satisfied with that explanation. They want to learn about the detailed pathophysiologic chain of events which leads to such tormenting abdominal pain, even in the absence of physical disease. Therefore, we present our disease model and our explanation for the patients and their parents here:

"The whole of the intestines, stomach included, are muscles. The stomach's task is to break up the food into small pieces both mechanically and chemically (with the help of stomach acid) in order to allow the food to pass through the intestines. The bowel is a very long foldxed tubular muscle located just

> beneath the umbilicus and ending at the anus. As with all our muscles, those of the stomach or the bowel react to hormonal stimuli provoked by all kinds of stress. One of those stimuli is the stress hormone adrenalin. The bowel is especially sensitive to those stimuli that exaggerate its motility, or lead to constipation or increased flatulence (meteorism). Both strong muscular contractions and extension are very painful. In many anxious children just the idea of separation or anticipating a class test lead to abdominal pain. By no means is such abdominal pain just imagined or pretended. In fact, in such a situation abdominal pain is a normal reaction of the body to the emotional state. Hence, it may accompany fear of any origin, and the use of measures such as physical rest or passive pain coping don't make any sense since the intestinal muscles are not "exhausted", needing time for rest. On the contrary, only active pain coping (where the child will gradually learn to influence his/her reactions to emotions) will help."

The different types of primary abdominal pain are discussed in detail in Sect. 4.6.2.

In spite of this evidence, an endless number of different diets are recommended in the treatment of abdominal pain. This approach is contradictory to the explained cause and background and also contradictory to current scientific knowledge. Diets rich in fiber show only a small positive therapeutic effect in a minority of children and adolescents with complaints clearly dependent on the type of food consumed, such as constipation (Huertas-Ceballos et al. 2008). A diet rich in fiber is identical to the normal nutritional "diet" recommended to all children and adults anyway.

The presence of a directly observed relationship between consuming a certain kind of food and subsequent abdominal pain is the only reason to change a child's diet. In such a case, it may be advisable to try the diet for a few days (*not weeks*) and meticulously record nutritional intake and symptoms. In children with intolerance to specific foods, we can typically observe an increase in abdominal pain and accompanying symptoms (e.g., nausea (sometimes), meteorism, increased bowel motility or diarrhea) right after consuming the respective food.

While changing nutritional intake, the child should be closely guided by a paediatrician experienced in gastroenterology; otherwise, there is the great risk of unbalanced nutrition and unnecessary restriction in the child's quality of life. In our outpatient department, we have seen many children on a diet free of lactose or fructose as recommended by friends, relatives, or even physicians without having undergone medically indicated tests for food allergy or intolerance. It is not only the family's increased financial burden but also the child's impaired quality of life that is inacceptable. In such cases, the benefit of a diet free of lactose or fructose is minimal (if there is any benefit at all) and is seen as a slight and mostly insignificant decrease of abdominal symptoms, but this "success" will perpetuate the diet. Since the child on a diet has to focus on his/her body and the pain in order to get to know which food in the individual case actually has any impact on the pain, pain sensitization is one of the possible adverse effects of all those diets.

Most parents who consent to such a treatment refuse to abandon their previous explanations. Therefore, we usually arrange (together with the – in most cases – thankful patient) a nutritional "challenge" in which the patient (not accompanied by his/her parents) eats the food he/she has been avoiding for a long time. The child can check afterwards on his/her own by means of a questionnaire to see if the impairment expected by the food actually occurred. In most cases, the re-implementation of a standard mixed "diet" rich in fiber (along with being allowed to eat sweets) *doesn't* result in an increase in pain or any symptoms at all; quite the contrary indeed, it results in a better quality of life.

4.6.2 Paediatric Dysfunctional Chronic Abdominal Pain

In the past, chronic abdominal pain was named "recurrent abdominal pain" (RAP; Apley 1958). However, that terminology didn't allow for a differentiation of the various types of primary abdominal pain. Therefore, in 1999, dysfunctional abdominal pain was classified according to the criteria defined by the ROME II conference (an international meeting mainly on gastroenterology). Those criteria were updated in 2006 (ROME III), and dysfunctional chronic abdominal pain now by definition is present if abdominal pain is (1) observed for more than 2 months, (2) observed more than once a week, and (3) cannot be explained by any underlying physical disease (e.g., Crohn's disease, or ulcerous colitis).

According to the ROME III criteria, we differentiate (1) functional abdominal pain from (2) irritable bowel syndrome, (3) abdominal migraine, or (4) dyspepsia (for more information on definition, background, and differentiation from secondary abdominal pain, see the review by Bufler et al. 2011).

4.6.2.1 Irritable Bowel Syndrome
According to ROME III criteria, the symptoms typical of irritable bowel disease are as follows:
1. Abdominal pain of changing intensity and localization
2. Irregularities in bowel movements (diarrhea, constipation)
3. Meteorism
4. Bloating (after a normal-sized meal)
5. Food "intolerance" (e.g., in acid or spicy food)
6. Expanded stomach
   Irritable bowel syndrome can only be diagnosed by exclusion (Sect. 4.6.1).

A large twin study ($n = 4,480$) proved that both the environment and learned behavioral patterns contribute to the development of irritable bowel syndrome (Mohammed et al. 2005). Mainly psychological factors perpetuate or amplify the disease (Mohammed et al. 2005).

From a biological viewpoint, the intestines of a patient with irritable bowel syndrome are more sensitive to distress, nervousness, worries, and fears, and react rather with cramps and rectal tenesmus compared with healthy people (Mohammed et al. 2005). Rectal tenesmus may become urgent in that many children with irritable bowel syndrome are afraid of not finding a toilet in time. Those patients benefit from education in relaxation techniques combined with psychotherapeutic pain interventions (Sect. 6.4).

4.6.2.2 Dysfunctional Dyspepsia

Dysfunctional dyspepsia is a repetitive upper abdominal pain independent of defecation or constipation. Attendant symptoms are bloating, premature feeling of satiety, nausea, or vomiting. The estimated prevalence in childhood is 2.5 % (Devanarayana et al. 2011). Its main cause is presumably impaired intestinal motility with delayed emptying of the stomach. In children, the speed of emptying is significantly correlated with the severity of symptoms (Devanarayana et al. 2012). Often, affected children suffer rather from nausea, occasionally accompanied by vomiting, or from reflux than from upper abdominal pain. Affected children seem to have an increased risk of developing anxiety disorders with a resulting reduced quality of life (Rippel et al. 2012). We feel that those children benefit from therapeutic interventions aiming at improving coping abilities in stressful situations in combination with biofeedback, relaxation techniques, or interoceptive exposure techniques (Sect. 6.4.6).

4.6.2.3 Abdominal Migraine

As in dysfunctional dyspepsia, pain related to abdominal migraine is independent of bowel movement or defecation. The pain is periumbilical, has severe to very severe pain intensity, and arises in attacks (similar to a headache migraine attack). Typically, pain is so severe that it is impossible for the patient to continue his/her everyday activities. Pain is accompanied by at least two of the following symptoms: loss of appetite, nausea, vomiting, headache, photophobia, or paleness. Sometimes the child awakes from severe abdominal pain. Duration of an episode can range from less than one to more than 24 h.

This rare disease is most frequent in children aged 5–9 years (Rasquin et al. 2006). Of 600 children aged 1–21 years with chronic dysfunctional abdominal pain, only 4–5 % have a confirmed diagnosis of abdominal migraine (Carson et al. 2011). Frequently, classic migraine is reported in the family. With increasing age, the symptoms of abdominal migraine will change, abdominal pain moving into the background, and symptoms of classic migraine arising. This disease course suggests that abdominal migraine might be a precursor of classic migraine (Carson et al. 2011). Medical and behavioral treatment approaches are similar to the ones for classic paediatric migraine.

In a female adolescent reporting cramp-like severe abdominal pain similar to the symptomatology of abdominal migraine and starting at the age of 13, one should be cautious with the diagnosis of abdominal migraine especially if the patient's history is free of former abdominal pain attacks. In these adolescents, a history of traumatic events will often be revealed (Seng et al. 2005; Sansone et al. 2006) (Sect 6.5.2).

4.6.2.4 Dysfunctional Abdominal Pain

Following the somewhat bizarre wordings and definitions of the ROME III criteria, dysfunctional abdominal pain is a distinct entity, being a sub-diagnosis of dysfunctional chronic abdominal pain. More or less a diagnosis by exclusion, dysfunctional abdominal pain is characterized by periumbilical pain independent of defecation habits. Apart from an increased sensitivity to body signals and a close relationship to both psychological and psychosocial factors, an enhanced visceral sensitivity seems to contribute to increased pain perception (Eccleston et al. 2009).

4.7   The Basics on Paediatric Back and Joint Pain

In 90 % of adult cases, chronic backache is "unspecific." Radicular pain is assumed to be of somatic origin in a complex interaction of neurogenic or muscular processes and inflammation (Deyo et al. 1992). In childhood, underlying simple somatic causes (e.g., degeneration of an intervertebral disc) are very rare. Lacking a better explanation, the weight of the child's school backpack was often in the past held responsible for childhood back pain; nowadays, we know that this is *definitely wrong* (Kovacs et al. 2003). However, we still sometimes see children in our outpatient clinic who use a trolley instead of their school backpack due to their back pain – a useless attempt often inducing teasing by peers.

While the theory that a deficit in physical activity results in muscular deficits and chronic back pain seems more reasonable, this assumption has also so far not been proven (Balagué et al. 1996; Kovacs et al. 2003). Not only too little activity but also competitive sports increase the risk of the development of chronic paediatric back pain. The link may be the increased frequency of injuries (Kovacs et al. 2003). Many patients presenting at our clinic with back or joint pain practice serious sports. Besides the enormous physical stress, the psychological pressure to succeed may lead to back pain. As in* headache or abdominal pain, any underlying disease should first be excluded.

4.7.1   Secondary Back Pain and Joint Pain

Secondary backache and joint pain is rarely seen in childhood. Even in adults no more than 10 % of the cases suffer an underlying physical disease (Deyo et al. 1992). Section 3.2.3 pinpointed what to look for in order to exclude secondary diseases.

Even if one of the physical, biochemical, or other investigations turns out to be pathologic, that seemingly underlying disease is not necessarily the only cause of pain. Carragee et al. found only a weak correlation between somatic findings in adults (MRI) and pain symptoms, both at the beginning of the disease and during its course (Carragee et al. 2005). In children free of back or joint symptoms/complaints, 26 % showed degenerative changes, a number *not* significantly different to that in children with back pain (Tertti et al. 1991). In the healthy group, the most frequent pathological findings were spinal disc protrusion or degenerative changes of the upper and lower elements of the vertebral bodies. A slipped disk with a shift of the inner nucleus into the spinal canal constricting the nerves is very rare in children. And even in those few cases, microsurgery is indicated only under special circumstances, i.e., if the pain or the poor posture continues for more than 3 months even with optimal physiotherapy.

Spondylolisthesis is prevalent in about 5 % of the general population. Many of the affected people have no symptoms at all. Severe spondylolisthesis with pain triggered repeatedly in a similar manner is frequently seen in adolescents who train to excess in gymnastics or javelin. Therapy consists of pausing their sports and doing physiotherapy to build up the muscles.

Scheuermann's disease is a juvenile impairment of growth primarily of the thoracic and less frequently of the lumbar vertebral bodies (anterior wedging) resulting in Scheuermann's kyphosis. An X-ray reveals the so-called Schmorl's nodes. On physical examination we find a thoracic hump. Thirty percent of the affected adolescents suffer back pain; complaints are more frequent in the lumbar type of the disease. Treatment options are physiotherapy, posture training, or regular swimming. Surgery is rarely needed.

Childhood backache may also be caused by benign tumors or tumor-like changes, or malignant tumors. In such cases, imaging (X-ray, computed tomography, MRI) always reveals pathologic findings.

4.7.2 The Origin of Chronic Back Pain

Next to psychological factors (Sects. 2.2 and 2.3), passive (= avoiding) pain coping strategies add to pain perpetuation or increase it (Vlaeyen and Linton 2000; Asmundson 2012).

4.7.3 Implementing Active Pain Coping Measures

Chronic back pain or joint pain lasting more than a few weeks – no matter if it is primary or secondary – should *always* (even after slipped disk) be treated with active pain coping. Medical diagnostic procedures mainly serve to check the indication for analgesics (analgesics are indicated, e.g., in rheumatic inflammatory disease or in neuronal irritation in neuropathic pain) and for physiotherapy.

4.8 Gain from Illness: Fact or Fiction?

Sometimes during the course of treatment of pain disorders, the parents or the professional helper system ask if there is any gain from illness (e.g., "The only reason for the child's pain is that he/she doesn't want to go to school."), or for the underlying cause (e.g., "What is your *real* problem?," or "There is something wrong within the family! Right?"). We think such an attitude originates from the First Thought Trap and *is a no-go* in the therapy of children with chronic pain.

Certainly, chronic pain may develop in a child with separation anxiety if he/she is separated from his/her parents; and certainly there are children with acute school aversion who use their pain as a reason not to attend school. But a child with a pain disorder suffers pain even after the disliked situation is over. Not to forget, many of our patients and their parents communicate plausibly that many of their psychological problems developed in the course of the pain disorder.

Admittedly, it would not be wise to suppose that any child suffering severe pain will not try to get the most benefit out of this situation (don't forget that for the child the pain seems nearly unmanageable in demanding situations). Why would any child opt of his own free will to behave and feel worse than necessary?

It becomes clear that the concept of "gain from illness" as a cause of (simulated) pain is detrimental. It causes the interruption of treatment because the child and his/her parents do not feel taken seriously. Finally, we should refrain from entertaining that idea since it puts all children with chronic pain under general suspicion (Sect. 7.4).

In our experience, there is occasionally a child in whom "gain from illness" is indeed an issue. But, since these children are a minority of the population of children suffering chronic pain (Sect. 7.4), we don't recommend favoring this explanation model at the beginning of therapy. Otherwise the probability is high that the patient or his/her parents will not continue treatment, which will benefit neither the patient nor his/her family or therapist. On the contrary, this would be another step contributing to chronicity.

4.9   Therapeutic Attitude

"Why did you become a therapist, when you like to laugh so much?" – Patricia (15 years) during her final therapeutic reflection

Irrespective of the psychotherapeutic approach used and actual symptomatology, therapeutic attitude is an important part of successful therapy. There are some peculiarities with respect to the therapeutic attitude in pain disorders which are recapitulated here.

1. Pain is never of pure psychological or somatic origin.
2. Pain is the result of body signals, degree of distraction, emotional state, complex somatic reactions, and pain memory.
3. It is the child who defines what is "the correct" pain perception and not his/her parents or therapist.
4. Sometimes, analgesics are necessary and useful provided they are medically indexed (e.g., in paediatric migraine) and dosed correctly.
5. Quite apart from the pain, the concomitant helplessness in itself results in a pronounced reduction in the child's and his/her family's quality of life.
6. Many emotional and interaction problems are direct or indirect results of the pain disorder. Problems that already existed before the pain disorder may have a

negative impact on symptomatology but should not be erroneously regarded as the only cause of the pain disorder.

7. A child never feigns pain in order to achieve something.
8. Sustained pain reduction cannot be expected unless active pain coping strategies are applied.
9. A humorous therapeutic attitude focusing on resources and problem solving is helpful, independent of the severity of (comorbid) symptomatology.

References

Anttila P (2006) Tension-type headache in childhood and adolescence. Lancet Neurol 5(3):268–274

Apley J (1958) A common denominator in the recurrent pains of childhood. Proc R Soc Med 51(12):1023–1024

Asmundson GJ (2012) Do attentional biases for pain depend on threat value of pain and competing motivation toward non-pain goals? Pain 153(6):1140–1141

Balagué F, Nordin M, Dutoit G, Waldburger M (1996) Primary prevention, education, and low back pain among school children. Bull Hosp Jt Dis 55(3):130–134

Bigal ME, Lipton RB, Winner P, Reed ML, Diamond S, Stewart WF, AMPP advisory group (2007) Migraine in adolescents: association with socioeconomic status and family history. Neurology 69(1):16–25

Bufler P, Gross M, Uhlig HH (2011) Recurrent abdominal pain in childhood. Dtsch Arztebl Int 108(17):295–304

Carragee EJ, Alamin TF, Miller JL, Carragee JM (2005) Discographic, MRI and psychosocial determinants of low back pain disability and remission: a prospective study in subjects with benign persistent back pain. Spine J 5(1):24–35

Carson L, Lewis D, Tsou M, McGuire E, Surran B, Miller C et al (2011) Abdominal migraine: an under-diagnosed cause of recurrent abdominal pain in children. Headache 51(5):707–712

Claar RL, Simons LE, Logan DE (2008) Parental response to children's pain: the moderating impact of children's emotional distress on symptoms and disability. Pain 138(1):172–179

Devanarayana NM, Mettananda S, Liyanarachchi C, Nanayakkara N, Mendis N, Perera N et al (2011) Abdominal pain-predominant functional gastrointestinal diseases in children and adolescents: prevalence, symptomatology, and association with emotional stress. J Pediatr Gastroenterol Nutr 53(6):659–665

Devanarayana NM, Rajindrajith S, Rathnamalala N, Samaraweera S, Benninga MA (2012) Delayed gastric emptying rates and impaired antral motility in children fulfilling Rome III criteria for functional abdominal pain. Neurogastroenterol Motil 24(5):420–425

Deyo RA, Rainville J, Kent DL (1992) What can the history and physical examination tell us about low back pain? JAMA 268(6):760–765

Dobe M, Zernikow B (2013) How to stop chronic pain in children: a practical guide. Carl-Auer-Verlag, Heidelberg

Dobe M, Hechler T, Behlert J, Kosfelder J, Zernikow B (2011) Pain therapy with children and adolescents severely disabled due to chronic pain: long-term outcome after inpatient pain therapy. Schmerz 25(4):411–422

Eccleston C, Crombez G, Scotford A, Clinch J, Connell H (2004) Adolescent chronic pain: patterns and predictors of emotional distress in adolescents with chronic pain and their parents. Pain 108(3):221–229

Eccleston C, Palermo TM, Williams AC, Lewandowski A, Morley S (2009) Psychological therapies for the management of chronic and recurrent pain in children and adolescents. Cochrane Database Syst Rev 15(2), CD003968

Flor H, Diers M (2007) Limitations of pharmacotherapy: behavioral approaches to chronic pain. Handb Exp Pharmacol 177:415–427

Hechler T, Kosfelder J, Vocks S, Mönninger T, Blankenburg M, Dobe M et al (2010) Changes in pain-related coping strategies and their importance for treatment outcome following multimodal inpatient treatment: does sex matter? J Pain 11(5):472–483

Hechler T, Martin A, Blankenburg M, Schroeder S, Kosfelder J, Hölscher L et al (2011) Specialized multimodal outpatient treatment for children with chronic pain: treatment pathways and long-term outcome. Eur J Pain 15(9):976–984

Hermann C, Hohmeister J, Zohsel K, Ebinger F, Flor H (2007) The assessment of pain coping and pain-related cognitions in children and adolescents: current methods and further development. J Pain 8(10):802–813

Huertas-Ceballos A, Logan S, Bennett C, Macarthur C (2008) Pharmacological interventions for recurrent abdominal pain (RAP) and irritable bowel syndrome (IBS) in childhood. Cochrane Database Syst Rev 23(1), CD003017

Kovacs FM, Gestoso M, Gil del Real MT, López J, Mufraggi N, Méndez JI (2003) Risk factors for non-specific low back pain in schoolchildren and their parents: a population based study. Pain 103(3):259–268

Logan DE, Engle LB, Feinstein AB, Sieberg CB, Sparling P, Cohen LL, Conroy C, Driesman D, Masuda A (2012) Ecological system influences in the treatment of pediatric chronic pain. Pain Res Manag 17(6):407–411

Loggia ML, Mogil JS, Bushnell MC (2008) Empathy hurts: compassion for another increases both sensory and affective components of pain perception. Pain 136(1–2):168–176

Merlijn VP, Hunfeld JA, van der Wouden JC, Hazebroek-Kampschreur AA, Koes BW, Passchier J (2003) Psychosocial factors associated with chronic pain in adolescents. Pain 101(1–2): 33–43

Mohammed I, Cherkas LF, Riley SA, Spector TD, Trudgill NJ (2005) Genetic influences in irritable bowel syndrome: a twin study. Am J Gastroenterol 100(6):1340–1344

Perquin CW, Hazebroek-Kampschreur AAJM, Hunfeld JAM et al (2000) Pain in children and adolescents: a common experience. Pain 87(1):51–58

Piazza F, Chiappedi M, Maffioletti E, Galli F, Balottin U (2012) Medication overuse headache in school-aged children: more common than expected? Headache 52(10):1506–1510. doi: 10.1111/j.1526-4610.2012.02221.x

Quiring J, Ochs M, Franck G, Wredenhagen N, Seemann H, Verres R, von Schlippe A, Schweeitzer J (2007) Parent satisfaction with a child and family-centered treatment program for primary headache in childhood and adolescence. Prax Kinderpsychol Kinderpsychiatr 56(2): 123–147

Rasquin A, Di Lorenzo C, Forbes D, Guiraldes E, Hyams JS, Staiano A et al (2006) Childhood functional gastrointestinal disorders: child/adolescent. Gastroenterology 130(5):1527–1537

Rippel SW, Acra S, Correa H, Vaezi M, Di Lorenzo C, Walker LS (2012) Pediatric patients with dyspepsia have chronic symptoms, anxiety, and lower quality of life as adolescents and adults. Gastroenterology 142(4):754–761

Sansone RA, Pole M, Dakroub H, Butler M (2006) Childhood trauma, borderline personality symptomatology, and psychophysiological and pain disorders in adulthood. Psychosomatics 47(2):158–162

Seng JS, Graham-Bermann SA, Clark MK, McCarthy AM, Ronis DL (2005) Posttraumatic stress disorder and physical comorbidity among female children and adolescents: results from service-use data. Pediatrics 116(6):e767–e776

Tertti MO, Salminen JJ, Paajanen HE, Terho PH, Kormano MJ (1991) Low-back pain and disk degeneration in children: a case-control MIR imaging study. Radiology 180(2):503–507

Vlaeyen JW, Linton SJ (2000) Fear-avoidance and its consequences in chronic musculoskeletal pain: a state of the art. Pain 85(3):317–332

Zeeberg P, Olesen J, Jensen R (2009) Medication overuse headache and chronic migraine in a specialized headache centre: field-testing proposed new appendix criteria. Cephalalgia 29(2): 214–220

When to Decide on Inpatient Pain Therapy?

5

Michael Dobe and Boris Zernikow

Contents

Abstract

Many children suffering chronic pain can be effectively treated in an outpatient setting. With pain disorders severely affecting the patient's and his/her family's life (frequently missing school, social withdrawal), however, we have found the most effective treatment is multidisciplinary inpatient pain therapy. In this chapter, we first discuss the criteria used to determine the need and usefulness of inpatient pain therapy. Then we discuss contraindications.

M. Dobe (✉)
German Paediatric Pain Centre (GPPC), Children's and Adolescents' Hospital,
Witten/Herdecke University, Dr.-Friedrich-Steiner Street 5,
Datteln 45711, Germany
e-mail: m.dobe@kinderklinik-datteln.de

B. Zernikow
German Paediatric Pain Centre (GPPC), Children's and Adolescents' Hospital,
Witten/Herdecke University, Dr.-Friedrich-Steiner Street 5,
Datteln 45711, Germany

Chair Children's Pain Therapy and Paediatric Palliative Care,
Witten/Herdecke University, School of Medicine,
Datteln 45711, Germany
e-mail: b.zernikow@deutsches-kinderschmerzzentrum.de

M. Dobe, B. Zernikow (eds.), *Practical Treatment Options for Chronic Pain in Children and Adolescents*,
DOI 10.1007/978-3-642-37816-4_5, © Springer-Verlag Berlin Heidelberg 2013

Severe pain disorder has considerable negative impact on the psychological or psychosocial development of the affected child. Often, outpatient treatment (from treatment in less severe cases by a general practitioner to individual or group treatment of more severe cases by specialised outpatient institutions) is sufficient (Palermo et al. 2010). If the pain disorder reaches a point at which quality of life is severely affected as reflected by a substantial number of days missed at school as well as a high emotional burden for the child and his/her parents, an outpatient therapeutic approach will probably fail and inpatient pain therapy is indicated (Eccleston et al. 2003; Hechler et al. 2009; Dobe et al. 2011). If not treated properly, chronicity into adulthood can occur (Brna 2005).

5.1 Criteria Used to Decide on Inpatient Therapy at the German Paediatric Pain Centre (GPPC)

Our way of examining the need for inpatient pain therapy in children with chronic pain is a procedure long proven in clinical practice (Dobe et al. 2006, 2011; Hechler et al. 2009). Inpatient therapy is recommended if (1) pain-related impairment of quality of life is severe (as judged by the pain therapist), (2) the child and his/her parents are motivated for therapy, (3) they agree on at least one weekly family talk, and (4) three of the following five criteria apply as checked in a previous outpatient contact (Dobe et al. 2006):

1. Pain duration ≥6 months.
2. Mean intensity of constant pain ≥5 (numeric rating scale (NRS) 0–10).
3. Pain peak with an intensity ≥8 (NRS 0–0) with a frequency of ≥2 times/week.
4. Missing school on >5 days during the last 4 weeks.
5. The patient *feels* severely impaired in his/her daily life (Paediatric Pain Disability Index, P-PDI-Score ≥36/60; Hübner et al. 2009).

5.2 Contraindications for Inpatient Therapy

Children suffering (atypical) anorexia nervosa, psychotic symptoms or severe depression are not appropriate for the inpatient therapy programme as described in this manual (for details, see Sects. 7.2 and 7.7). If the child has a history of self-harm, endangering self or others or drug abuse, the patient and his/her parents should be specifically informed of the institutional rules to be followed before inpatient therapy can start. In particularly difficult cases, we found it helpful to invite the patient to write a letter on her/his motivation for therapy, testing her/his personal goals for pain therapy and declaring his/her consent to keep the institution's rules before starting inpatient therapy (see Sect. 6.8.3 for detailed instructions).

5.3   Advantages and Disadvantages of Inpatient Pain Therapy

Without a doubt, any inpatient therapy severely interferes with the life of both the patient and his/her family. But if the pain disorder has led to a severe deterioration of life, this is the most reasonable treatment option (Hechler et al. 2009, 2011). The necessity for inpatient treatment is indicated less by the pain itself than by the fact that passive pain coping strategies have been followed for such a long time that it has become impossible for the child to master a normal daily routine without substantial support. Often the circadian rhythm of day and night activities is out of order due to physical rest and inactivity, resulting in pain enhancement and perpetuation. Also, the family interaction mainly focuses on pain. In such a vicious cycle, increased demands of whatever type – even those that must be met for successful outpatient therapy – result in deterioration. There is a high risk that arrangements made in an outpatient setting will or not fully be followed in everyday life, adding feelings of guilt to the worries already present.

Moreover, quite a few children and their parents are stuck in one or more of the three thought traps. One should not underestimate the difficulties inherent in changing the increased and fearful body awareness of patients with pain disorder, even if the patient and his/her parents are highly motivated for therapy. Mental comorbidity (e.g. adjustment disorder) may have a disease-perpetuating effect. With this complex mixture of conditions, along with all the daily phone calls to be expected, e.g. the patient is missing school and he/she is physically/emotionally not doing well, an outpatient therapy will quickly reach its limits. However, in many cases, inpatient pain therapy is no substitute for a continuing outpatient therapy. But by giving the patient and his/her family a new structure to their everyday life and guidance for active pain coping, the premise for attending the outpatient therapy later on is created.

Unfortunately, some features of inpatient pain therapy are disadvantageous to the child and his/her family.

Inpatient therapy with all its travelling costs and time spent in travelling to the institution means a substantial financial and time burden to the family. In most cases, the families do not live close to an institution specialising in paediatric pain treatment. During the course of inpatient therapy, it may well be necessary for the parents to visit the institution several times (Family Talks – see Sect. 6.6.1–6.6.4; Stress Tests – see Sect. 6.6.6). The patient's brothers and sisters frequently may feel neglected during the course of treatment (that is why they should be integrated into inpatient therapy, e.g. in family talks).

Inpatient treatment will lead to the child missing a substantial number of days from school, a deficit which needs to be addressed. The belief that missed content can be made up during inpatient therapy is an illusion. After having finished inpatient treatment, the first 4–6 weeks of school are especially strenuous, as the child must write all the missed class tests in addition to attending school as usual.

This additional emotional burden is a critical test of the newly learned strategies and arrangements.

As the mentioned disadvantages are a deterrent, they have to be discussed with the child and his/her parents before inpatient therapy begins in order to allow them to make a rational decision.

References

Brna P, Dooley J, Gordon K, Dewan T (2005) The prognosis of childhood headache: a 20-year follow-up. Arch Pediatr Adolesc Med 159(12):1157–1160

Dobe M, Damschen U, Reiffer-Wiesel B, Sauer C, Zernikow B (2006) Three-week multimodal inpatient treatment of children with chronic pain. First results of the long-term follow-up. Schmerz 20(1):51–60

Dobe M, Hechler T, Behlert J, Kosfelder J, Zernikow B (2011) Pain therapy with children and adolescents severely disabled due to chronic pain: long-term outcome after inpatient pain therapy. Schmerz 25(4):411–422

Eccleston C, Malleson PN, Clinch J, Connell H, Sourbut C (2003) Chronic pain in adolescents: evaluation of a programme of interdisciplinary cognitive behaviour therapy. Arch Dis Child 88(10):881–885

Hechler T, Dobe M, Kosfelder J, Damschen U, Hübner B, Blankenburg M et al (2009) Effectiveness of a three-week multimodal inpatient pain treatment for adolescents suffering from chronic pain: statistical and clinical significance. Clin J Pain 25(2):156–166

Hechler T, Martin A, Blankenburg M, Schroeder S, Kosfelder J, Hölscher L et al (2011) Specialized multimodal outpatient treatment for children with chronic pain: treatment pathways and long-term outcome. Eur J Pain 15(9):976–984

Hübner B, Hechler T, Dobe M, Damschen U, Kosfelder J, Denecke H et al (2009) Pain-related disability in adolescents suffering from chronic pain. Preliminary examination of the Paediatric Pain Disability Index (P-PDI). Schmerz 23(1):20–32

Palermo TM, Eccleston C, Lewandowski AS, Williams AC, Morley S (2010) Randomized controlled trials of psychological therapies for management of chronic pain in children and adolescents: an updated meta-analytic review. Pain 148(3):387–397

Pain Therapy in Childhood and Adolescent Chronic Pain

6

Michael Dobe, Rebecca Hartmann, Holger Kriszio,
Tanja Hechler, Jürgen Behlert, and Boris Zernikow

Contents

M. Dobe (✉) • R. Hartmann • H. Kriszio • T. Hechler • J. Behlert
German Paediatric Pain Centre (GPPC), Children's and Adolescents' Hospital,
University Witten/Herdecke, Dr.-Friedrich-Steiner Street 5,
Datteln 45711, Germany
e-mail: m.dobe@kinderklinik-datteln.de

B. Zernikow
German Paediatric Pain Centre (GPPC), Children's and Adolescents' Hospital,
Witten/Herdecke University, Dr.-Friedrich-Steiner Street 5,
Datteln 45711, Germany

Chair Children's Pain Therapy and Paediatric Palliative Care,
Witten/Herdecke University, School of Medicine,
Datteln 45711, Germany
e-mail: b.zernikow@deutsches-kinderschmerzzentrum.de

M. Dobe, B. Zernikow (eds.),
Practical Treatment Options for Chronic Pain in Children and Adolescents,
DOI 10.1007/978-3-642-37816-4_6, © Springer-Verlag Berlin Heidelberg 2013

Abstract

This chapter focuses on the therapeutic approach to pain therapy in children with a pain disorder, as well as the organizational and structural premises of this approach. We present the evaluated inpatient pain therapy program of the German Paediatric Pain Centre, which is suited to children suffering from a monosymptomatic pain disorder, as well as those with a pain disorder coupled with mental or severe somatic comorbidities. Besides the program's organization and structure, we present several case studies to elucidate specific aspects of our education program. We also present various clinically approved pain coping strategies and approaches. Finally, we present practical hints on how to integrate therapy into the family system, as well as procedures to follow in case of crisis, relapse, or any other unexpected difficulties.

Having discussed the scientific background, diagnostic tools, basics of successful treatment, and criteria for inpatient treatment, we will now present the organizational and structural premises as well as the therapeutic approach for paediatric pain therapy. In so doing, we will focus on our inpatient therapy program. Many of its elements, however, could be successfully integrated into the outpatient setting as well. The program suits both children suffering from a pain disorder alone and those with mental or somatic comorbidities. Although this program is no substitute for the treatment of the aforementioned comorbidities, pain therapeutic interventions as described in Sect. 6.4 (module 2) often contribute to the amelioration of mental disorders. These interventions also aim at changes in cognition, emotion, somatization, and attention processes. In Sect. 6.5 (module 3), we discuss some other interventions which may – combined with pain therapeutic interventions – result in a reduction of the symptoms of depression, fear, and emotional distress caused by psychological trauma. General aspects of combined therapy aiming at the pain disorder and comorbid mental disorder are discussed in Chap. 7.

When implementing the therapeutic program, we recommend a solution-oriented approach; the child and his/her parents are already "trained" well enough in focusing on problems. We are always astonished at the joy and enthusiasm children (and their parents) show when finding their way out of their pain disorder with the help of a lively, humorous, and positive therapist. Patients and families are willing to share their thoughts and fears when they feel accepted, internally strengthened, taken seriously, and buoyed by renewed laughter. From then on, phenomena like "resistance," "missing motivation," and "gain from illness" are rather the exception than the rule. Children visiting the GPPC for inpatient pain therapy do not attend school regularly, if at all. They have already undergone many different outpatient treatments, and in most cases at least one inpatient treatment. Previous physicians or psychotherapists sometimes describe them as being unmotivated and not accessible. In our experience, most of the children with a pain disorder – and also families with a strong somatic focus at the beginning of the program – are highly motivated for treatment as long as the physicians, the NET, and the psychotherapists understand and convey this therapeutic attitude.

Finally, we want to point out that children prefer a direct and transparent style of communication, although this opinion is not commonly held. As a consequence, treatment plans, therapeutic hypotheses, clinical observations, and family talks should be reviewed and discussed *together with the child*. When the child's perception (or the child's "gut feeling" or "inner wisdom") is different from the psychotherapist's, the working hypotheses should be reanalyzed. Nearly all children appreciate being seen as equal partners in these discussions, since they also experience themselves as equal partners in treatment. Such an approach will take time (and rattle nerves) and depends on a primary psychotherapist being informed of all aspects of treatment. It is well worth the effort, though, as it will decrease splitting of the team, discontinuation of treatment, and lack of motivation.

6.1   Organization and Procedure of Inpatient Admission

Before a child is admitted to the inpatient program at the GPPC, he/she will have visited the outpatient department at least once. Generally, the first contact with the outpatient clinic is by phone. At times, parents will contact the GPPC after having heard about it from friends, acquaintances, on the television, or on the Internet. Often the patients are referred by other Paediatricians, general practitioners, neurologists, orthopedic physicians, or fellow hospitals. After contact is established, diagnostic questionnaires for the child and the parents are mailed to the family.

An appointment for the first personal contact is arranged once the questionnaires are completed and returned to the clinic. Families are informed that it is advisable for both parents/custodians to attend the first appointment. The battery of question-naires includes (for a detailed description of the questionnaires see Chap. 3):

1. German paediatric pain questionnaire
2. Anxiety questionnaire for children and adolescents (AFS)
3. Depression inventory for children and adolescents (DIKJ)
4. Questionnaire on pain-related cognitions in childhood (FSBK-K)
5. Health questionnaire for children and their parents (Kidscreen-27)
6. German version of the Pain Coping Inventory (PPCI-R)
7. Parents' version of the Parental Pain Catastrophizing Scale (PCS-P) (mother/father)
8. Inventory for Pain-related Parent Behavior (ISEV) (mother/father)

The appointment at the outpatient clinic lasts between 1 and 2 h and is co-led by a paediatrician and a paediatric psychologist. During this appointment the develop-ment and maintenance of the pain problem is discussed with the child and his/her parents (or custodians). We present the criteria for inpatient pain therapy and value the child's and family's previous efforts in dealing with the pain. Then we discuss the essentials of our program: 3–4 single psychotherapy sessions per week, one weekly mandatory therapeutic session with the patient's family, two Stress Tests (see Sect. 6.6.6) whenever possible including attendance at the home school, daily routine with normal activities, one Stress Day, and active pain coping irrespective of mood and pain intensity. Since their previous efforts were not satisfactory, the patient and his/her family find it even more challenging to experience their worldview turned upside down by this pain therapy and the demands of considerable therapeutic efforts. Since the child's motivation for therapy is dependent on having realistic expectations, it is essential in this first appointment to give the child a realistic impression of the efforts required and the successes to expect during and after inpatient pain therapy.

In case both the patient and his/her parents are interested in inpatient pain ther-apy, they visit the ward together with a member of the inpatient nursing and educa-tional team (NET) in order to become familiar with the layout of the ward and the structure of the 3-week therapy (visiting hours, leisure time activities, own bed-clothes, posters, stuffed animals, toys, musical instruments, mobile phone/smart-phone allowed, portable gaming consoles allowed only during visiting hours). The ward visit takes between 10 and 15 min, during which their questions are addressed. The family is told to indicate within the next 24 h if they are interested in participat-ing in the inpatient program, and if so, they will be placed on a waiting list of approximately 6 weeks. When a place is available, parents are informed 7–10 days beforehand, and a date for admission is confirmed.

6.2   Structure and Organization of Inpatient Pain Therapy

This manual aims to help interested inpatient institutions get familiar with the work-ing structure of the GPPC. Hence, in this section we present some detailed structural aspects, beginning with the team structure of the pain ward of the GPPC. Then we describe the premises, daily schedule, organization of daily routine, structure of the ward round, and the organization of standard inpatient follow-up.

6.2.1 Location

The inpatient treatment ward can accommodate 20 patients. During the 3-week therapy program, patients live in two or three bedrooms. There are no single rooms available – not even on special request – in order to not perpetuate or reinforce the tendency for social withdrawal often observed in children with chronic pain. Interaction problems arising from the accommodation (children of different ages, social background, or social competence together in one room) are utilized for diagnostic purposes and are worked on in the various group therapy sessions. It is the child's responsibility to individually decorate the room. Patients are encouraged to bring posters, photographs, books, paintings, their own bedclothes, toys, musical instruments, mobile phone/smartphone, portable gaming console, etc. in order to create some familiarity within the setting. Such an atmosphere facilitates faster familiarization and is of benefit in light of the rather short stay. Apart from the patients' rooms on the ward, there is a large dining room with integrated cooking facilities, a playroom, a time-out room equipped with a punching bag, and a living room with television, PC with Internet, and gaming consoles.

6.2.2 Team Structure

The nursing and educational team (NET) of the Lighthouse ward has 12.5 established posts including nurses and two educators (or teachers). They work in a three-shift schedule, nurses doing the night shift. In addition, nurse trainees support the NET. Apart from the NET, paediatricians and paediatric psychiatrists (3.5 established posts) as well as paediatric psychotherapists (3 established posts) are part of the permanent ward team which is supported by a secretary (0.5 established post). The team is supervised by the head of the department and if absent by the senior physician. Psychological diagnostics are performed by specifically trained psychologists (requiring 12 h per week). The team is supplemented by members of other pedagogic or therapeutic disciplines not exclusively working for the inpatient pain therapy of the GPPC (see Sect. 6.7 for detailed information on the various disciplines):
1. One musical therapist, one art therapist, one body therapist, one social worker.
2. There is good cooperation with the physiotherapy department. They work with the children up to twice a day according to the patient's individual needs (mostly patients with chronic backache, musculoskeletal pain, or CRPS type I or II).

The patients are cared for by the NET following a primary nursing approach. Thus, for each child in each shift, there is one contact person within the team. This team member is also the contact person for the patient's family, psychotherapist, and physician. The contact person is responsible for collecting all information concerning the patient, accomplishing the daily therapeutic interventions together with the patient, and documenting and transferring all relevant information to the next shift.

The work of the NET includes taking part in the admission session, the family – and discharge – talks, care within the therapeutic daily life context, and support in active pain management. Some team members are qualified in biofeedback or in supporting imaginary interventions (see Sects. 6.4.2 and 6.4.4).

6.2.3 Daily Routine and Organization of Everyday Life on the Ward

The daily routine includes high-frequency intensive pain therapy with the following main elements:

Four single psychotherapy sessions per week (during weeks without prolonged Stress Tests (see Sect. 6.6.6) including attendance at the home school) or three single psychotherapy sessions per week (during weeks with holidays or short Stress Tests, see below):

1. One family therapy session per week.
2. Two group therapy sessions per week.
3. Two Stress Tests (if possible with attending home school). Depending on the distance of the family's home to the clinic, the Stress Test will last between 1 and 3 days.
4. One observation day for one parent on the ward once per stay.

Depending on the individual case, a child may undergo supplemental medical (e.g., blood work) or psychological investigations (e.g., intelligence test), use graduated schemes (e.g., to increase activity or mobility), attend the clinic school (2–4 h daily), or visit physiotherapy sessions. In addition, the child has to take the time to accomplish his therapeutic homework and practice new therapeutic techniques, TENS or biofeedback.

Those appointments are embedded in a well-structured daily routine with fixed times for getting up, morning and evening rounds, "beef rounds" (where children can express complaints), as well as five meals. In order to not lose the overview, every morning each child will get a note with all his/her individual appointments. It is mainly the child's responsibility to organize the appointments. If the child turns out to be overburdened with this organization, this is an important diagnostic hint with respect to the management of both the demands of everyday life and stressors. Those potential deficits can then be worked on in additional interventions (interventions aimed at improving organizational skills are presented in Sect. 6.5.3).

Table 6.1 presents a prototypical daily schedule excluding the various therapeutic appointments (the latter are individually scheduled and the exact times are given every morning).

Table 6.1 Prototypical daily schedule on the ward (without single or family therapeutic appointments)

Monday	Tuesday	Wednesday	Thursday	Friday	Saturday	Sunday
6:30 h Getting up	6:30 h Getting up	6:30 h Getting up	6:30 h Getting up	6:30 h Getting up	7:30 h Getting up	8:00 h Getting up
7:25 h Morning round	7:25 h Morning round	7:25 h Morning round	7:25 h Morning round	7:25 h Morning round	8:00 h Morning round	8:30 h Morning round
7:30 h Breakfast	7:30 h Breakfast	7:30 h Breakfast	7:30 h Breakfast	7:30 h Breakfast	8:15 h Breakfast	8:45 h Breakfast
8:00 – 11:30 h School	8:00 – 11:30 h School	8:00 – 11:30 h School	8:00 – 11:30 h School	8:00 – 11:30 h School	9:00 – 10:00 h Tidying up ward Cleaning room changing sheets	9:00 – 16:30 h Visiting time
09:15 – 10:15 h Psychomotoric training	9:00 – 10:00 h Swimming	09:15 – 10:15 h Psychomotoric training	9:30 – 10:30 h Swimming Or	12:10 – 13:00 h Group therapy session	10:00 – 11:30 h Cooking	
11:30 h Lunch	10:45 – 11:30 h Musical therapy	12:30 h Musical therapy or Group therapy session	10:00 – 10:45 h Musical therapy	13:15 – 14:00 h Break. Time spent in the patient's room	13:00 h Start Stress Test	
13:15 – 14:00 h Break. Time spent in the patient's room	12:10 – 13:00 h Group therapy session	13:15 – 14:00 h Break. Time spent in the patient's room	12:30 – 13:15 h Psychomotoric training	14:00 h Sports	13:00 – 18:00 h Visiting hour	
14:00 – 15:30 h Art therapy or 14:00 h Sports	13:15 – 14:00 h Break. Time spent in the patient's room	14:00 h Sports	13:15 – 14:00 h Break. Time spent in the patient's room			

(continued)

Table 6.1 (continued)

	Monday	Tuesday	Wednesday	Thursday	Friday	Saturday	Sunday
	15:30 h Snack	14:30 h Snack	14:30 h Snack	14:30 h Snack	14:30 h Snack	14:30 h Snack	14:30 h Snack
	16:00 – 17:00 h Gym	15:00 – 18:00 h Visiting hours	15:00 – 18:00 h Activity planned by NET	15:00 – 17:30 h Activity planned by NET	15:00 – 17:30 h Visiting hours		16:30 h End of visiting hours or Stress Test
							17:00 – 18:00 h Swimming
17:45 or 18:00 h Dinner							
	19:00 h Organizational round	19:15 h "Beef round"	18:30 – 19:30 h Visiting hours	18:00 – 19:30 h Visiting hours	18:15 h Sports/self defence		
	19:30 h Evening round	19:30 h Evening round	19:30 h Evening round	19:30 h Evening round	19:30 h Evening round	19:30 h Evening round	19:30 h Evening round
19:45 h (every day) Night meal							
	Sleep/quiet time	Sleep/quiet time	Sleep/quiet time	Sleep/quiet time	Sleep/quiet time	Sleep/quiet time	Sleep/quiet time

6.2.4   Grand Rounds

Twice a week there are grand rounds lasting 2 h each. On the other 5 days, rounds are considerably shorter.

Apart from the permanent ward team (Sect. 6.2.2), the various therapists partici- pate in the grand round. To work time-efficiently, the optional therapists participate partially, joining at individually prescheduled times (i.e., Thursday the physiothera- pist participates from 9:30 to 10:00 a.m. while the grand round lasts until 11:00 a.m.). Grand round serves to extensively discuss all new referrals. Biopsychosocial and family background is presented using genograms (Sect. 6.6.1). Initial discussion of a new patient takes about 20 min; discussing the other patients is significantly shorter. All planned interventions are recorded in the meeting notes.

A small round is held every other morning. The NETs and the ward physicians participate in the small round to cover nursing and medical interventions. If any questions regarding therapeutic interventions arise, the psychotherapist in charge is called in.

6.2.5   Follow-Up Care

Strictly speaking, despite the Stress Tests during the stay (Sect. 6.6.6), inpatient pain therapy is nothing but a first preparation for the "real" pain therapy starting with the patient's discharge. Discharge day marks the step from the safe inpatient setting with all its daily social, therapeutic, structural, and medical support into the stresses of everyday life. It is in everyday life that the child and his/her family have to stand the test of the successful implementation of the newly learned active pain coping strategies in family life, with friends, in their daily activities, or at school. In most cases they succeed, but this is not always the case (for treatment evaluation, see Sect. 6.8.2). Generally, patients visit the outpatient clinic 3 months after dis- charge for reevaluation. Since the child and his/her family often establish a thera- peutic relationship with the primary psychotherapist, this therapist will *always* participate in the follow-up appointments. During those appointments the child and his/her parents can decide how useful a further follow-up appointment at 6 or 9 months after discharge would be. If the child and his/her family have implemented the learned therapeutic interventions into everyday life well (Sect. 6.8.2), most fam- ilies decide on another outpatient appointment in the event of pain escalation.

In the event of a relapse after inpatient pain therapy, patients can get an appoint- ment on short notice after talking to their primary psychotherapist (there is a quota of emergency appointments provided at the outpatient clinic). Often a second inpa- tient treatment can be prevented since therapists know the individual problems, pain symptomatology, and family dynamics and can, for instance, refresh the strategies proven helpful during inpatient treatment. If indeed a second inpatient treatment seems necessary, motivation for therapy and readiness to change should be tested beforehand using the interventions outlined in Sect. 6.8.3 (special case: readmission).

6.3 Inpatient Pain Therapy: Module 1 (Presentation, Setting Goals, Education)

"Stupid brain!" – Linja (12 years) during her education

This section presents various approaches, adapted to the patient's age and knowledge, for setting realistic goals as well as education on biopsychosocial aspects of chronic pain, supplemented by hints on how to reduce somatic fixation. One section will focus on how to normalize an exaggerated body awareness arising from pain-related fears.

Education in the biopsychosocial model of chronic pain is a basic module of pain therapy. Starting with further interventions is not useful until the patient has understood this basic concept. This does not usually take more than two sessions.

When the education session starts, the child's primary psychotherapist should address the patient by his/her first name and introduce himself/herself giving his/her full name, age, professional development, and experience; it may also be appropriate to give information on the psychotherapist's family situation and his/her main professional interests. A reserved stance has a negative impact on therapy (Kuttner 1997). We therefore recommend that none of the professionals involved in therapy takes a reserved stance towards the child. From the very beginning, staff members should interact with the child, being the main client, in the way of professional service persons, and this is not only because it is ethically demanded but also because it enhances the motivation to cooperate. Taking such an attitude has an impact on cooperation since it requires certain rules to be followed: It is expected that the child will do the therapeutic homework as best he/she can. It might be helpful if the psychotherapist outlines his/her therapeutic attitude in order to give the child a chance to adapt to it or express concerns.

Example: Clarifying the Therapeutic Setting

"You should know that working with me also means laughing and I also like talking about your personal strengths. On the flipside I would like to be honest with you. If you can accept this, it has the advantage that you don't have to bother wondering what I might mean. At the same time, it might be quite strange for you to hear someone else's honest opinion about you. Finally, you should know that doing your therapeutic homework regularly is a prerequisite for successful pain therapy. If you don't do your homework, the next scheduled session will be canceled, and you will lose time. If that happens several times (usually more than twice) we have to conclude that you are lacking motivation at this time, and unfortunately that would mean that we will have to discharge you before finishing the inpatient program."

Some psychotherapists will find such an attitude too strict, especially clarifying the respective points within the first few minutes of the first patient contact on the ward. However, our experience with that is solely positive so far. Such an approach can also be advantageous for children with ambivalent motivation since it will soon be an issue and thus can be addressed early in therapy.

After the psychotherapist has introduced him/herself and the goals of treatment are clarified, we ask the child for any positive and negative experiences with previous pain treatment. Based on this experience, the child can express his/her idea of the therapeutic interaction and the therapy process. Often children prefer to avoid using set phrases such as "I understand this…" or "Gee, that is horrible." Or they express the wish "not to have to lie down on a mattress and close my eyes." Many of the children expect to be informed about the therapeutic methods so that they really understand what is happening. Some children state plainly what can be expected to be a common wish: to be taken seriously. Usually all these points can be easily clarified, so that in the next step the therapeutic goal can be (Sect. 6.3.1) checked in order to educate the child on the background of chronic pain. In most cases all that has been written so far is part of the first therapeutic session (generally taking place on the first day after admittance).

6.3.1   Setting Realistic Goals

"The pain should vanish forever." – Nina (9 years)

Nina's wish is understandable. But, if uncritically adopted for therapy, this would be a classic error in treatment, right from the start, for the following reasons:

The experience of pain is unpleasant but nevertheless universal. And not to forget, pain as a warning signal is indispensable for survival. While this can be easily understood for acute pain, it is not obvious at first glance for chronic pain. But even pain due to a pain disorder can be seen as a warning signal.

> *First*, the chronic pain is not or at least not alone signaling a somatic impairment. However, it is a hint that the patient's life is developing in an undesirable direction and that something has to be done in order to change it (e.g., changing to a more active way of life or better coping with stressors).
>
> *Second*, if not tolerating any pain, the patient will perceive even the slightest pain as very disturbing, since "the pain is still there." This will make a sustained change in body awareness very difficult. Thus, the goal of reducing pain presumably cannot be met unless the patient has achieved a more realistic attitude of acceptance.
>
> *Third*, setting the goal to the total absence of pain is related to being stuck in the third "Thought Trap" ("The pain has to vanish, no matter what it takes" – see Sect. 4.1). In consequence, any success in treatment is perceived as smaller than it actually is, and therapy might be devalued by the patient or his parents ("Therapy was unsuccessful since my child is still tortured by pain."). As a consequence the child's and parents' next step might very well be to get really stuck in the third "Thought Trap" and follow the radical and potentially harmful approaches arising from it.

In the small number of studies regarding this issue, it is assumed that a reduction of pain intensity by 2 points (NRS, 0–10) is perceived as a significant success by the child (Hechler et al. 2009). This data in mind, we recommend negotiating with the child *and* the parents to aim for a 2-point reduction in pain intensity during episodes of pain.

6.3.2 Education: The Vicious Cycle of Pain

It may be necessary to first explain the difference between acute pain (e.g., due to a contusion) and chronic pain before starting with the education on chronic pain. The following explanation will be understood by any 13-year-old adolescent with average intelligence.

> **Example: Education in Acute Pain**
> "We all know pain. Mostly, pain is a sign of injury or contusion, or of another illness (e.g. common cold; flu) or inflammation (e.g. infected wound; otitis media). Usually this pain will vanish even without any effort, since the body can heal small injuries or infections. Sometimes analgesics are helpful (e.g. with a flu). This kind of pain is referred to as acute pain. It is triggered by external or internal damage to the body."

Although pain arises from simple physical damage, it is important for the child to understand that *only* our brain generates pain perception. Even with a burning pain in our hand when touching a hot stove, the perception of pain is exclusively in one specialized cerebral area. The following explanation directed to the child illustrates that pain perception is performed exclusively in our central nervous system.

> **Example: Introduction of the Pain Center**
> "In our example of the hand touching the stove, the pain signal is transmitted along neural tracts in our hand via the spinal cord along other neural tracts to the brain. This process is comparable to a telephone line. Much simplified, the pain signal is conducted via several hubs to a type of "pain center". In this center the whole body, from head to toe, is mapped like a topographic map, and the area is named "somatosensory cortex". The somatosensory cortex comprises multiple subareas. Each of them is connected to one distinct part of our body. The more important a body part is or the more complex the tasks it performs, the larger the cerebral area representing it. For instance, a pain signal originating in the hand is associated with the area of the pain center representing the hand. In conjunction with other cerebral regions, that part of the brain triggers the perception of pain. Even when the pain signal is still at the spinal level (before you perceive any pain), specific neural connections will make your hand retract, and you will become more careful in future. As you can see, due to this acute pain you only get a minor blister instead of a serious burn wound."

Having given that more or less detailed explanation – depending on the age and knowledge of the patient – it is time to discuss any questions or misunderstandings that arise. If the child has no questions, the psychotherapist should continue.

"Now you know how acute pain is generated. But still, there is no explanation for how it is possible that you perceive pain even if there is no hot stove around anymore, or no appendicitis and no brain tumor. Chronic pain doesn't signal acute danger; indeed, it is no warning signal at all. Factors triggering the pain can no longer be identified, but the pain continues, and in the end pain perception is poorly correlated with other factors. The origin of chronic pain is best explained with the help of the following chart."

Now hand the chart "the vicious cycle of pain" over to the child and start explaining (Fig. 6.1).

"The chart "The Vicious Cycle of Pain" provides a schematic description of the mechanisms generating chronic pain. Let us start at the top. In the beginning there is an acute pain signal sent to our brain. If it is strong enough, or if we just focus on our body, it is "important" enough to our brain to be consciously perceived. This means that there are a lot of pain signals we are never aware of. Certainly you can remember an evening you suddenly noticed a bruise or a small scrape without having noticed when it occurred. This may

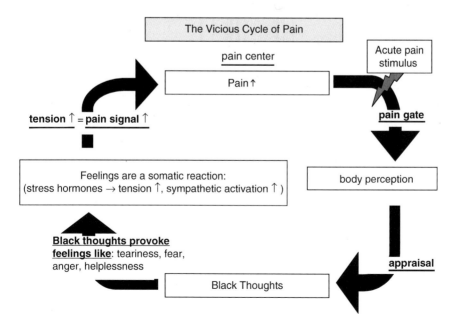

Fig. 6.1 The vicious cycle of pain (Modified from Dobe and Zernikow (2013). Reprinted with permission)

even be the case with more severe pain signals. Think of football players being injured during a game and how they shortly afterwards focus on the ball and their opponent again, even though their body is still sending strong pain signals to the brain. I am sure you can imagine other situations where the pain signal is reaching the pain center only weakly, or not at all (ask the child for one or two examples). The most important question is: How is this possible? And why is this important to your pain?"

At this point you should carefully check that the child fully understood everything. Some of the children have their own interesting ideas concerning the last question. This is a good way to get to know and validate the child's resources. But, since most children are not that familiar with the mechanism underlying chronic pain, it is advisable that the psychotherapist answers the question himself.

"Pain inhibition is possible because the brain is able to choose to focus on or ignore processes. The more attention we pay to our body, the stronger the body perception and thus the pain perception, and vice versa. Imagine you rush to school in the morning and bash your knee on your desk. Most probably you won't notice it. If you lie down with severe pain, doing nothing else but focusing on the pain, you will perceive your pain more intensely than when listening to music or watching TV. Everyone who's had the flu knows that. This is how it should be under normal circumstances. However, having a pain disorder makes everything different.

This is what happens: Although you are distracted (you are meeting friends or playing games), you more or less continuously perceive the pain. You may even wake up in the morning and know for sure that you had pain even while you slept - even if you actually slept through the night. In children with a less severe pain problem, permanent pain is susceptible to external factors (e.g. class test; quarrel; home cinema with friends) or distractions (e.g. music; movie; games). In severe pain disorders, pain is perceived as unchangeable by any situation or thought. It is important that you know that this process can easily be explained, though not when a severe bacterial or viral infection, inflammation, cancer, or other severe somatic disease is the cause of pain. Actually, we know that exactly the opposite applies: The more pain cannot be influenced by any external factor and the longer the pain persists, the more probable that it is not caused by one of those underlying somatic diseases (infection, inflammation, cancer, etc.).

There was a point in your life when your pain began. And at the beginning of a chronic pain condition we can often identify an infection, inflammation, other disease, muscular tension or an accident (note: here you should show an interest in what might have been the patient's biologic trigger). But those somatic processes tend to either worsen or heal. Viruses, bacteria, and inflammation could certainly not permanently cause pain over several months or years while not showing up in medical tests. Acute pain caused by infection or inflammation is extremely accessible to factors such as distraction or posture.

Before I proceed with chronic pain, I would like to ask you whether you have any questions. What about you? Can your pain still be manipulated or has it already become inaccessible? By how many points can you lower your pain intensity in the very best circumstances (great movie in the cinema; holiday with your best friend; going for a horseback ride in the forest; thrilling computer game; etc.)? Are you still worried that a so-far-unknown somatic disease is underlying your pain and complaints?"

After all questions are satisfactorily answered, we summarize what we have learned so far on the vicious cycle of pain.

"To what extent can chronic pain be explained? As you see on the chart (Fig. 6.1), the pain has started somehow. It doesn't come out of nowhere just to bother you. As you know by now, the degree of body awareness is of great importance. Depending on what you are focusing on, you perceive your pain as more or less severe, or you may not notice it at all. That mechanism can be compared to a gate. Let us call it the "pain gate". If you are well distracted, the gate is kept closed or opens just a little bit. But if you aren't distracted or if you focus on your body, the gate is wide open, and you perceive your pain more easily. You are here because you feel your pain nearly all the time. Why doesn't the pain gate close anymore? How did it happen? In order to understand what's going on we should proceed with the details of the vicious cycle up to the step marked "appraisal" (see chart). What does that mean? Human beings tend to think a lot, maybe too much sometimes. We evaluate everything that happens. We think about anything that comes to mind, our pain included.

I suppose you worry about your pain a lot, and you don't think "Hey, it's fine. I finally am in pain, I longed for it so much". Otherwise you wouldn't be sitting here with me right now, would you? (Wait for the child's – in most cases – unambiguous reaction). Okay. I don't know you well, but many of the patients report thinking "Why me?"; or "Oh no, not again! Will it ever stop?"; or "With the pain, there is no joy left in my life"; or "I can't stand it any longer"; or "If I don't lie down, the pain will certainly increase". Maybe you know those or even worse thoughts (wait for the child's reaction). As you have already noticed, those thoughts don't make things better. As time goes by, there are often more and more of those even more negative thoughts – we call these "Black" Thoughts. Many of our patients describe this as a feeling of falling into a pain "pit" where they probably can't get out by themselves. Typical thoughts are "All this doesn't make any sense"; "Damn, no matter what I try I can't focus anymore"; "I can't go on like this"; or "It makes me mad".

Our brain is programmed to compare things to similar ones. Therefore, it is likely that irrespective of our pain, further Black Thoughts become associated with other negative thoughts that are already present. The additional Black Thoughts could be related to our pain (e.g. former painful injury or surgical procedure) but do not necessarily have to be related. Actually, severe pain combined with Black Thoughts may well trigger stressful and traumatic life events *and vice versa, if experienced*. It is essential how we appraise our pain. If you have already experienced any stressful or traumatic life events, according to our experience, it is likely you will remember them together with the Black Thoughts during episodes of severe pain. If this happens repeatedly this will result in classic conditioning, i.e. memories, thoughts and pain mutually trigger and perpetuate pain. Have you personally had similar experiences?"

This is the time to check if the child reports on associations of Black Thoughts or memories and increased emotional distress resulting from these thoughts. If this is the case (even if the child simply nods with an inward gaze), we recommend responding, "Yes, you seem to know," then proceeding with the education and exploring the associations in the next session. Otherwise, this bears the risk of losing the focus of the so-far successful education.

The next part of the education deals with the associations between thoughts, appraisals, emotions, and the resulting somatic responses.

"Black Thoughts alone don't cause severe pain, otherwise there would be many people in the street screaming in pain. That is not the case. However, if Black Thoughts accumulate, our mood tends to darken, and depending on individual appraisals, helplessness, fatigue, anger or fear may become the predominant feeling(s). This means that Black Thoughts result in negative feelings. Feelings are named feelings because you can feel them, which means even a feeling as a bodily sensation is always a physical response. For instance, if you are totally relaxed with your heart beating smoothly and regularly, this shows you are free of fear. But you can't feel happy if your body is tense or if you frown and look angry."

A fun and lucid way to do this part of the education is to try together with the child to provoke feelings contrasting the bodily situation: sit down very relaxed – also relax your belly – and smile, and simultaneously try to get angry but stay relaxed or try to think about happy experiences while frowning and clenching your fists. The next section will show us how the resulting stress reaction leads to intensified pain.

"In the end, all those negative feelings are based on a physical stress reaction which will arise whenever something jeopardizes our personal well-being. Sometimes it may be enough to not be in the mood to perform an activity (e.g. housework or homework) and to have to force oneself to get it done. This stress reaction will be even stronger when negative thoughts or bad memories are present, or even when you have negative appraisals. Of course, stress reactions differ in their intensity. It is essential to understand that *each* Black Thought and *each* negative judgment will result in somatic reactions from small to large depending on the intensity of the thought. In conjunction with other somatic reactions, feelings arise which may be fear, helplessness, fatigue or anger. Black Thoughts and brief somatic stress reactions are totally normal; all people have their daily Black Thoughts.

However, much more problematic than *isolated* and *brief* Black Thoughts or brief stress reactions are *prolonged* ones. Pain itself will contribute somewhat to a stress reaction. It is, however, essential to see that not the pain signal itself but the appraisal of the pain is the main cause of the stress reaction. What makes a prolonged stress reaction so unfavorable, apart from the increased muscular tension, is its ability to cause pain sensitization. What does that mean?

It means that the same physical pain signal will be perceived as more intense. This indicates that "sensitization" has taken place. The sensitization can be compared to a highway being broadened from two to three lanes in order to make the traffic (=pain) flow better (=processing of the pain signal). In the pain center the enhanced pain signal provokes an intensified pain perception. Former pain experiences may lead to a further increase in pain.

From that point on, everything depends on how much I anticipate my pain, or how much I see the pain as a threat. The more I anticipate my pain, the easier the pain gate opens, and the more I worry about my pain, the more pronounced is the resulting physical reaction. In the end, the result is the same: pain is perceived more strongly due to the increased activity of the pain center. We are alarmed.

Chances to focus even more on the painful area of the body increase, opening the pain-gate wider. Consequently, body awareness will increase, and all fears and worries (Black Thoughts) are realized. The next round of the vicious cycle has begun."

At this point, the child should summarize the education program's essential points in his/her own words. Most patients already know the vicious cycle from their own experience; therefore, the task is not too difficult, and they will not need to ask many questions.

In the last section of the education program, we sketch the mechanism rendering chronic pain a pain disorder affecting all areas of life.

"If the vicious cycle repeats itself (3 months with pain on most days will suffice), pain memory starts to be consolidated. The same way our brain stores memories of a wonderful holiday, foreign language vocabularies, memories of a funeral, or the result of 100 minus 53, it will also store (learn) pain – and this rather effectively. Once pain memory is established it doesn't matter anymore at which point of the vicious cycle the process starts. Your mother or grandmother asking, "Are you in pain?" will be sufficient to start the vicious cycle, even if up to that moment you were free of pain, or not aware of it. Negative feelings (anxiety, teariness) or muscular tension due to distress or physical (in)activity may activate the cycle, even if they are not associated with the pain. Slowly the body awareness will increase and at the same time your ability to be distracted will decrease. In the end, the pain is permanent and very strong, and is no longer accessible to any ameliorating factors.

In addition, parents or friends worry about you and will ask you about the pain, always reminding you of your pain. Recommendations to relax or lie down improve the experience. The search for a somatic cause of the pain along with many doctor's appointments and various investigations make you more and more focused on your body. And since the one and only "cause" cannot be found, both Black Thoughts and passive pain coping become more frequent. Moreover, many patients worry about their parents, suffering from having a child in pain. Or the family atmosphere becomes tense and unhappy. Naturally, all this has an added impact on Black Thoughts and body tension."

At this point you should review and discuss with the child how far his/her pain disorder has advanced. A lot of information was given, and you should offer time for further questions. If the child has no questions, the psychotherapist should ask, and answer, the most important question of all: "Will this pain processing remain unchanged, or can we do something to change it?"

"No, this pain processing does not have to remain the way it is now. It can change, since our brain has the ability to change. Fortunately, you are still young. Your brain is learning much faster than that of an adult as you may have already seen with your parents. The premises for change are that you understand that chronic pain is a disease on its own, which you can influence by altering attention processes, appraisals and physical reactions. The result is that in conjunction with active pain coping (doing a lot of activities irrespective of pain intensity) your intrinsic cerebral pain-inhibiting system is activated, and distraction and periods free of pain become possible again."

If some of the older children (especially if gifted, above average, or very concerned about their body) wish more detailed education, we recommend explaining neuroanatomy with the help of figures (e.g., see Fig. 2.1 or Kuttner 2010).

At the end of the education program, the children should be familiar with the biopsychosocial dimensions of the vicious cycle of pain. Interestingly, knowing this background makes it possible for many children to step back from their dualistic world view (somatic vs. mental pain) and the three Thought Traps. All in all this education takes approximately 30 min, but the time needed varies of course with the age and giftedness of the child. If the child is somatic fixated, much more time is needed (up to 3 sessions, in rare cases even more) (see Sect. 6.3.3).

After this first education session, the child's homework is to summarize the theory in his/her own words. This is essential in order to have a good idea of what was really understood. A basic understanding of the topic is an absolute prerequisite for a successful sustained treatment. According to our experience, even children with learning difficulties or dyslexia will do their homework if it was discussed at the very beginning of the education (Sect. 6.3). In addition, the child should make brief notes on what he/she tried so far to distract him/herself from pain (→ interruption of body awareness), which colorful thoughts he/she tried (→ interruption of Black Thoughts), or which technique he/she tried to relax (→ interruption of muscular tension).

The child is explicitly told to note all efforts undertaken irrespective of their effectiveness. That homework is a good basis for deciding which pain coping strategies (Sect. 6.4) are the best to begin with in this patient and also for evaluating therapy motivation.

The following written summary is the homework of Rabea, 14 years old, average intelligence (IQ: 105), and illustrates the amount of information a child can learn in one session.

> **Example: Rabea (14 Years), Pain Disorder, Underlying Migraine**
> "Pain results from transduction of a stimulus. The pain signals reach the brain along neural tracts and have to pass a gate where they either recoil or pass. The gate determines the intensity and the amount of pain being let through. How much pain will pass depends on current awareness of the body. When we focus on our body, pain is stronger than when we are distracted. Pain may be blunted or enhanced by joy, anxiety, good memories or bad ones, as well as by muscular tension or relaxation. All this happens simultaneously and the pain is generated within the brain, in its pain center. The pain center memorizes the pain. So, if the same pain signal more or less reaches the brain repeatedly, the brain will assume that it is much easier to continuously produce pain than to transmit the signal, impulse by impulse. This is how chronic pain is generated, even if no pain signal reaches the brain anymore."

6.3.3 Somatic Fixation: Pain-Related Fears and Anxiety Sensitivity

"But I do feel that there is something real. This can't be just imagination." – Mirjam (16 years)

By means of the education session, as described in Sect. 6.3.2, most children and their families will be reached and motivated for pain therapy irrespective of the severity or chronicity of symptoms. However, in families with pronounced somatic fixation, education is a big challenge, as they have a selectively distorted perception of body signaling as a malign somatic pain producing process.

People with a tendency towards somatic fixation do not necessarily doubt the truth of the education or the process of modulating pain, since the relations are familiar to the child and the family from everyday life experiences. Rather than having a problem with the pain itself, they worry that the pain is a symptom of a threatening somatic process. As long as the child and the parents are stuck in that assumption, pain therapy doesn't make sense and will not be successful. The following chapter is on the special educational needs and measures necessary to build up a trusting relationship with a child and his family with somatic fixation.

6.3.3.1 Supplemental Background Information on Chronic Pain

Acute pain alerts the body. It serves to make us quickly realize potential threats and initiate action to eliminate the cause of pain and reduce the pain. Hence, pain is always accompanied by feelings of fear and threat. In a child, the degree of increased pain-related anxiety is determined by three processes. These are attention to the pain, the amount of pain-related catastrophizing, and pain-related behavior. The most important facts underlying the biopsychosocial model of chronic pain are summarized as follows:

1. As a potential threat, most acute pain stimulus result in increased *vigilance* and attention to that signal. Thus acute pain signals in most cases will interrupt the attention to signals simultaneously present (Crombez et al. 2005). Crombez et al. investigated the construct of hypervigilance towards pain signals extensively and concluded that both hypervigilance and pain signals are outside conscious control, occurring early in case the threat is perceived as high, the anxiety system (= part of the limbic system) is activated, and the individual tries to escape the situation to avoid pain.

2. People differ as to how much they direct their attention to painful stimuli. Supposedly, *on the one hand early pain experiences* may determine sensitization to and focusing on painful stimuli (Hermann et al. 2006; Hohmeister et al. 2010). According to our experience, on the other hand children whose limbic system is already activated by a *high emotional burden* sense pain more easily and as more threatening.

3. *Catastrophizing* – the habitual and fast appraisal of a situation as extremely catastrophic has become one central construct for the understanding of cognitive processing in patients with chronic pain. In many investigations it was a significant predictor of perceived pain intensity and functional or emotional impairment (Sullivan et al. 2006). In studies on children and adolescents, patients with

increased catastrophizing on a painful event reported more severe pain and impairment (Crombez et al. 2003).

4. Not only the child's but also his/her parents' catastrophizing has a great impact (Goubert et al. 2006). The latter is significantly correlated with the patient's pain perception and impairment. Perhaps parental fears lead to increased parental distress and that reaction is interpreted by the child as a warning signal ("If my parents are concerned, the situation must be precarious."), resulting in increased anxiety and impairment of the child. According to Eccleston and Crombez (2007), the *daily worry* about existing pain is also important for therapy. These authors see these worries as a chain of negative thoughts and the precursor of catastrophizing.

The degree to which pain-related behavior predicts the pain perception of children or adolescents is explained by the "fear-avoidance model" of Vlaeyen and Linton (2000) which was recently hypothetically adapted to paediatric pain (Asmundson et al. 2012). Pain as a potential threat leads to increased anxiety and tension. Cognitive processes such as fear of pain may result in situations or movements being erroneously considered as threatening. Those appraisals make the patient avoid certain situations or body movements in order to evade the pain. Especially in patients with backache, such behavior will result in increasingly restricted mobility and even more pain in the long run. According to the theory of Vlaeyen and Linton (2000), the fear of pain has more impact on the patient's life than indeed the perceived pain itself. The patient's fear of pain is dependent on the extent to which he/she is able to fearfully perceive physical processes in his/her body (*anxiety sensitivity*). Increased anxiety sensitivity is closely associated with fear of pain. In a study of 21 children and adolescents suffering from chronic pain, Martin et al. (2007) were able to demonstrate that premorbid anxiety sensitivity is a predictor of fear of pain. Presumably, anxiety sensitivity is associated with maladaptive interoception. Thus, anxiety sensitivity modulates pain perception to a considerable degree and has a strong impact on pain-related behavior (see Sect. 6.4.6.1 for a detailed account of the theoretical background of fear of pain and anxiety sensitivity).

What are the practical consequences of all this theory for the education session?

6.3.3.2 Education for Families with Increased Somatic Fixation

It is important for children and parents with a somatic fixation that all their perceptions and fears are taken seriously. From a psychotherapist's viewpoint, it is important to evaluate the somatic observations but at the same time refuse the underlying irrational assumptions. This may be a challenge since every child knows cases from the family, the newspaper, or TV – and even if it is just one case – in which a malignant disease was not recognized on time. Counteracting these fears by recognizing them as being normal may help to avoid any dysfunctional conflict about the "right" perception. Most patients will usually be ready to follow the pain education supplemented by the information above. Asking the child to explicitly scrutinize that information with respect to his/her own case will motivate him/her to continue work. As a next step, we discuss the child's own biological concept of permanent pain. If he/she has a sense of humor, it is quite easy to quickly find a common basis, as the following example will illustrate:

Case Report: Dustin (Age 15 Years), Pain Disorder with Abdominal Pain

"I mean… how could it be possible? There cannot be viruses or bacteria agreeing to "Let us only reproduce and spread so much that we permanently cause the same amount of pain". Then it can't be a tumor or an inflammation. What kind of tumor or inflammation would not grow or spread? Any tumor grows, increasing in size, causing more and more pain. Any inflammation either gets worse if the body can't stop it, or is extinguished or at least attenuated by the body's immune system. Sometimes inflammations may change like waves. But they will never remain at the same biological level for long, provoking stimuli of constant intensity. Did you ever think about that? And to be honest, your body would fight against it and not just wait while thinking "How lovely, a tumor or inflammation!" Of course it is true what you say or perceive. But there are many reasons why the body could react the way it does and why pain is perceived in the brain. Even if the highly improbable is true and there is still a small, undetectable inflammation in the body – did the search for it so far help you in any way to better deal with the pain? Was the benefit worth the effort? Or wouldn't it be better to at least be able to alter the pain irrespective of its cause?"

Questions aiming at the cost/benefit ratio are easy to understand by the affected children.

"Do you think it would hurt you to leave "the search for the origin of your pain"? Various investigations have currently shown that your body does not seem to be endangered."

Even if no question about the child's physiologic processes and their interaction with body signals were left unanswered, we have to acknowledge that there will never be 100 % security in life, as some of the smart children will point out. In those cases it has always been helpful to ask the child to make a list of pros and cons with respect to a so-far undetected severe somatic disease being responsible for the pain. This task ends with a decision as to which way to go and which way is worth living. This decision should be taken solely by the child (or if too young, together with the family) taking all the facts into account – try to leave your personal opinion out. If the decision is not to give up the search for "the" one and only cause (the still undetected disease), pain therapy doesn't make sense and should be stopped. The psychotherapist should never be hurt by such a decision. Instead, he should offer to start pain therapy when the child and the family are ready.

6.4 Inpatient Pain Therapy: Module 2 (Pain Coping Strategies)

"The pain is always there, no matter what I do." – Mirco (15 years) at admission

In the following chapter, we describe the pain coping strategies we use for inpatient pain therapy at the GPPC. Starting with the vicious cycle of pain (Sects. 6.3.2 and 6.3.3), there are several points where the cycle may be interrupted. Distraction aims at altering body awareness, cognitive restructuring aims at minimizing Black Thoughts, systemic interventions aim to reduce the feeling of guilt or the burden of pain on family life, and relaxation training targets muscular tension. Various types of exposure techniques aim at reversing the process of chronicity and sensitization by trying to decrease the fear of pain and pain catastrophizing or to decondition negative emotions and related pain perception. You will need 6–10 therapeutic sessions to teach those strategies. Transcutaneous electrical nerve stimulation (TENS) and biofeedback therapy is applied to all children (except in abdominal pain: only biofeedback) from the very beginning of inpatient treatment and is performed by specially trained staff of the NET. Pain provocation, as a technique of interoceptive exposure (see Sect. 6.4.6), won't be offered until the end of the stay and not before at least one pain coping strategy has been successfully implemented.

Having clarified all questions with regard to the education sessions or therapeutic homework and having appropriately complimented the child, a decision is made by the child whether he/she wants to first learn a strategy to reduce pain awareness (e.g., distraction technique), to influence Black Thoughts or a relaxation intervention. For this decision we use the list of pain coping attempts applied in the past which was put together by the patient. Although the child has not learned the first pain coping strategies before the third day of the stay, an active daily routine (in vivo exposure) irrespective of pain is pursued by the NET starting from day one.

6.4.1 Techniques That Alter Body Awareness

"Try to distract yourself!" – A mother prompting her child with chronic pain (This is a typical but not very helpful intervention in families with children suffering from chronic pain.)

Although this prompt may seem helpful, from the child's point of view it is not. It may be an expression of the parents' helplessness or temper. Why is that prompt not experienced as being helpful?

Distraction, i.e., a decrease in attention towards acute painful stimuli in acute pain resulting in pain inhibition, belongs to the standard repertoire of human behavior. Fearfully increased pain-related body awareness combined with passive pain coping and an exaggerated tendency to catastrophize make it more and more difficult to actively diminish attention towards physical processes. With severely prolonged pain, even the best distraction technique (e.g., watching a thrilling movie together with a best friend) will only cause a very small pain reduction. If a child tells us that the pain was unchanged during the movie, this is no lie of a wailing child trying to get attention, but probably an adequate description of his/her experience. With less prolonged pain, "positive" activities like horseback riding, playing, or being with friends result in better distraction and pain reduction.

Before working on a new distraction strategy, you should ask your patient about his/her current ability to distract himself/herself and how strong the distraction could be at most. An 11-step numeric rating scale (0=no distraction at all; 10=maximal possible distraction) serves this purpose best. You may ask:

> "Well, Jenny, how much do you think you are currently most able to distract yourself? As I know, you like to go to the movies with your friend, or you like to listen to loud music. Imagine you are sitting in the cinema together with your friend, you are thrilled, and the music is as loud as it can be: tell me how much your maximum distraction is then? Please use the scale from 0 to 10 that you are already familiar with."

What is the significance of the child's feedback for the therapeutic process? If a child reports a degree of distraction of 8 or higher, his body awareness and pain perception can still be modulated. With a degree of 4, however, even a massive stimulus satiation will probably have little or no impact on the pain perception. In such a case it may be advisable to introduce elements of acceptance-based techniques early in the therapeutic process (Sect. 6.4.3.3), since a fast change in pain perception (be it due to a comorbid depression or a prolonged chronicity of body awareness) may be impossible. Before such a decision is made, the child should be asked for his/her estimate of how helpful the reported distraction was for the pain, because for some of the children sometimes even a degree of distraction as low as 3 can be helpful.

Besides external methods of distraction (games, friends, etc.), there are in principle two different approaches to reducing body awareness:

1. Mindfulness-based approach
   First, we can reduce body awareness of pain by increasing our current focus on sensory perceptions (mostly with regard to sight and hearing, but partly also feeling as it applies to unaffected body parts) that are incompatible with the perception of pain.
2. Distraction-based approach
   Secondly, we can also achieve a reduction in body awareness by an increased focus on cognitive or imaginative tasks or themes that are also incompatible with the perception of pain.

6.4.1.1 Mindfulness-Based Techniques

Body awareness may be reduced by focusing on sensory perceptions incompatible with pain perception. Focusing on sensory perceptions (external or internal stimuli) is also well suited to the regulation of emotions and for controlling stressful memories (e.g., for experiencing flashbacks of traumatic or critical life events; Sect. 6.5.2). Hence, those techniques are also used in trauma therapy.

One version of a mindfulness technique is the adapted version of the 5-4-3-2-1 technique and can be found in Chap. 9 (instructions included; Chap. 9, Worksheet #8).

In this technique the child focuses first on five different things he/she sees, then on five things he/she hears, and then finally on five different bodily perceptions (incompatible with pain) that he/she can feel. Then the child begins again, but concentrates each time on just four different things. In the next round, the child concentrates on only three things, and so on. The child's ability to concentrate on that which he/she really perceives is crucial to the success of the exercise. Some children do better when they recite each of these perceptions out loud to themselves. Some children love to run through this exercise quickly; others take a lot of time with it and enjoy the quiet and relaxation it produces or use the technique to get to sleep at night. It often happens that a child will experience the bodily perceptions as rather unpleasant, as the increased attention to interoceptive stimulus results in stronger pain perception. In this case the child will be encouraged to focus on sight and hearing (possibly on smell). Finally, many children reject the given structure (5-4-3-2-1). But the exact structure of the technique is not significant to its success. This is rather determined by the extent to which the child is able to concentrate on the present sensory stimuli. Alternating between sight and hearing (1-1), for example, without focusing on feeling, can also work well, as can closing the eyes and concentrating exclusively on various noises that are perceptible in the moment. Increased practice will reveal which variant of the technique best suits the child, whether it be slowly concentrating exclusively on hearing and feeling, the 5-4-3-2-1 or another structure. In the instruction in the 5-4-3-2-1 technique, it is very important to portray the described structure as just one possibility which can be changed to suit the needs of the child. Children should therefore try out various variants in order to be able to decide which suits them best.

This technique is especially suitable for children aged 13 years and older. You should plan on 30 min for giving the instructions as well as teaching the technique and another 10–20 min in upcoming appointments to discuss with the patient what was good and what was difficult. In order to decide whether this technique is suitable for the child and which part of it is especially suitable, the child should practice it well – at least three times a day. He/she should make a table with three columns, i.e., the time, which variant was used, and how successful it was. The procedure is illustrated in the next case report.

Case Report: Marlies (15 Years), Pain Disorder with Backache
Marlies reported that the exercise did not work that well (version: alternating sequence of seeing, hearing, feeling; speed: fast; describing the sensations out loud to herself). When exploring the exercise it turned out that especially the seeing part didn't work (degree of distraction: 3), while hearing (degree of distraction: 7) and feeling (degree of distraction: 9) worked well. Whenever Marlies focused on viewing she was "catapulted" out of the concentration which made the whole technique less successful (degree of distraction: 4 to 5). In consequence, we decided on a change, i.e., to cancel the "seeing" part. Practicing the modified technique, a distraction of 7 was reached.

6.4.1.2 Distraction Techniques

Body awareness can be reduced by focusing on topics incompatible with pain perception. As often practiced in everyday life or in the treatment of acute pain, in its simplest form this technique may comprise remembering one's birthday or great holidays or doing simple counting exercises. But, this is often not enough to reach an elevated distraction score as needed in the treatment of pain disorders.

Of course the exercise should be neither too demanding nor too simple so that its cognitive requirements don't render it unsuitable to some children. The distraction-ABC exercise that we have developed has turned out to be especially beneficial to children from about the age of 8, as it can be adapted in endless variants in order to be suited to each child's age and abilities. This technique involves searching for words beginning with each letter of the alphabet within certain preset themes. These could be, for instance, animals – or horse breeds – (much loved by female children), or car words-ABC, or sentences-ABC, in which each succeeding sentence begins with the next letter of the alphabet. At higher levels of complexity, some of the children's favorite sensory channels are included. For example, some older adolescents love the juke box version, in which songs are played in their heads (for approximately 10–20 s), also in alphabetical order. Even more complex is music video in which a music video is played through along with its corresponding song. These more complex levels of the exercise require the patient to be able to imagine the relevant sensory channel, be it sight, hearing, or feeling. We usually get indications of the preferred sensory channels during the education sessions and evaluation of diagnostic resources (see Chap. 9, Worksheets #1–6). Of course, we can always simply ask the patient ("Do you know music well enough to be able to play it in your head?").

The distraction-ABC may be roughly categorized into four degrees of complexity:

1. Grade I. Animals, automobiles, horse breeds, single sentences (each sentence has to start with the next letter), and short stories in which the keywords start with next letter.
2. Grade II. For this level of complexity we add another sensory channel. In the "juke box," for example (the first 10–20 s of a song are imagined, with the title or artist in alphabetical order), a grade I distraction-ABC is combined with the auditory channel. It goes without saying that with those higher degrees of complexity, the child must be well able to imagine the respective sensory channel(s) which usually becomes obvious in a resource-oriented exploration during the first two appointments. Imagining touching one's house pet (or most loved animal) is another popular scenario, as are films or video clips watched in alphabetical order. Some children love to imagine painting pictures of words chosen in alphabetical order; still others imagine forming the word out of plasticine.
3. Grade III. The distraction-ABC with two additional sensory channels is even more complex. The favored version is the "music video" where not only some music but also the respective video clip must be played in alphabetical order (grade I distraction-ABC + auditory channel + visual channel). Other possibilities are to play clips from various favorite films or scenes (with images and sound) from books, all also in alphabetical order. A grade III distraction-ABC can also involve swimming in the ocean and touching plants and fish, imagined in alphabetical order.

4. Grade IV. The distraction-ABC is mostly combined with or integrated into other imaginative techniques. For instance, the child and an imagined helper (e.g., a magical animal) have to perform a distraction-ABC together at a "Safe Place" (see Sect. 6.4.2 for a description of "Safe Place").

In Chap. 9 (Worksheet #7) you will find instructions for the technique and several examples. Adolescents especially love the numerous possibilities and are eager to develop their own distraction-ABC. The examples presented here represent only a fraction of the many variants that have so far been developed by the children themselves. Therefore, the distraction-ABC is one of the most powerful interventions for treating even children with severely chronified pain disorders.

6.4.1.3 Combining Mindfulness and Distraction

The 5-4-3-2-1 technique and the distraction-ABC may well be combined. Such a combination is especially suited to children with general anxiety or hypervigilance due to trauma. An external focus increased by anxiety predisposes a child to the 5-4-3-2-1 technique, but the effect of this technique alone is sometimes not strong enough. In the combined version the child searches for visual or auditory clues (viewing, hearing, *not* feeling) in alphabetical sequence (A=hearing an automobile, B=seeing the beard of a therapist, C=seeing a computer, D=hearing the barking of a dog, E=…). Some children love to do this without an alphabetical sequence (i.e., S=snack, G=glasses, a=…).

6.4.1.4 Modification for Younger Children or Children with Learning Disabilities

The distraction techniques presented here are not ideal for children younger than 8 years or with a pronounced learning disability. Simpler versions of the distraction-ABC are better suited, e.g., variations of the game "I spy with my little eye" or the search of the surrounding area for a certain number of things with a certain color or shape ("Find 10 blue objects, then 10 red objects."). Another technique is to imagine stories on a given subject, e.g., the favorite doll.

Depending on the degree of pain chronicity, body awareness and pain perception may initially only show a weak and brief modification (seconds). But with ongoing practice, the effect is less transient. This is the reason why the child has to practice several times daily apart from the therapeutic sessions.

6.4.2 Imaginative Techniques: Better Mood

"Whenever I'm down I visit my Caribbean island" – Jana (age 12 years)

All imaginative techniques aim at the regulation of emotions and thus the conscious modulation of one's mood for the better. For this reason, imaginative techniques are used in pain therapy.

For inpatient pain therapy, the standard procedure is to teach the "Safe Place" in an age-appropriate way. For the youngest children, we use a variation of imagination techniques called "Pet on my Belly" or "Pain Fighter" (see below).

We teach other imagination techniques like "screen technique" or the "Safe" (see Sect. 6.5.2) only if in addition to chronic pain, there is a substantial emotional burden caused by stressful or traumatic memories. Those two techniques will be presented in detail in Sect. 6.5.2.

6.4.2.1 Safe Place

The child is invited to imagine a place (a real place from the past or present or an imaginary place) with as many sensory qualities as possible (seeing, hearing, feeling, smelling, tasting). For the individual child this "Safe Place" should be associated with feelings of security and safety. Mediated by the evoked positive physiologic reaction of relaxation, the aim is to positively influence both mood and body awareness and possibly also negative memories, thoughts or perceptions.

Depending on the patient's feeling of familiarity with imagination techniques and his/her ability to visualize, we need 2–4 single sessions lasting between 10 and 40 min to teach and discuss the respective techniques. The first session is used to explain the exercise and its goal. When the child fully understands all information, explore his/her ability to evoke vivid imagery (use questions like "Can you imagine things in pictures?" or "If you imagine your last holiday, do you *see* any pictures with your inner eyes?"). Most patients will react unambiguously (e.g., intense thinking with a frown vs. "Sure, everybody can do that."). If children with a vivid imagination agree to do the technique, the next step is to find a suitable "Safe Place." It could be a real place from the last holiday, the patient's room, a fantasy, or a fantasy construct from the movies (e.g., Lord of the rings or Twilight). Any place is allowed as long as the child associates security and safety with it. Having identified a suitable place, the patient's homework is to write down in short descriptions what precisely he/she is seeing, hearing, feeling, smelling, or tasting at his/her "Safe Place" (Chap. 9, Worksheet #12).

In most cases no real people should be present at the "Safe Place" (animals and fictitious people are allowed, i.e., from movies, games) in order to avoid transferring relationship problems with a real person to the "Safe Place" which would then make it unhelpful. Sometimes a child wishes to also have a beloved person in his/her "Safe Place." If this person is associated with feelings of security and is not ill, it is worth a try. It is no obstacle if the child is unable to describe the "Safe Place" with all the mentioned sensory qualities. In case the child spontaneously names two "Safe Places," he/she should try a detailed description using all sensory qualities for both places. Usually the child will know intuitively which one is better suited. In the next therapeutic session, only one "Safe Place" is practiced.

Instruction on the "Safe Place"

The child is asked how much he/she is satisfied with his/her notes (or if anything should be added or omitted) and how well he/she could already imagine the "Safe Place" while making the notes (scale 0 to 10; 0 = I couldn't imagine it at all; 10 = I *visited* my "Safe Place"). A score of 4 or less should trigger the question concerning what exactly the difficulty was (e.g., too loud, impossible to *picture* the place, bad memories, or body feeling). Generally, all difficulties arising during the task should be taken seriously. Usually any difficulties are important aspects for pain therapy. If the child can imagine the "Safe Place" well and any difficulties can be overcome, the child is instructed to sit in a comfortable position, eyes open or closed – just as he/she likes. He/she is told to listen to the psychotherapist reading out the list of cues exactly as they were written down. Having finished, the child is asked how well he/she could imagine the "Safe Place," if anything should be added or omitted, and if reading speed and intonation have been pleasant. The technique is practiced in this and the following sessions (don't forget the homework (see below)) until the degree of imagination is at least 8.

For homework the child is asked to practice the "Safe Place" and to document the degree to which he/she achieves clarity of imagination each time. In addition, a talented child may paint his/her "Safe Place" in order to establish another emotional approach to the exercise. Asking this of a child without talent risks devaluing the exercise, due to the tendency towards overachievement and self-criticism often found in children with chronic pain. Since it is not the aim of the exercise to discuss the patient's dysfunctional thoughts, you should ask the child in advance if he/she feels confident in painting the "Safe Place" in a way that will satisfy him/her. If the "Safe Place" is a real place and photographs of this place exist, it makes sense to look at them while doing the exercise.

6.4.2.2 Pet on My Belly

A special version of the "Safe Place" is described by Seemann et al. (2002) ("children with headache," only available in German language). They name it "Pet on my Belly." Instead of a place, an animal is conveying safety and security. This version is less dependent on the ability of abstract thinking and is thus well suited to younger patients. However, the child must be able to imagine emotions and touch. Since the exercise is meant to be a relaxation technique and the setting is predefined in the instructions, we modified this technique. Especially younger children who see their pet as a source of comfort are very susceptible to exercises involving their pet. Also children with a strong imagination who like animals but do not have a pet themselves often enjoy imagination exercises with animals as a central anchor. The pet involved should not be sick or very old such that its death is foreseeable, a point that should be determined explicitly. Especially younger children like to repress those facts. To maintain the positive features of animal imagination independent of the context, biography, and the child's abilities, we recommend a procedure following that of the "Safe Place." In younger children it is helpful if the psychotherapist collects the cues together with the child and the psychotherapist writes them down (Chap. 9, Worksheet #12). Often a numerical rating scale (NRS) is too abstract for children younger than 9 years. In this case you may substitute the numeric imagination score by verbal denotations such as "excellent," "good," "moderate," and "bad."

6.4.2.3 Pain Fighter

Imagining a Pain Fighter or a creature from fairy tales is supposed to reduce the child's helplessness by supporting the child in his/her efforts to cope with the pain. In accordance with the previously presented imagination techniques, the child is instructed to imagine with as much detail as possible. Together with the child the psychotherapist should consider in which way the Pain Fighter could support pain coping. Please find below three examples:

1. The Pain Fighter has magical power and will transfer the power necessary for active pain coping to the child.
2. The Pain Fighter is a huge eagle, carrying the child through the sky to easily escape his/her severe pain.
3. The Pain Fighter is a tall knight who puts the malicious pain monster to flight with his sword.

This imagination technique is trained and practiced the same way as the "Safe Place" or "Pet on my Belly." The technique especially suits children younger than 12 years. The Pain Fighter arises from a very infantile fantasy in which the pain is considered an opponent. This technique – at least as presented – is not recommended for children aged 13 years and older. In those patients it should not be the primary aim to fight the pain as an enemy. It is sometimes difficult to explain this to the younger child. For older patients we recommend the "internal helper" well-known from trauma therapy (Reddemann 2005; only available in German language).

6.4.3 Cognitive Strategies: Seeing Things Differently

"My therapy includes evaluating my thoughts. By now I'm confident that a life with pain is possible, and I am much more relaxed in many situations. I would have never thought that in the beginning." – Maria (age 15 years)

The approach for children aged 8–12 years tends to differ from that for older patients. The former will benefit from classical positive self-instructions and can generally modify their thoughts more easily. Approaches where thoughts are extensively discussed are of only limited use in children aged 10–12 years and not suited at all for younger children.

There are two fundamentally different approaches to dysfunctional thoughts and appraisals perpetuating pain symptoms. Dysfunctional thoughts and appraisals are either modified or replaced by more helpful thoughts (cognitive restructuring). Otherwise, the patient has to learn to accept and observe the various dysfunctional thoughts, appraisals, and cognitions in a neutral way and direct his/her behavior towards longer-term positive targets, independent of dysfunctional thoughts and perceptions (acceptance-based approach). In less severe pain disorders pain is not yet that chronic that it is perceived as unalterable. In our experience, cognitive restructuring is the best strategy for those cases. In severe pain disorders it may, however, be advisable to apply an acceptance-based approach. Importantly, this approach is less suitable for children aged 13 years and younger. Their pain symptoms are still accessible to modification, and a worldview based on change works better.

First, we present several methods of cognitive intervention in which children with dysfunctional cognitions challenge and dispute their cognitions in order to be able to use more helpful thoughts and appraisals in the future. If applicable, we point out age-specific peculiarities. Then we present an acceptance-based approach, suited for older patients with long-standing constant pain symptoms, where cognitive interventions aiming at modification are less promising.

6.4.3.1 Methods for Cognitive Restructuring

Usually children are very quick to spot dysfunctional thoughts and change them with the appropriate support. As with adults, cognitive restructuring is a multistep approach:

1. Development of an age-appropriate cognitive model
2. Extraction of dysfunctional cognitions and assumptions
3. Questioning of old dysfunctional cognitions and creating functional new ones
4. Practicing the new functional thoughts.

In this chapter, we simply focus on describing the implementation of this cognitive restructuring in pain therapy. For a comprehensive presentation of approaches to cognitive restructuring in children, see Stallard (2005) or Schlarb and Stavemann (2011).

Step 1: Creating an Age-Appropriate Cognitive Model

It is fundamental to any cognitive approach that the child understands why examining his/her thoughts is a significant part of therapy. This understanding will motivate him/her to search for dysfunctional patterns in his/her thoughts. The basic assumption of the cognitive approach is that dysfunctional thoughts, assumptions, and cognitive schemes result in negative feelings and behavior.

A prototypical dysfunctional pain-related cognition is the set of assumptions underlying somatic fixation. If a child believes that the physicians did not search long and hard enough for a physical cause of the pain, he/she will be fearful or insecure and ask for further investigations. Those additional investigations will in most cases yield no pathological findings, thus confirming the child's thoughts ("They're not finding the underlying cause."), or will deliver results with pathological findings which are, however, not to blame for the symptoms and are thus irrelevant (e.g., a slightly conspicuous EEG or an increased C-reactive protein) but further increase the fear.

It is best to start informing the child about dysfunctional thoughts and their significance during psycho-education. The "ABC scheme" (according to A. Ellis) has proven helpful in the search for dysfunctional thoughts (A = activating experience, B = belief system, C = consequences).

For cognitive therapeutic interventions, the child must be able to examine his/her thoughts and name his/her feelings. Often, practicing those abilities is the first therapeutic step. Patients commonly do not initially succeed in differentiating reliably between levels of the cognitive model (thoughts vs. feelings) (e.g., "…then I think I am sad."). If this is the case, the psychotherapist should work with the child on the identification of the child's feelings first, using picture stories, comics, or photographs illustrating various emotions. Alternatives are tasks such as "charade of emotions."

Charade of Emotions
"I would like to start this session with a game called "Charade of Emotions" which works as follows: On this sheet I have written down feelings (e.g. sadness, anger, happiness). Can you think of any other feelings? Now let us put the notes into that box, and in alternating sequence one of us will take out a note and do a pantomime representing the indicated feeling. This means you try to express that emotion without words."

Since some children may feel insecure or awkward doing this, it is very helpful if the psychotherapist is the first to act in order to create a relaxed, humorous atmosphere.

The "Mood Barometer" is another tool to train the child's ability to differentiate between various feelings.

The Mood Barometer
The child writes down feelings that are relevant to him/her and puts them in a hierarchical sequence (similar to a thermometer or barometer) or clockwise order. With the help of a slider or watch hand, the child informs the NET about his/her current feelings and at the same time become aware of them. Two to three times a day, one of the staff prompts the child to assess his/her feelings using the Mood Barometer. If the child has difficulty answering, the NET may give some feedback or pose a hypothesis ("Your shoulders and your gaze are down. I assume you are sad."). Then this observation is discussed with the child.

Gradually the child will learn to recognize and to express feelings. Many children show great difficulty differentiating between various feelings and tend to repeatedly express similar or the same feelings. Those are the children in need of reflection with and detailed feedback from the NET.

If the child is sufficiently trained to recognize his/her feelings, the psychotherapist may start to query him/her about his/her dysfunctional thoughts ("What did you think about in this situation?"). Then together with the child a simple ABC-model is created (Table 6.2). With younger children the psychotherapist should be more active and give input, i.e., suggestions that the child understands well, such as thoughts closely connected with behavior. The older the child, the more elaborate the chains of thought that can be worked on.

Table 6.2 Prototype of an ABC-model

Activating experience (A)	Belief system (B)	Emotion and behavior/consequence (C)
Boy sitting in a bus and smiling at me	Decent boy. Maybe he also goes to my school. I think I should speak to him	Emotion: curiosity Response: looking into his eyes and speaking to him
Boy sitting in a bus and smiling at me	Oh dear, why is the boy laughing? I don't know him. Maybe there is still some jam on my face. Certainly he is laughing at me	Emotion: insecurity Response: quickly passing by and taking a seat somewhere else

The following case illustrates our practical approach to create an ABC-model in a child with chronic pain.

> **Case Report – Maria, 15 Years, Pain Disorder (T = Therapist, C = Child)**
>
> T: When we discussed the vicious cycle, I explained how thoughts may have an impact on the pain experience. Every appraisal of a situation has some impact on what and how we feel. Can you still go with that? Or are there any questions left?
>
> C: Well, I am often under the impression that I do not think at all. I just feel helpless when I am in pain.
>
> T: Right. Thoughts often are ultra-fast, as quick as lightning, being nearly unrecognizable for us. This is the reason why they are called automatic thoughts. I'd like to illustrate the significance of thoughts with a little story. Imagine, holidays are over and you are getting on the school bus for the first time again. A boy you have never seen before looks at you and smiles. In that moment you think: "Nice boy. Maybe he also goes to my school? I think I should speak to him." How do you think you feel?"
>
> C: I would be curious.
>
> T: What will you do?
>
> C: I think I will sit next to him and talk to him.
>
> T: Okay, let's write that down (T: makes a note on the ABC-model template). Now imagine, the same situation, the same boy, exactly the same smile. But, in this moment you are thinking "Oh dear, why is the boy laughing? I don't know him. Maybe there is still some jam on my face." How do you feel, and what will you be doing?
>
> C: I suppose I am insecure. I would probably go and sit somewhere else in the bus.
>
> T: Great. Could you please write this down in the template? What did you learn from this example?
>
> C: Depending on what I'm thinking there will be different emotions.
>
> T: That is correct! Do you mind if I ask you about your feelings and thoughts while you are experiencing pain every now and then in the upcoming sessions?

By means of the newly created ABC scheme, you can now work on the patient's pain-related examples. Admittedly, the given example is somewhat prototypical. Mostly, the analysis of relationships between situations, thoughts, and feelings is not that simple. But with some support most patients will quickly recognize the given interrelations. Often it is advantageous to ask the patient about the thoughts he/she had in former stressful situations. Then the patient's homework is to fill in his/her worksheet with his/her observations, for example, as a "diary of thoughts." To prepare the worksheet, use a white sheet with three equal columns with the headlines "A," "B," and "C." The child is asked to write down any stressful or unpleasant situation, a detailed description of Black Thoughts arising in this situation and the physical response to them.

Step 2: Distilling Dysfunctional Cognitions and Assumptions

Once the model is finalized and all negative thoughts are documented, the second step aims to identify the stressful thoughts that should be reviewed. It cannot be the goal of cognitive therapy to change all negative thoughts or feelings. Instead, we focus on those that are particularly stressful and dysfunctional. The following questions proved helpful in the identification of automatic thoughts (for a fuller discussion, see Stallard 2005 or Schlarb and Stavemann 2011):

1. *Basic question – "What were your thoughts in this situation?"*
   (a) The basic question may be asked if the patient's mood changes during the session.
   (b) The therapist may ask the patient to describe a difficult situation and then to ask the basic question.
   (c) The therapist may initiate a visualization of the depicted situation and then ask the basic question.
   (d) Have the patient re-experience the situation in a role play, and then ask the basic question.
2. *More questions to identify automatic thoughts:*
   (a) "What do you think you were thinking about?"
   (b) "Is it possible that you were thinking about _____ or _____?" (therapist proposes a plausible alternative)
   (c) "Did you imagine something that could happen, or did you remember something?"
   (d) "What meaning did this situation have for you?"
   (e) "Did you think: _____?" (therapist proposes the opposite of the assumed answer)
3. *An alternative approach is indicated if there are any problems with the implementation of the previous approaches:*
   (a) With a child having great difficulty with the approach described under 2) or children too young to have the required cognitive ability for reflection, it may be helpful to name several examples of Black Thoughts and ask directly if the child has ever had that specific thought.

(b) It goes without saying that in addition to what is proposed in paragraph 2), it is also possible to go over those Black Thoughts most often mentioned by children with chronic pain. Those are:

- "When I am in pain I can't perform well in school."
- "I can't do anything about my pain."
- "I can't control my pain. The pain is controlling me. I lose control!"
- "Perhaps the physicians did miss something after all?"
- "Why me?"
- "I can't stand any more pain."
- "Being ill is awful."
- "Nobody can help me."
- "A life with pain is futile because I can't achieve anything."
- "Nobody believes that I am in pain."
- "I hate my body for its pain."

When several dysfunctional appraisals and cognitions have been identified, the child may choose one cognition that should be checked first for its relationship to reality. It is not always advisable to start with the "Blackest" Thoughts (i.e., "My mother hates me." or "Awful things will happen to me."). It is better to begin with thoughts that are more easily scrutinized in order to make the child see the success of the exercise.

Step 3: Scrutinizing Old and Dysfunctional Cognitions and Creating New and Functional Ones

Some of the pain-related Black Thoughts (e.g., "I can't do anything about my pain.") may already start to change after the first few days of inpatient pain therapy. This can occur due to learning from other patients or due to the experience that pain is not as inalterable as previously thought. This is a typical patient report:

> "I used to think I couldn't do anything about my pain. Now I know that with the help of various techniques (e.g. distraction-ABC) I will be able to manage my pain in such a way that I can go to school."

In case a child reports this, you should point out that he/she has performed a reality check on his/her own, without any instruction, and compliment him/her for that. Since the child proved by himself/herself the mutability of Black Thoughts, he/she will be highly motivated to continue working on other Black Thoughts. Sometimes it may be helpful to ask for previous positive exceptions from Black Thoughts in order to emphasize the modifiability of thoughts and appraisals. Regarding dysfunctional cognitions, we use the following disputation techniques:

1. *Proof/counterproof (logical disputing)*: First, the child is prompted to describe his/her Black Thought in detail ("Could you please describe exactly the Black Thought that made you scared and lose control? What would it mean to you if

you didn't actually pass the exam? What would that tell us about you?"). Then the child's task is to prove the soundness of this Black Thought to the psychotherapist. Typically this technique will work only with children who show the necessary ability for reflection and abstraction. With Black Thoughts affecting the child's mood or causing stress, it may well be that the child cannot generate any ideas. In this case the psychotherapist could give the child one or two obvious ideas as to how to counterprove the thoughts.

2. *Querying catastrophes* (*balancing out*): Children with chronic pain are usually prone to pain-related catastrophizing ("While I'm in pain, I can't concentrate."). If this is the case, we start searching for the worst-case scenario together with the child ("I will have to leave school before graduation, and I will have to live on the street in winter."). Then we describe the best scenario imaginable ("Pain will have totally vanished soon, and I will perform very well all the time."). Finally the child should depict the most probable scenario ("Sometimes it will be difficult to perform well while in pain. But sometimes I will perform as well as I did before my pain problem began."). Then the psychotherapist asks the child to search for reasons in favor of the most probable scenario.

3. *How much does your Black Thought help you?* (*hedonistic disputing*): We instruct the child to make a cost/benefit analysis of his/her thought and its associated behavior, differentiating between short-term and long-term consequences. Table 6.3 gives an example of a hedonistic disputing of the thought "Being in pain is awful."

Table 6.3 Hedonistic dispute of the thought "Being in pain is awful"

	Cost	Benefit
Short-term	I start getting anxious and tense, which makes the pain worse	When I complain I get help from other people
		When I am not feeling good my teachers are less strict
Long-term	I don't search for solutions but keep on complaining	There is no long-term benefit
	This way my pain disorder won't get better	

4. *Extending the ABC-model*: In order to work on new cognitions, the ABC-model may be extended. Having explored a stressful situation, the psychotherapist asks: "How would you like to feel in that situation, and what would you like to do?" During the following brainstorming session where the child and his psychotherapist find out which thought might be necessary for an emotional or behavioral change, a change of viewpoint may be worthwhile ("What would your girlfriend think about that?"). Then the patient's task is to search for arguments proving the alternative thought. This may be supported by a short role play where the psychotherapist is taking the child's point of view. In the discussion that follows, the patient should find arguments in favor of and some against his/her new point of view.

5. *Behavioral experiments* (*empirical disputing*): Dysfunctional thoughts may also be tested against reality by means of formal reality tests (behavioral experiment), a stepped procedure more suited to children aged 12 years and up:

(a) Isolate the thought to be tested (e.g., "While in pain I can't do anything."). You may use the cognitive techniques mentioned before (e.g., proof/counterproof) in order to increase the child's motivation to undergo a behavioral experiment.

(b) Depict a detailed scenario suited to testing the thought (e.g., "While in pain I can't play the piano."). Then make an exact plan of all the variables to be tested during the behavioral experiment (e.g., "For how long would you have to play the piano in order to have a counterproof?")

(c) Accomplishing the behavioral experiment.

(d) Drawing a conclusion and working on a new functional thought (e.g., "I can't play the piano as long as before, but I can play for some time, and this means a lot of fun for me.").

Children younger than 12 years benefit from a much reduced disputational approach. Typically their thoughts are less complex, and often a dichotomous distinction (black vs. colored) is sufficient:

(a) The psychotherapist is working on Black Thoughts about pain. For hedonistic disputing it is only necessary to pose the simple question "Does it help you to think like that?"

(b) As a next step, we search for Colored Thoughts together. The psychotherapist may make his/her own suggestions in order to facilitate the process.

(c) In the course of treatment, those new Colored Thoughts should be practiced with the child (see Step 4).

Step 4: Practicing the New Functional Thought

Towards the end of this exercise the child will have acquired one or more functional cognitions. These new thoughts should be phrased in the child's own words, use the "I" mode and be as detailed as possible (a bad example would be "Everything will be okay."). Unfortunately, just gaining insight isn't enough to have a long-lasting positive effect on the child's experience. The psychotherapist should inform the child of this ("It is the same as with learning vocabulary. It is not enough to read the words once in order to be able to reproduce them in an exam."). It is essential to regularly apply the new helpful cognitions and evaluate them for their effectiveness. To this end, behavioral experiments may be used (Step 3). In addition, the following training methods have proven effective:

1. *Creative techniques.* The patient creates a collage using the notes on the functional new thoughts. Depending on the patient's creativity, he/she may write or paint a comic around those helpful thoughts together with the psychotherapist. Painting a Pain Fighter (Sect. 6.4.2) is the combination of a cognitive and an imaginative technique. The collage should be placed in a prominent location to be seen in every-day life. Together with the psychotherapist, the child decides how those thoughts portrayed in the collage could also be practiced in everyday life (e.g., starting a list of thoughts on a sheet of paper fixed to the cover of the child's school book).

2. *Role play and flashcards.* Functional thoughts may also be practiced in a role play in which the child is using functional thoughts in a difficult situation and rates their effectiveness. The child may write down the new functional thoughts on an index card (flashcard) in order to read them during the role play. These flashcards may also be used in everyday life. Any further favorable thought may

be recorded on an extra flashcard, with the positive experience from it on its back ("lesson passed ☺," "distraction techniques were applied successfully," etc.).

3. *Imagination*. If the child has the ability to imagine scenes, the psychotherapist may encourage him to imagine these helpful scenes during an imaginary experience, such as guided imagery or hypnosis.

4. *List of thoughts/interruption of thoughts and positive self-instruction*. Creating a list of Black Thoughts may be used to instruct children to pay more attention to actually applying Colored Thoughts. One possible way of doing so is to interrupt a Black Thought whenever it is noticed (e.g., by saying out loud *STOP*) and replace it with a Colored Thought. When the child has succeeded in doing so, he/ she should mark this on the list of thoughts (tally list) (bar on the list; other sign like a paper clip changing from the right to the left jean pocket).

6.4.3.2 Three Letters

Some patients are not that happy with a purely cognitive approach. They don't really like to extensively dispute their thoughts. These patients (of course this approach fits for the other patients as well) might be suited to writing down the "Three Letters" before deciding to learn more cognitive interventions or to learn a more acceptance-oriented approach.

This technique will work only if the child has the necessary cognitive ability (typically from 13 years and up) and is willing to take on the required homework.

The psychotherapist asks the child to write three letters (for a detailed instruction, see Chap. 9, Worksheet #17). The third letter should be written immediately after the second letter is finished (only a short break is allowed). Each letter should comprise about one written page. Some of the children will pack all necessary information into a letter of no longer than half a page; others will need 2 to 3 pages each:

1. *Letter 1*. In this letter the patient describes how his/her life will be for the next 2 years *in the best case* (alternatively, until his/her next or the next but one birthday, 18th birthday, other significant future event, …) after this therapeutic session (alternatively, inpatient treatment program, outpatient psychotherapy, …). With this exercise the challenge is to write the letter from a future and first-person perspective to oneself in the present ("Dear Martin, two years have passed since you opted for the inpatient pain therapy. Since then, …"). For the intervention to be effective, it is important that the patient describes his/her development in *all* relevant aspects very precisely (i.e., not just concerning pain but also friends, relationships, school, family, leisure activities) and comments on which decisions, judgments, and behavior contributed to steering life into just that direction (*incorrect*: "I won the lottery, and suddenly everybody was overwhelmingly nice to me." *Correct*: the child is supposed to focus on *his/her own* efforts and changes).

2. *Letter 2*. The second letter is the counterpart of the first one. As in the first letter, it is written from the future to oneself living in the present and reports about the worst imaginable course of the pain condition (same formal criteria as for letter 1). The letter should describe precisely the writer's *own* behavior, appraisals, and decisions contributing to that disastrous course. It should be emphasized again how important it is to continue with writing letter 3 immediately after the second letter and *not* to pause; otherwise, there is the risk that the negative feelings

evoked by writing letter 2 will result in a negative trance that may have a negative impact on the pain and the mood for days.

3. *Letter 3*. Most patients regard this letter as the one most difficult to write. While it is quite simple to imagine the best possible or the worst possible course, it is a challenge to imagine a realistic one, *taking into account one's own personality and perception of abilities*. And that is exactly the aim of letter 3: to find a *realistic* course; somewhere between the extremes described in letters 1 and 2 regarding the patient's *own* behavior, appraisals, and decisions.

These letters are well suited to gaining an overview of all relevant parts of the child's life, his/her own perspectives of change, important resources, and critical (cognitive) factors relevant for therapy. It is then quite easy to filter all important negative cognitions out of the Three Letters together with the child. Often you will find those written down word by word. An invaluable benefit of that intervention is that it will help the child analyze his/her situation more clearly. Reaching this clarity by his/her own effort will make the child proud. Writing the Three Letters allows the child to ponder all relevant areas of life, presumably for the first time.

This intervention should be avoided with children with a current depressive episode. If suicide is the only solution given at the end of letter 2, the child should be complimented for his/her courage in writing down his/her worst fears. This information should then be made known to the psychotherapist for immediate attention. Any real current danger of a suicide attempt may reflect a depressive comorbidity which will require further action.

6.4.3.3 Acceptance-Based Methods

At the end of the last chapter, we explained a technique ("the Three Letters") that allows for the elaboration of pain-related desires and goals. That intervention is also well suited as a preparation for the work with acceptance-based cognitive techniques that do not focus on the modification of thoughts. Research results offer preliminary support for the view that an acceptance-based approach is effective in both adults and children with severe chronic pain (Wicksell et al. 2009, 2011). In children with a pain disorder, the acceptance of pain may result in a better quality of life (Feinstein et al. 2011). Pain acceptance seems to have an inverse relationship to emotional impairment and pain intensity (Wallace et al. 2011).

What exactly is the difference between a cognitive and an acceptance-based approach? And how can the difference between acceptance and resignation be explained to the patient and his parents?

Contrary to the cognitive approach, the focus of an acceptance-based approach is not to teach alternative appraisals or lines of thought concerning pain but to reach the goals important to the patient in the intermediate or long-term future, irrespective of pain intensity. The focus of pain therapy shifts from pain reduction to a meaningful and happy life even if it is still painful (Wicksell et al. 2007). As mentioned before, the Three Letters can be the first step to identifying the long-term goals of the child.

The advantage of an acceptance-based approach is that pain is no longer regarded as an enemy that should be modified, reduced, or circumvented. Thus, the *symptom distress* of the whole family system arising from the pain-reduction battle can be eased. This approach is especially helpful if long-standing chronic pain makes quick pain reduction seem improbable. Because of their severe impairment in school, these children are at high risk of dropping out. Therefore, action is badly needed although options for change are minimal. The acceptance-based approach can be implemented in four steps.

Step 1: Understanding the Idea of the Acceptance-Based Approach

The acceptance-based approach aims to build mindfulness towards, and acceptance of one's own situation and to value one's own abilities. It also changes the language-based context provided by dysfunctional thoughts by increasing the neutral distance to cognitive processes (*cognitive defusion*, see below). The procedure should be discussed with the parents and their child in advance, because many families are somatic fixated and thus antagonistic towards psychological pain treatment. If not fully informed, they may misunderstand this approach as a sign of resignation, which may lead to a premature termination of treatment. The first step is to make the patient and his/her family familiar with the specific idea of the acceptance-based approach and the differences between acceptance and resignation.

> **Exercise: Getting Familiar with the Acceptance-Based Attitude**
> "Today I'd like you to write down all your thoughts about your pain on index cards. When you are done please stand up in front of me. I will throw the cards at you one by one. You should try not to let the cards touch you. After this we will do a second exercise. This time you will just stand there and hold your hand in front of you, palm up. I will place the cards in your hand, and the only thing you have to do is look at them."

Having finished the exercise, the psychotherapist will ask the child which one of the exercises was more exhausting and took more effort (usually it will be the first one – avoiding the cards – if the psychotherapist is a good pitcher). Psychotherapist and child will figure out the essentials of an acceptance-based approach together and discuss whether it seems suitable for the child. It is essential to clarify the difference between an acceptance-based approach and resignation. For many children acceptance is not that different from resignation. The difference may be illustrated as follows:

> **Example: Explanation of the Difference Between Acceptance and Resignation**
> "With an acceptance-based approach I choose a life following my own goals, irrespective of the existence of one, two, or more aspects of life that bother me. In other words, with active pain coping I can achieve all those things in everyday life that I planned for a pain-free life. Resignation is if I give up the battle against pain out of exhaustion or desperation, assuming my life will never change for the better, and could even deteriorate."

This shows that acceptance and resignation are very different attitudes based on different ideas, and although the word "acceptance" is suggestive of passivity, the acceptance-based approach is an *active* coping approach. An acceptance-based approach contributes to the disconnection of emotional distress and pain perception (Wicksell et al. 2009, 2011).

Step 2: Training a Neutral and Mindful Perception

Once the patient has recognized the difference between an acceptance-based and a resignation-based attitude, he/she should understand that the thoughts and appraisals ("If in pain, I can't attend school.") and perceptions of body signals (i.e., pressing pain on the forehead, a pulling intestinal pain, shallow breathing) that so far have determined everyday life are nothing more and nothing less than – thoughts, appraisals, and perceptions. This can only be fully understood if the child is aware of his/her thoughts, appraisals, and perception of body signals.

Mindfulness is one central idea of acceptance-based therapy and describes an active process of perception and an attitude of neutrality and freedom from judgment. This concept is often conveyed by a spiritual attitude. In this book mindfulness is defined as consciously noticing what is going on in the here and now. In the beginning, this is not a simple task, for children or adults. Thus, it is important to practice mindful perception, using the 5-4-3-2-1 technique (Sect. 6.4.1) or several other perception exercises (e.g., to focus on one's breathing, to carefully focus on what is sensed with one's own sensory channels in this moment, body scan).

Step 3: Cognitive Defusion

If a child succeeds in being aware of his/her thoughts, appraisals, and feelings, Step 3 is to *just* perceive one's thoughts, appraisals, and body signals from the position of a mindful observer. This implies that thoughts, appraisals, or perceptions of body signals are neither devalued nor followed; instead, they are observed from a distance (like clouds passing by). This mental state is called *cognitive defusion*. The aim is not to change the content of the thoughts, appraisals, or perceptions but to create some sort of inner distance (metalevel: I *have* a thought or feeling, but *I'm not* the thought or feeling). Cognitive defusion creates a distance from one's own experience (this is, e.g., comparable to various distancing techniques used in trauma therapy) and enables a reduction of the emotional burden.

Case Report: Caroline (Aged 17 Years), Pain Disorder with Backache

"First of all now you know the basic ideas contributing to a happy life irrespective of the pain. By observing your thoughts you have learned that most of them follow a simple logic: "I can't do _____ because I am in so much pain. Therefore I will never achieve _____ and will stay unhappy." Now it's time to introduce a small modification to this logic. Instead of "I can't do _____ because I am in so much pain", please think "I have the thought that I can't achieve _____ because of my severe pain". Do you feel a difference in your thinking and feeling? Please write down how often you could change your thoughts in this way and if you could feel a difference."

A variant of verbal cognitive defusion is to give names to one's thoughts (e.g., "pain monster"). This may be done in a humorous way. Maybe the child could even tickle his pain monster or find other methods to attain greater inner distance by externalizing his thoughts.

Another variant of cognitive defusion is to alienate the dysfunctional thoughts. This is achieved by repeating a thought in your head with a distorted voice, or with a modified speech melody, as soon as you notice the dysfunctional thought. Even if "pure neutrality" can't be achieved, this exercise will create an inner distance to those thoughts.

Step 4: Departure into a New Life

Once the child has learned how to attain some distance from his/her thoughts, he/she will start to identify important *goals* for his/her future life and essential *inner values* that they are based on (i.e., honesty, discipline, self-confidence). Finally, we will reflect on how the patient's behavior (e.g., passive pain coping) matches those goals and if the goals can be met by sticking to that behavior. In case the patient decides that his/her behavior (e.g., not attending school when in pain) has so far not helped him/her, the child can explore with the psychotherapist future steps to reach the desired goals (e.g., active pain coping). This is usually a lengthy process. So, it is essential to regularly practice these exercises and record their success for the next therapeutic session.

In closing, we would like to report an interesting clinical observation from children who have successfully practiced mindfulness techniques for a long time. They unanimously report that at first they perceived their pain as less stressful but of unchanged intensity. Within a short time, however, their pain perception was reduced. In many children, with further practice it was reduced to such a degree that they felt (nearly) pain free. They "just stopped thinking about" their pain. This clinical observation is in accordance with the findings of Wicksell et al. (2011) who detected a major decrease in pain perception in children with chronic pain when using an acceptance-based approach.

6.4.4 Techniques to Reduce Muscular Tension: Stay Cool!

"Great! I can watch my body relax." – Chris (14 years) during a biofeedback session

Procedures reducing muscular tension are of great importance in pain therapy. Their use with children is well investigated (Palermo et al. 2010). Based on these studies, relaxation techniques are recommended as a procedure of choice in chronic paediatric pain. But unfortunately these studies do not take into account the fact that the meta-analyses in most cases are based on investigations of children with migraine or tension-type headache with only moderate pain-related disability. In many studies the participants were recruited via newspaper advertisements – thus, some of the participants were not pain *patients* with significant pain impairment or disability but children with pain who neither felt that ill nor *suffered* from pain, pain-related fears, or impairment in everyday life. We believe that it is not advisable to confer those results to children with severe chronic pain without some precaution. In our experience in the treatment of paediatric chronic pain patients, both autogenic training (AT) and – to a lesser degree – progressive muscle relaxation according to Jacobson (PMR) may even have a *negative* impact on the patient.

How can this discrepancy be explained? Children with severe chronic pain have an increased body awareness, often accompanied by fear. Furthermore, many of these children know that severe pain may be associated with stressful memories or thoughts. In these patients, calm or relaxation often results in increased interoceptive pain perception and/or exposure with aversive thoughts. Thus, they experience an increase in *tension* instead of relaxation. Hence, classical relaxation techniques should only be used after detailed education and when the technique seems to be suitable for the patient.

Consequently, during inpatient pain therapy, some children don't want to be trained in classical relaxation techniques. But all are trained in TENS therapy (with the exception of children with abdominal pain) and biofeedback. Those techniques provide the effect of relaxation as well as increasing one's distance from interoceptive stimuli. Irrespective of which technique is trained, the education in relaxation techniques has three goals:

1. To learn self-initiated and voluntary relaxation in stressful situations
2. To gain active control of physiological activity in order to decrease pain
3. To strengthen the patient's belief in self-efficacy

Training in those relaxation techniques takes several sessions. The patient should practice daily and record his/her success, especially during stressful situations (scale 0 to 10).

6.4.4.1 Progressive Muscle Relaxation According to Jacobson (PMR)

Applying this technique, groups of muscles are tensed and then relaxed in a predefined sequence, always starting with the large muscles of the extremities and proceeding to the trunk muscles and finally to the small muscles of the face:

1. Activation of the muscle group
2. Sensing the muscular tension
3. Gradual relaxation of the respective muscle group
4. Focusing one's attention on the feeling of relaxation within the relaxed muscles

The children receive a CD with auditory instructions (partially supplemented with music) for their daily exercises. Apart from the extended instructions (45 min) found on PMR CDs, some also contain short versions (15 min). We recommend exclusively using the short versions since the patients' adherence to the extended version is low. Muscle relaxation techniques may be used before, during, or after stressful situations as well as to fall asleep. Many children with chronic pain are mentally but not physically exhausted in the evening due to their established passivity and inactivity. PMR will help to (re)establish an adequate daily schedule including active pain coping. Many children consider PMR helpful but dislike the accompanying music. In this case they should do the exercises without music.

6.4.4.2 Autogenic Training (AT)

In its simplest form, AT comprises a sequence of six exercises. In the first two exercises, set verbalizations (e.g., "My right arm is becoming pleasantly warm.") combined with imaginations directed towards the respective sensory perception (heaviness: lying beneath a pleasantly heavy blanket; warmth: the sun is shining on the respective part of the body). Not every child has the necessary ability to visualize.

Exercises:

1. Heaviness: hands, arms, feet, legs, neck, shoulder, whole body
2. Warmth: hands, arms, feet, legs, neck, shoulder, whole body
3. Breathing exercise
4. Sensing one's heartbeat
5. Exercise for the solar plexus/abdominal organs
6. Sensing the coolness of the forehead

In pain therapy, these exercises are frequently supplemented with positive self-verbalizations aiming to modify pain perception. Compared to progressive muscle relaxation (PMR), the time needed to get acquainted with AT is longer, the technique is less concrete, and it is less suited to daily use. Although AT is often practiced in paediatric pain therapy and is very popular with psychotherapists, so far only one controlled study has shown that AT is effective in the induction of relaxation in children suffering from chronic headache (Labbé 1995). We feel AT is less suitable for paediatric inpatient pain therapy. The main problem with AT in paediatric pain therapy is that one has to become calm and focus on interoceptive signals. Many children in need of an inpatient pain therapy dislike focusing on their body due to a rise in pain perception. Besides, premises such as liking calmness, the ability to visualize, as well as experience interoceptive signals comfortably are a rare combination in children suffering from chronic pain. If however these premises are met, AT can provide a worthwhile contribution towards pain therapy.

6.4.4.3 Relaxation for Smaller Kids: Telling a Story

A relaxation story is an abbreviated version of PMR or AT presented as a story for use in children up to 11 years – older patients may not feel taken seriously when applying this technique (For example, one could tell the story of an underwater adventure in which the patient has to do the most important PMR exercises in a wet suit in order to progress through the story). A relaxation story aims to accustom the child to relaxation techniques in a narrative and age-appropriate way. Its narrative character enables the patient to focus on the story and to be less flooded with interoceptive stimuli or memories compared to AT. On the other hand, it is difficult for a child to perform a relaxation story on his/her own. Thus, normally the child depends on an adult to perform the relaxation. A relaxation story can be easily performed by the patient's parents. Its narrative character makes the relaxation story well suited to combination with hypnotherapeutic elements. If the psychotherapist is trained in hypnotherapy, such a combination is a very useful addition.

6.4.4.4 Favorable Place: A Place to Experience Relaxation and Comfort

An alternative to telling a relaxation story is a guided imagination exercise to an imaginary place where the child can relax and feel well. This technique is usually used as part of a hypnotherapeutic intervention in which, using the child's language and inner world, a relaxed and pleasant condition is created that is incompatible with pain perception. Becoming familiar with the child's language, metaphors, and desires at the start makes it much easier to accompany him/her with these metaphors and this language on the journey to the Safe Place. If this technique is used in a hypnotherapeutic intervention, additional positive suggestions can be worked in which relate, for instance, to pain perception or to changing certain dysfunctional thoughts (see Kuttner and Culbert 2003 for an overview). The success of this exercise depends on the psychotherapist's ability to coordinate his/her language and the procedure with the child's present state of mind. For this reason, psychotherapists trained in hypnotherapy can achieve more beneficial effects on the exercise.

6.4.4.5 Biofeedback Therapy

Biofeedback therapy is both a mental and a physiological training technique, usually giving the patient visual feedback on a physiological process not accessible to direct perception (e.g., muscular tension, skin resistance). The continual perception of biological processes helps the child learn to control these processes (e.g., to reduce muscular tension). Biofeedback is a scientifically sound, well-validated, and approved technique in pain therapy.

In most cases, electromyographic (EMG) biofeedback is used to train the child to positively control muscular tension in areas where it is often increased. It enhances body awareness of and early intervention against distress-induced muscular tension. Meanwhile, biofeedback is used to control a plethora of physiological processes and even the modulation of EEG patterns. Provided instruction and technical implementation are age appropriate; even a 7-year-old child is able to learn the technique. Biofeedback has proved highly effective in children with recurrent headache or abdominal pain (Weydert et al. 2003; Trautmann et al. 2006). Biofeedback is also well suited for training strategies in the regulation of stress and emotions (Kuttner 1997, 2010). Children get a direct reading of their current stress gauge (for instance, during a "Stress Day" or when they are momentarily excited) via biofeedback. Or they can immediately experience the relationship of bodily and psychic events when imagining especially stressful situations, such as school work or arguments with their parents (see also Kuttner 1997, 2010). The technical design of the biofeedback paradigm fits well with the media-technical-dominated world and is accepted exceedingly well by the children. It often takes the first two biofeedback sessions to convince many children of all elements of the education and to get them better involved with their pain therapy. Biofeedback has so far not been evaluated as part of inpatient multimodal therapy in children with a pain disorder.

During their inpatient treatment, most children finally succeed in down modulating their sympathogenic activation (measured as muscular tension of the forehead or neck, electrodermal activity, warmth, or heart rate variability). In accordance with recent studies (Liedl et al. 2011), we also use biofeedback for the evaluation of therapy, meaning that children will undergo a biofeedback session, for instance, during their "Stress Day" (Sect. 6.4.5.3) in order to evaluate the effectiveness of their learned therapeutic strategies. This will strengthen their perception of self-effectiveness.

6.4.4.6 Transcutaneous Electrical Nerve Stimulation (TENS)

TENS has its roots in behavioral medical treatment. In TENS, a weak alternating current stimulates neuromodulatory stimuli resulting in muscular relaxation, increased perfusion, and pain inhibition (Kuttner 1997). Electrical stimuli stimulate peripheral nerves, muscles, the skin, or the subcutaneous tissue, respectively, inducing both spinal and central reactions of the nervous system which are thought to result in a segmental spinal pain inhibition. Typically, the devices provide 10–14 different programs. It is advisable to follow the manufacturers' recommendations for which program to use, and it should be tested for two to three sessions. To encourage compliance, let the child try several programs until he/she has found the most suitable one. The application of TENS is indicated for most paediatric pain conditions (Kuttner 1997, 2010).

The electrodes are placed as near as possible to the painful area, which is often quite sensitive to touch. TENS is recommended for two to five sessions a day, each lasting 20–50 min. Many children perceive TENS as beneficial from the very beginning and use it regularly. In most cases, however, the effect is not lasting. TENS can be easily integrated into the therapeutic setting as an additional module. It is a good additional module because even light relaxation and pain reduction will support pain therapy and reduce both fear of pain and pain-related helplessness.

A promising variant of TENS therapy is gradual stimuli exposure in children with a pronounced fear-associated body awareness combined with advanced pain sensitization. In this case TENS is not used to achieve relaxation but as an exposure technique to reduce pain sensitization (see Sect. 6.4.5.4).

6.4.5 Exposure Techniques: In Vivo/Graded Exposure

In pain therapy we differentiate between *in vivo/graded* and *interoceptive* exposure.

Following a daily routine with all its rules and duties irrespective of pain intensity and mood can be challenging for a child suffering from a pain disorder. The next step in the inpatient setting after the end of the second or at the beginning of the third week is to implement a "Stress Day" during which the patient is confronted with strict time pressure while accomplishing various tasks (see Sect. 6.4.5.3 for a detailed description). For a child whose pain makes walking very far without crutches or a wheelchair difficult, a gradual *in vivo exposure* may be necessary. After consulting the physiotherapist, the final goal of meeting the demands of everyday life may be subdivided into several consecutive but smaller tasks ("graduated scheme"). Since fear of pain due to fear-associated increased body awareness is of central importance to all children in maintaining pain symptoms, pain therapy also includes *interoceptive exposure techniques* (in sensu exposure) for the control of pain and reducing helplessness and body awareness (see Sect. 6.4.6).

6.4.5.1 In Vivo Exposure: Scientific Background

"What? You expect me to go for a long walk? I'm here to reduce my pain so that *after* that I can walk longer distances again."

"Why should I increase my pain? I want my pain to diminish or vanish forever."

Some interventions, such as cognitive and distraction or relaxation techniques, are easily explained to the affected child and his/her family. However, it is not obvious to the patient why he/she should expose himself/herself to increased pain in the first place. According to the fear-avoidance model (Vlaeyen and Linton 2000), pain-specific fears play a central maintenance role in chronic pain. The model postulates that increased fear of pain arises due to catastrophizing appraisals of the pain experience. Those affected show pronounced avoidance behavior in order to escape further pain as much as possible. The results of this are a reduction in physical fitness, sharp limitations to everyday activities and consequently, worse pain (Asmundson et al. 1999; Turk and Wilson 2010). In view of this it is understandable that only exposure with the avoidance behavior on the behavioral level can make sense (in vivo exposure). The fear-avoidance model has been extensively researched in the last 10 years, and its effectiveness in musculoskeletal pain, especially in adults, has been confirmed (for an overview, see Crombez et al. 2012). Asmundson et al. (2012) recently suggested an adaptation of the model for children with chronic pain.

In vivo exposure is based on the assumption that with direct (and gradual) exposure to fear-associated body movements and confronting those fears, the patient's fear of painful body movements will decrease. The patient will gradually be able to increase activity, quality of life will improve, and in the long run the pain will more or less disappear (Bailey et al. 2010). The effectiveness of such a technique is experimentally proven in adults suffering musculoskeletal pain (Bailey et al. 2010; Leeuw et al. 2008). The evaluated inpatient treatment programs for children with musculoskeletal pain describe in vivo exposure as a central technique and connect their success partially to this technique (Sherry et al. 1999; Eccleston and Malleson 2003). In children with pain disorders in other locations (e.g., head or abdomen), it is not specifically the fear of painful movements but rather a mixture of general fear of pain and fear-associated perception of somatic signals leading to avoiding activities and a decreased quality of life (Simons et al. 2011; Sect. 6.4.6).

6.4.5.2 In Vivo Exposure: Active Coping with Everyday Life

Many children with chronic pain are debilitated so that they gradually cease to engage with their peers, attend school, and are physically less active due to their pain or their fear of an increase in pain. Consequently, they are easily exhausted and generally feel asthenic. Furthermore, a phase shift in the circadian cycle and a less restful sleep can be observed in many children. In such a situation, it may make sense for the patient to participate in all everyday life activities irrespective of pain intensity (untreated acute migraine attack excluded) and mood. This requires highly competent NET staff and considerable time to motivate the child. Sometimes patients do not openly show their aversion to this tedious and unaccustomed approach, but inform their parents instead, who will often try to achieve a rest for their child. Since the family agreed to the therapy conditions before admission, such a conflict delivers important diagnostic clues, such as conflicts between autonomy and dependency, or parents supporting ambivalent therapy motivation. This conflict can be attenuated by a telephone call between parents, physician, and psychotherapist, in which the parents' cooperation in therapy can be reestablished. Lack of cooperation from the parents, even when the concept of therapy is repeatedly explained to them, can endanger successful therapy and result in premature discharge from hospital. Cases like this point out the necessity of explaining the specific demands of inpatient pain therapy to the parents in advance.

In case of premature discharge, it should always be explicitly pointed out that readmittance is possible. To this end we offer another outpatient appointment where the child and the family have the chance to decide in favor of a second inpatient admission. In such a case, the child and his/her parents have to present their motivation and aims in written form (see Sect. 6.8.3). If sufficient motivation is not given, readmittance does not make sense after having aborted treatment due to noncompliance.

For children with a musculoskeletal pain disorder who are dependent on crutches or a wheelchair or who demonstrate extensive resting and avoidance behavior, the therapeutic approach must be modified. Together with the patient and in agreement with the physiotherapist, we put up a stepped plan with gradually increasing tasks and activities depicting not only the single steps (e.g., Step 2: to walk without crutches for 1 h; Step 10: to walk without crutches all the time while on the ward) but also the final goal (Step x: the day when there is no need to use the crutches anymore). Even these severely impaired children are encouraged to follow active routines and coping strategies, and resting time is confined to a normal amount (1 h at midday) while the child is encouraged to read, play, or listen to music instead of taking a nap.

6.4.5.3 In Vivo Exposure: Stress Day

If the child succeeds in active coping and in performing the daily routine, the inpatient therapy also includes a Stress Day lasting from about 6:30 a.m. to 8:00 p.m. In the morning the child receives a plan for the day including a detailed list of all the tasks he/she is expected to do on that day. A Stress Day usually includes doing all routine duties on the ward, planning and organizing several tasks, performing meaningful as well as senseless tasks, and engaging in several social situations, from simple to complex (for examples, see Chap. 9, Worksheet #14). The Stress Day is discussed with the patient and his parents in advance and has to be affirmed by the child and his parents. The child receives a certain number of "time-out cards" which the child may use to pause for 10 min at any chosen time, for instance, to practice a stress or pain reducing technique. The child is allowed to interrupt the Stress Day at any time, so that he/she is always in control of the situation. It is important to underline that with this control and these options, the child is in a position to challenge himself/herself and discover his/her resources and deficits regarding stress coping.

The Stress Day is an experiment in behavior therapy, and due to its similarity with behavioral experiments in cognitive therapy (Sect. 6.4.3), it may well be combined with the testing of dysfunctional cognitions. The Stress Day helps to answer the following questions:

1. How will my body react to severe time pressure?
2. Will my pain actually increase during or after the Stress Day as forecasted by the psychotherapist and person in charge?
3. How will I cope with senseless or boring tasks?
4. When will I begin to react stressed or annoyed?
5. How many of the time-out cards will I use?
6. Should the persons in charge (NET team member) notify me if they think I need a time-out?
7. Will I notice somatic stress signals early, or will the pain need to be severe in order to notice stress?
8. Which thoughts or appraisals contribute to my perception of stress on such an artificial Stress Day?
9. Will the various techniques practiced during a time-out help me?

Those questions are on the agenda of the preliminary discussion with the child, to evoke curiosity and ambition. The best time for the Stress Day is the end of the second week of the stay. At this point, the child will already be familiar with several pain coping techniques. The psychotherapist should discuss his anticipation with the child, e.g., "I believe that it will be difficult for you to do boring tasks. Thus I ask you to intensely observe how you and your body will react. Do you agree? Or do you rather think this won't be a difficult task for you?" It is helpful to preschedule both a single therapeutic session and a biofeedback session for the Stress Day. The single therapy session serves to discuss any acute difficulties or queries regarding stress or pain coping, while biofeedback will directly show the child the current stress level and give the opportunity to directly observe how well the learned therapeutic techniques work.

The day after the Stress Day is the time to reflect extensively on the Stress Day with the above-mentioned questions in mind. Any implications arising with regard to the child's future pain therapy are discussed. For instance, a high increase in the pain score and the need for many time-outs show that the child still has difficulties coping with even artificial daily "hassle." Consequently, repetition of the Stress Day might be worthwhile as could be exposure with the child's dysfunctional appraisals.

On the ward the newly admitted patients get the opportunity to observe how time pressure impinges on mood and somatic symptoms in their fellow patients. In children with mental comorbidities (i.e., anxiety disorder, adjustment disorder, depressive episode), the Stress Day may be modified (Sect. 6.5.1).

6.4.5.4 In Vivo Exposure: Gradual Stimulus Exposure Using TENS

Patients with excessive fear-related increased body awareness experience even the slightest TENS stimulus – not even noticeable in most people – as painful. This finding substantiates the diagnosis of a pain disorder and should be discussed with the child. Thus, TENS can be used to gradually increase stimulus intensity, using the lowest possible level for 20 min daily until the patient can withstand it and not perceive it as painful anymore. Then intensity is increased by one step. Note that progress with regard to the tolerated stimulus intensity may well differ between electrode locations (e.g., after 1 week of practicing, Lisa (15 years) perceived a stimulus level of 1 with the electrode placed on the left side of her neck as just bearable. After a week of daily training, Lisa succeeded in raising the tolerated stimulus level from 1 to 5 (TENS apparatus level). With time she became even less pain sensitive. It is of utmost importance to inform the child that the pain will not diminish. The goal is for the body to gradually become desensitized and for stimuli that is usually not painful, such as a light touch, to eventually cause no pain.

6.4.6 Interoceptive Exposure: To Face the Fear of Pain

The vast majority of children with a pain disorder suffer from head or stomach pain, while a few of them suffer from pain associated with movement of the musculoskeletal system. It can be assumed (Simons et al. 2011) that the vicious cycle of pain and avoidance in children with head and stomach pain is not triggered by fear of movement but by the fearful perception of bodily signals, such as, for instance, with strain or pressure. As a result of this fear, the children direct their attention to their bodies to check which bodily signals can predict the occurrence of further pain (Rief and Broadbent 2007; De Peuter et al. 2011). De Peuter et al. (2011) call this interoceptive conditioning of fear of pain. Therefore, some new pain therapeutic interventions aim at decreasing fear of pain through interoceptive stimulus exposure (Hechler et al. 2010). In the next chapter, we explain when the perception of interoceptive signals becomes maladaptive. Then we provide a short overview of the state of scientific research in this field and introduce a procedure for exposure to interoceptive stimulus (pain provocation).

6.4.6.1 Maladaptive Interoception in Chronic Pain

There is growing evidence (De Peuter et al. 2011; Vlaeyen and Linton 2012) that, besides fear of pain and pain avoidance (see Sect. 6.4.5.1), interoceptive conditioning processes also play an important role in the emergence of fear of pain. Analogous to fear disorders (Domschke et al. 2010), other stomatoform disorders, and hypochondria (Rief and Broadbent 2007), a fearful heightened sensitivity to the perception of bodily processes (anxiety sensitivity) as well as a distorted interoceptive perception and negative appraisal of these processes (maladaptive interoception) is assumed (De Peuter et al. 2011). The classification of these increased bodily perceptions can then succumb to a fear-ruled bias, for instance, through certain negative experiences and corresponding expectations, memories, or traumatizations (Pagé et al. 2013; Rief and Broadbent 2007; Rief and Barsky 2005). Meulders et al. (2011) verified within the framework of an experimental study that fear of pain can become conditioned to interoceptive stimuli. The perception of muscle tension plays a special role here, since it not only contributes to the occurrence of pain but also plays an important role in proprioception of movement. Meulders et al. (2011) showed that the coupling of movements with light pain stimuli in healthy people can effectively lead to a fear of movement conditioning (Meulders et al. 2011). Thus, interoceptive stimuli become associated with fear of pain (interoceptive conditioning of fear of pain), and therefore, the perception of interoceptive stimuli can trigger fear of pain and avoidance behavior (De Peuter et al. 2011).

Fear of Pain

Numerous studies have concurrently shown the meaning of fear of pain in adult patients with chronic pain (for an overview, see Turk and Wilson 2010). The studies verify increased fear of pain in patient populations compared with healthy people, increased tendency to catastrophize, and increased impairment in those who show strong fear of pain. Moreover, experimental studies that investigated the interference in capacity for concentration due to fear of pain in adults with chronic pain found greater impairment in concentration in those who reported stronger fear of pain (Crombez et al. 2005; Eccleston et al. 1997). As with adults, those children and adolescents with chronic pain who cite a heightened fear of pain show greater impairment (Martin et al. 2007; Simons et al. 2011; Turk and Wilson 2010). Martin et al. (2007) were able to verify that anxiety sensitivity constitutes a modulating variable. In the following pages we describe how it is possible that anxiety sensitivity, maladaptive interoception, and fear of pain influence each other.

Maladaptive Interoception

Maladaptive interoception is distinguished by definition from body image and body schema. Body image is defined as the conscious visual perception of the outward appearance of the body (Haggard and Wolpert 2005). Body schema refers to the perception of the representation of body parts in space (Haggard and Wolpert 2005). Maladaptive interoception is characterized by a distorted or one-sided perception of interoceptive stimulus. Gregory et al. (2000) showed using self-reports, in the Somatosensory Amplification Scale (SSAS) (Barsky et al. 1990), that, in comparison with healthy people, adult patients with head and stomach pain showed a greater maladaptive perception of body-specific processes. Scholz et al. (2001) investigated in an experimental study the question of whether people with a pain disorder perceive their muscle tension more precisely and intensively. In fact, affected people did perceive the stimulus more precisely, but not more intensively. Katzer and colleagues (2012) found a more sensitive perception with tactile stimuli in patients with a pain disorder. Witthöft et al. (2012) found that students showed that the stronger they were fixated on body symptoms, the stronger was their impressionability to aversive tactile stimuli. Unfortunately no studies exist at the moment on maladaptive interoception in children with pain disorders. The fact that children with chronic pain report heightened fear of pain in connection with anxiety sensitivity (Martin et al. 2007) and are more impaired allows us to simply presume that children with pain disorders also tend towards maladaptive interoception. Figure 6.2 summarizes the hypothetical relationship of the various factors with each other.

6.4.6.2 Studies on Interoceptive Exposure in Chronic Pain

As with fear disorders, the reduction of fear of pain is a central goal of therapy for people with chronic pain (Vlaeyen and Linton 2000; Bailey et al. 2010). There is

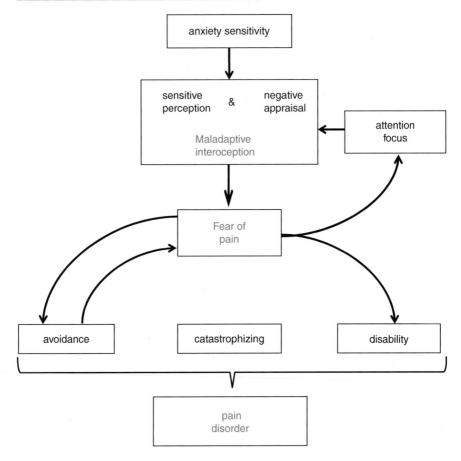

Fig. 6.2 Proposed model on pain-related fears and maladaptive interoception following the fear-avoidance model

growing evidence (De Peuter et al. 2011; Vlaeyen and Linton 2012) that interoceptive conditioning processes play an important role in the emergence of fear of pain. Thus, interoceptive exposure has recently been used in the treatment of the pain-specific fears of people with chronic pain (Wald et al. 2010; Watt et al. 2006; Flink et al. 2009; Craske et al. 2011). The checking of effect mechanisms in these interoceptive expositions in patients with chronic pain is however still to come. It is assumed that fear of pain can be reduced through interoceptive expositions of fear-related body-specific signals. The exact mechanism behind this change is however not clear. The studies on interoceptive exposure in patients with chronic pain so far have shown a reduction in maladaptive interoception (Craske et al. 2011), pain acceptance (Flink et al. 2009), and a reduction in fear components (Watt et al. 2006; Wald et al. 2010).

At the German Paediatric Pain Centre, children with a pain disorder learn a special variant of the interoceptive stimulus exposition ("pain provocation"). The pain provocation technique was introduced in detail in 2009 within the framework of a case report (Dobe et al. 2009). Its effectiveness was then checked within the framework of a case control study (Hechler et al. 2010 – see also Sect. 6.4.6.4). The course of the pain provocation technique will be described in the next chapter.

6.4.6.3 The Pain Provocation Technique (PPT)

The PPT was designed as a focused treatment strategy for adolescents severely affected by chronic pain. It integrates interoceptive exposure and implementation of pain-related coping to decrease pain intensity.

Prerequisites

Pain provocation cannot be started before the following four requirements are met:
1. The child is able to reduce the pain by 1 score on a numeric rating scale of 0–10 by means of a previously learned technique.
2. The child agrees upon a signal to interrupt the exercise if he can't increase or decrease the pain on his/her own. The child must be assured that he/she is in control and has the right to interrupt this technique at any time!
3. A way to proceed in case of interruption should be discussed in advance. In case the child cannot increase the pain, the standard arrangement is that the psychotherapist supports the child in focusing attention on his/her pain and memories by providing affective words (e.g., "Remember how awful your pain was when [insert situation]."). However, this is rarely the case and usually only observed in children who seldom suffer sever pain. A procedure to follow when the child is worrying about not being able to decrease the pain on his/her own should also be agreed upon in advance. In such a case, we recommend that the child and the psychotherapist practice one of the already learned distraction techniques together. Simultaneously, the psychotherapist should repeatedly – and in a humorous manner – reestablish the connection to reality using surrounding objects (e.g., the psychotherapist could ask: "How many objects starting with an 'A' do you see in this room?").
4. Before practicing pain provocation for the first time, the child should have expressed an opinion of how he/she would like the psychotherapist to behave during the exercise. For some children, especially traumatized children, it is important that the psychotherapist observes them closely in order to respond quickly. Other children prefer that the psychotherapist is involved with other things in the room or keeps his eyes closed and participates in an exercise on his own.

Practical Implementation

The child (mostly with his/her eyes closed) should focus on that part of his/her body currently or usually exhibiting the most pain. At the same time the child should evoke pain-related memories or Black Thoughts (e.g., any painful movements or thoughts of certain events to an increased distress level and thus severe pain, such as a quarrel, time pressure, or exam). In some children, concentrating on the pain is enough; for others just thinking certain Black Thoughts or evoking negative memories associated with pain is sufficient to provoke pain. Since the goal is to face the pain, it is not important by what means pain is enhanced. Having increased the pain by a score of 1 (NRS 1–10), the child should say aloud "STOP" (in order to give feedback to the psychotherapist, who cannot notice the increase in pain, and to make the child consciously recognize that he/she can control or stop his/her thoughts).

Directly afterwards, a trained pain coping strategy (e.g., distraction-ABC, or "Safe Place") is practiced until pain intensity has decreased by a score of 1. Then the child finishes the exercise saying aloud once more "STOP." In Chap. 9 we enclose written instructions for the introduction of pain provocation (Chap.9, Worksheet #18).

Further Procedure

Practicing the technique for the first time, the child usually does not need more than a few minutes for the exercise. Having finished, the child is asked how exactly he/she succeeded in increasing the pain intensity, if after calling "STOP" the pain ceased to increase, and how exactly he/she managed to finally reduce the pain intensity to where it was before the exercise.

The child is then asked to repeat the exercise in order to allow him/her to do an alternative procedure. Having done so, the child may decide on how often he/she will have to repeat the exercise until he/she feels able to do it as homework on his/her own (usually after practicing two to three times). We recommend practicing alone three to four times a day.

If the child has succeeded in the first step of pain provocation, the next step is to increase pain by a score of *two* and bring it down again. The following steps are to increase the pain by 2 scores and then minimize it by 3 scores (+2/−3) and +2/−4.

Successfully learning the method proves to the child that the biopsychosocial model used in the education sessions is not just theory but is indeed reality.

Contraindications

Pain provocation must not be used in children with a comorbid eating disorder, especially of the anorexia nervosa type, since their increased body awareness enables them to easily increase pain intensity, but hardly to decrease it later. Pain provocation is contraindicated in active/florid psychosis, since those patients' ability to organize and plan their actions is typically highly impaired. This will most probably also be the case with major depressive episodes.

Restricted Scope of Application

In children suffering dissociative symptoms or posttraumatic stress disorder, pain provocation should only be applied by an experienced psychotherapist familiar with these disorders.

The procedure is illustrated in the following example case (for a more detailed description, see Dobe et al. 2009).

Case Report: Malte (15 Years), Pain Disorder with Headache
Background
Malte had been suffering from chronic headaches for more than five years. Over the years, the headaches became more frequent. One year prior to admission, he suffered from continuing headaches of increasing intensity. Over the course of his pain experience, he underwent a number of outpatient and inpatient consultations without any beneficial effect. His helpless parents initiated numerous paediatric and psychological consultations and tried a variety of analgesics without any success. The diagnostic work-up consisted of two EEGs, one MRT, blood screenings, and neurological and rheumatological investigations. Taken together, there were no signs of an organic explanation for the continuing headaches. Half a year prior to admission, Malte stopped meeting with friends, refused to go to school, and spent most of the day lying in bed due to his pain. The parents had separated during the mother's pregnancy. The boy had rarely seen his father. The mother had been remarried for 8 years to a new partner who lived in the same household. The relationship between the boy and his stepfather was reported to be good. The loss of his grandmother who died from cancer two years ago was very disturbing for the boy. Inpatient therapy in the German Paediatric Pain Centre was recommended due to the boy's particular painful life circumstances. After some 6 sessions Malte was able to control his pain by means of two techniques ("Safe Place," 5-4-3-2-1 technique). Moreover, he was able to again take part in normal inpatient life under inpatient conditions. The prerequisites for learning pain provocation were therefore met. The following is an illustration of how Malte learned pain provocation.

At the first PPT session, the boy managed to increase and then decrease the pain by one point (on the NRS). He pointed out that focusing on the most aching body location together with thinking "Black" Thoughts (like "I am alone and nobody is interested in me!" or "Why has she died?") helped him to increase the pain level. Most helpful for him to reduce the pain to the starting level was the use of "Safe Place" in combination with a variant of the 5-4-3-2-1 technique. He pointed out that raising the pain level inevitably lead to thinking of his grandmother's funeral and of vivid memories at the time she was very ill (e.g., he always remembered lowering the coffin into the grave as the rain poured down, as well as the smell of the humid earth). The memories were accompanied by feelings of helplessness and fear as well as dizziness and nausea. In reducing the pain level, the symptoms disappeared. His homework was to practice this technique twice a day until the next meeting two days later. During the second session he increased and then decreased the pain by two points. The symptoms, memories, and feelings became even more prominent, but as during the first session, they disappeared when reaching the starting pain level. By the third session the next day, he had to again practice twice for homework. At the beginning of the third session Malte denied having experienced any difficulties exercising the technique. He then agreed to first increase the pain by two points and then to decrease it by three points. After accomplishing this he stated that he was somehow beginning to feel more lighthearted because his intrusive memories started to be less vivid. Again, he had to practice this technique twice a day for homework. At the beginning of the fourth session, he said that every time he successfully managed the technique, he felt more and more convinced that he had the ability to control his pain as well as to reduce his intrusive memories and feelings of helplessness. At the end of the fifth PPT session Malte was able to reduce the pain by 5 points (NRS). He pointed out that the distressing memories were starting to "go back in the past, where they belonged."

6.4.6.4 Effectiveness of the Pain Provocation Technique: Case Control Study

Our case control study aimed to investigate the effectiveness of the pain provocation technique (PPT) where adolescents utilizing PPT were compared to a group of adolescents matched for age, gender, and diagnosis, both groups receiving standard multimodal inpatient treatment. Primary endpoints were pain intensity, pain-related disability, and emotional distress. In line with previous studies into the effectiveness of graded exposure in adults, it was hypothesized that adolescents obtaining additional PPT would demonstrate a greater decrease in pain intensity, disability, and emotional distress.

Cases and Controls

Forty-four adolescents consecutively admitted to standard multimodal inpatient treatment between July and December 2006 were asked at admission to participate in the adjunctive PPT treatment (cases). Four participants declined to participate after commencement of the PPT, resulting in a sample size of 40 adolescents. Forty control subjects treated on the ward between January 2004 and June 2006 were selected according to matching criteria, i.e., age, gender, and leading pain diagnosis, by a random 1:1 match (1 case to 1 control) and formed the control group.

Results

Forty controls matched for age, gender, and diagnosis underwent standard multimodal inpatient treatment. At 3-month follow-up, data was obtained from 39 adolescents in the PPT group and 38 adolescents in standard treatment (the dropout rate was 2.5 and 5 % for the cases and controls, respectively).

Treatment Effects

Changes in pain intensity. Based on the results of the ANOVA, pain intensity decreased differently in the two groups from admission to 3-month follow-up. Specifically, patients in the PPT showed a more pronounced decrease in pain intensity 3 months after inpatient treatment compared to those in standard treatment ($F_{(1,75)} = 6.52, p = .013$).

Changes in pain-related disability (P-PDI) and school absence. These decreased significantly and similarly in both groups.

Changes in emotional distress (AFS, DIKJ). Only *school aversion*, i.e., a negative attitude towards issues related to school, decreased differently in the two groups from admission to 3-month follow-up, with patients in the PPT group demonstrating a more pronounced decrease in school aversion compared to those in standard treatment (significant interaction between time point and group: $F_{(1,57)} = 4.13, p = .047$).

Discussion

The findings of this study are in line with previous studies implementing interoceptive exposure in healthy participants and adult pain samples (see Sect. 6.4.6.2). Clearly, the therapeutic methods underlying the PPT and the contribution of each component need to be investigated in future studies (see Hechler et al. 2010 for a more detailed account of the study as well as the backgrounds).

6.4.7 Active Pain Coping

"It is impossible to get up. My pain is so bad, I can't bear it any longer." – Philipp (13 years)

We've already reported on the necessity of active pain coping irrespective of pain intensity. We discussed in depth how to best educate children about the background of chronic pain in order to make them motivated and cooperative and which strategies they should use to reduce their pain.

Regarding active coping, the NET plays a crucial role in developing the child's ability to return to the old daily routine and to implement active pain coping strategies. This means that after the first night on the ward, which may not be so refreshing for many patients, the NET will prompt the child in a polite, insightful, but insistent way to get up out of bed irrespective of his/her severe pain. The child's comments regarding the pain should be taken seriously but left uncommented upon. Especially children with pronounced passive pain coping and high school absence will have difficulties implementing active pain coping into their "normal" everyday life in the beginning of inpatient pain therapy. The NET may refer to the rules of the ward or the upcoming appointment with the psychotherapist or physician instead.

"Sure you suffer severe pain. Otherwise you wouldn't be here. But, staying in bed didn't help at home. And as you know from your outpatient appointment and the admission talk we are not allowed to make any exceptions to the ward rule. But I can offer to write a short note to your physician or psychotherapist telling him how difficult it is for you to get up, okay?"

The same applies to all prescheduled activities on the ward (meals, group meetings) as well as to the activities arranged by the child himself/herself. Regarding sports, the motto is to "participate at one's best." This hard-line attitude has proven effective. With the help of the NET, most children will successfully join the ward's daily routine even after months of passivity in everyday life at home. As pointed out, the NET will collect all sorts of complaints and behavioral observations and – mostly giving feedback to the child – hand them over to the responsible psychotherapist or physician. This close cooperation between NET, physician, and psychotherapist enables most of the children to actively cope with their pain from the very beginning and is essential for successful treatment.

To facilitate the NET's work, one should bear in mind the following aspects:

1. During the outpatient appointment in the pain clinic, before admission, the child and his/her family are informed of the importance of active pain coping, a normal everyday life, and the child's obligation to do his/her therapeutic homework. The child and his/her parents are told plainly that especially the first few days of inpatient therapy will be quite burdensome. If it then turns out that such an approach seems too rigorous for the child or his/her parents, it might be helpful to discuss their alternatives (which in most cases will be a variant of "Before my child can do that, the pain must decrease." In those cases it may be helpful to meet the family halfway (for an example, see Sect. 6.5.3)). However, the principles of active pain coping should never be given up. Only in the minority of patients do the demands of therapy seem too high for the family, and they will agree on admission but not under the premises of normal everyday life on the ward. In such cases it is better to abstain from admission and invite the family to contact the clinic when they are more open to the clinic's approach. After having successfully completed their pain therapy, many children report that it was precisely that rigid attitude of the NET and the therapeutic team that gave them security and hope.

2. If during the stay on the ward active pain coping is refused by the child, the parents should be informed and instructed how to support their child in developing active coping to manage everyday life. If the parents are not able to motivate their child, it is time to stop the inpatient pain therapy, since continuing would result in permanent frustration on the part of both the patient and the NET.

3. The close cooperation between the NET, physician, and psychotherapist on the ward is one of the prerequisites for successful support of the child in active pain coping. Each NET is able to support up to 8 children in coping with the demands of everyday life on the ward, provided that all participants cooperate closely (and the child recognizes this, i.e., he/she knows that the psychotherapist and physician are always well informed about the NET's behavioral observations), all patients are treated equally (suffering the same burden with their active pain coping), and there are no alternatives to active pain coping.

4. The NET should regularly update their knowledge on the treatment of chronic pain.

6.5 Inpatient Pain Therapy: Module 3 (Supplementary Interventions in Comorbid Symptomatology)

"Whenever I feel severe pain I automatically have to think of what "he" has done to me." – Lena (15 years)

Facing frequent mental comorbidity in patients with a pain disorder, it often becomes necessary to adapt the pain therapy program to the patients' needs to also be successful with children suffering comorbid anxiety disorders, depressive episodes, or adjustment disorders with depressive reactions, a limited ability to cope, lack of internal structure, or social fears.

6.5.1 Limited Stress Tolerance: The Stress Day

"How can you do this to me? You are doing it on purpose." – Melissa (16 years), during her Stress Day, focusing on conflict solving strategies

Arranging Stress Days is a huge challenge and takes a lot of time. However, passing the day successfully usually gives the child a great sense of achievement with the potential to change his/her chronic and dysfunctional behavioral patterns. The Stress Day described in Sect. 6.4.5.3 has to be modified if a comorbid mental disorder is present.

1. If the patient suffers from pronounced exhaustion combined with little ability to cope with stress (e.g., due to adjustment disorder with depressive reaction or mild depressive episode), the Stress Day may be shortened to some hours or half a day. The child will experience success and will be led by the NET to normal distress coping without the risk of symptom escalation (gradual exposure).

2. In case of substantial social insecurity or even social phobia, it has proven successful to integrate some smaller exposure exercises into the Stress Day, using whatever social abilities the patient has, e.g., making a phone call to a telephone hotline, setting up a travel plan with public transit, talking to a stranger (e.g., a salesclerk in a bakery), and holding a lecture for a small group of people.

3. Analogous to the approach used for social fears, there could also be a therapeutic focus on other specific fears or phobias present during the Stress Day.

4. The situation is different if the child tends to react impulsively and aggressively when feeling treated poorly or unfairly. These children will experience very intense distress, muscular tension, aggression, together with pain. For these children the Stress Day is a particular challenge. If he/she declares himself/herself ready to undertake a Stress Day under these circumstances, it should be made quite clear to him/her that he/she can take some time out at any time in order not to be overtaxed. Some of these children believe that a Stress Day constitutes a punishment. For this reason it can be worthwhile to explore this aspect during the education sessions in order to be able to clear this up, if necessary. In no event should a Stress Day for these children be arranged if there is a negative attitude towards the child among the team. A Stress Day during which the NET pushes the child in a harsh manner to do his/her tasks is an enormous challenge to that

child. Psychotherapists and the other team members should be aware that such a Stress Day, if not well prepared, carries the risk of substantial escalation. As a preventive measure, all children on the ward should be informed that it was the child that explicitly asked for an unfriendly version of the Stress Day. The affected child should·be able to stop the harsh treatment anytime and switch to a "normal" Stress Day's mode or to stop the Stress Day at all. The NET should repeatedly make that clear to the patient! On the other hand, if the NET has the impression that the child feels offended, they may interrupt the Stress Day for a brief discussion with the patient to reflect upon and discuss the situation.

5. A variant suited to children who previously experienced bullying or substantial disappointment regarding their social relationships is to confront the child with tasks and scenarios in which he/she has to do something for the staff of the NET or other children. Those variants of the Stress Day should also be fully discussed in advance with the child and everyone on the ward, to make the patient see the Stress Day as a chance for some changes in dysfunctional patterns and not to increase distrust towards a presumably hostile world.

6.5.2 Trauma Therapeutic Interventions and Methods for Stabilization

"It's over now." – Moritz (14 years), after having finished a trauma exposure

Not every stressful life event is a critical life event, and not every critical life event is equivalent to a traumatic experience for the patient. But it was only recently recognized that the term "traumatization" clearly defined in adults cannot readily be transferred to children or adolescents (e.g., Van der Kolk and Courtois 2005). In the child, both the current developmental age and the developmental age at the time of the stressful event are important factors for the understanding of the child's processing of a stressful, emotional experience. Children may experience a situation as traumatic which may not be so for an adult. The foreseeable loss of a grandmother after a long and severe disease may become a traumatic experience to the child if circumstances are unfavorable, for instance, if the grandmother was the only close attachment figure. The same may be the case when a family court judge asks a 10-year-old boy in the absence of his parents for his opinion on his parents' extreme conflicts and with which parent he would like to live in the future. Depending on how severe the parents' custody conflict is and what incidents have happened between the parents so far, such a questioning may be experienced by the child as a threat to his existence and (re)trigger traumatization.

A significant proportion of children with a pain disorder suffer from very stressful memories (visual, auditory, or kinesthetic). These memories may have their origin in surgery, an accident, a death, the sudden, severe mental disorder or physical illness of a beloved attachment figure, the experience of domestic violence, ambiguous parental behavior crossing the boundaries of personal space (i.e., the father standing up menacingly in front of his child, making him/her fear physical violence although there will be none), sexual abuse, alcohol excesses of a parent, bullying, or a conflict-loaded parental separation.

Especially if therapy-resistant chronic pain is caused by sports or traffic accidents, processing patterns that are in at least one aspect suggestive of traumatization play an important role. Some of these patterns are hypervigilance combined with high muscular tension, substantial problems with concentrating, and pronounced avoidance behavior. It is well-known that even the experience or witnessing of domestic violence (not necessarily as the victim) is predictive for the development of chronic abdominal pain (Sansone et al. 2006). In another study by Seng et al. (2005) on children aged 9–17 years, posttraumatic stress disorder (PTSD) was a risk factor for the development of chronic abdominal pain (odds ratios: simple PTSD = 4.5; complex PTSD = 14.9). Young Casey et al. (2008) showed that past traumatization had a significant impact on the development of acute backache to chronic pain. Depending on premorbid anxiety sensitivity, traumatic life events and chronic pain seem to mutually perpetuate and amplify each other (Asmundson et al. 2002; Liedl et al. 2011). This perpetuation is likely to be mediated by interoceptive conditioning (please see Sect. 6.4.6 for a detailed definition and description). Thus, simultaneous treatment of traumatic symptoms and chronic pain seems to make sense (Asmundson et al. 2002; Wald et al. 2010; Liedl et al. 2011).

Only some affected children strictly fulfill the diagnostic criteria of the common diagnostic manuals for PTSD. Far more patients suffer severely from their past experiences and their aftermath. Often these experiences continue to occur in the context of existing conflict-loaded family situations. While they do not fulfill the strict criteria of PTSD, they may meet the criteria of an adjustment disorder or the reaction to an unspecified trauma.

According to our experience it is best that all concurrently present pain and trauma disorders be addressed at the same time. This is true irrespective of the possible existence of any causal connection (i.e., accident) between the two disorders. In the education sessions, it is important to point out how much stressful or traumatic life events are associated with pain perception and that they mutually perpetuate and amplify each other. The following examples illustrate what this means in everyday life:

1. Justin (17 years, pain disorder, backache) developed chronic backache after a severe swimming accident causing incomplete spinal paralysis and dependency on a wheelchair and, eventually, very painful surgery. Remembering the surgery increased his pain perception by a score of 2 within seconds, with concomitant pronounced vegetative symptoms and difficulties in concentrating.
2. Judith (16 years, CRPS type I, left foot) told us that whenever she stressed her left foot to pain for some time, she became very exhausted, then suddenly very sad and hopeless, which triggered intrusive memories of a traumatic sexual assault that happened 3 years before. When she entered pain therapy, Judith had never told anybody about this sexual abuse due to her fear of the offender.
3. Mohamed (14 years, pain disorder, headache) reported that since being involved in a severe traffic accident 2 years ago (the perpetrator of the accident had died at the scene), he suffered severe chronic pain. Certain traffic scenes make his severe headache worse, while pain peaks also trigger memories of the traffic accident.

4. Whenever Patricia (14 years, pain disorder) had backache (for instance, after physical exercise), she suffered stressful memories from her childhood, which was dominated by family violence. In one of her memories her drunken father throws her so violently against the wall that her whole back hurts afterwards.

Pain therapy for these children is made more difficult by the fact that passive pain coping has so far been a solution to coping with stressful memories. Giving up on this passive pain coping means incurring an increased risk of stressful memories.

Many techniques presented in Sects. 6.4.2 and 6.4.3, especially the imaginative, distraction, and mindfulness techniques, are in principle suited to reducing the emotional burden caused by traumatic memories. More trauma-specific stabilizing techniques are the "Safe" exercise and distancing techniques like screening techniques. When planning treatment one should never forget that the prerequisite of successful pain therapy is a sufficient capacity for emotional stabilizing and inner distancing. Techniques for trauma-specific stabilization are described in the following paragraphs.

Trauma exposure or processing stressful life events are not necessary prerequisites for a successful start to pain therapy (although both are indicated in the subsequent outpatient psychotherapy). Our approach will take the mental and emotional pressures off children for whom trauma exposure is contraindicated in the foreseeable future (e.g., if there are insufficient safety measures present in everyday life or if contact with an offender cannot be avoided at the moment).

The responsible installation of stabilizing techniques helpful to the child requires special training and experience in trauma therapy. If the initial stabilization and the safety of the patient after inpatient therapy is guaranteed, pain therapy can be successful; it may contribute to further reducing the emotional burden and impairment of everyday life. However, only the successful treatment of the trauma disorder in the subsequent course of treatment will prevent reactivation of pain symptoms. The reason is that untreated trauma disorders result in severe muscular tension due to the concomitantly disturbed regulation of emotions and stress. Often the power of concentration is impaired, as is sleep behavior. Altogether, those symptoms bear the risk of reactivating the pain disorder.

We confine this discussion to a short description of two stabilizing techniques that are usually taught in trauma therapy training:

1. The "Safe" *exercise* will teach the child to lock stressful or traumatic memories into an imagined vault (alternatively: locked room, cabinet, locker, strongbox, secured location, …) in order to be less burdened by those intrusive memories in everyday life. A naturally given dissociative ability (e.g., the ability to "lock" thoughts, emotions, or memories) is used as a resource (for survival) and not regarded as problematic behavior. There should be enough time to experience the imaginative process in developing the "Safe," i.e., more than one therapeutic session. The child's spontaneous ideas should be allowed even if this will change the "Safe" several times. With gradually increasing stressful memories, the child may test step by step if the technique works. The more sensory channels (i.e., visual, auditory, haptic) are involved, the more precise the various steps that are practiced (locking, reopening, taking out or putting back the memory), and the earlier the child creates an icon of the vault (e.g., painting, collage, photograph), the better he/she will be able to perform that exercise.

2. The imaginative distancing techniques (also named "screening" techniques) follow a different approach. Their best known variant is the "screen" *technique*. With this technique, the emotional burden, due to intrusions, is blunted by having the child transfer his/her stressful pictures or movies onto a TV screen (big screen, monitor, DVD player, smartphone, etc.) installed in an imaginary room and view these intrusions from a distance. With the help of an imaginary remote control (alternatively: helper, magic abilities, …), the child may try to modify speed, play mode (forward, backward, fast forward, …), color mode (black and white, color), or tone (loud/quiet, distorted, etc.). The movie may be switched on or off; the child may insert breaks or create still pictures showing the more stressful situations. There is no limit to creativity (e.g., press the "comic" button and all voices change to Donald Duck character). As with the "Safe" exercise, stepwise installation is recommended, starting with the less stressful "films" or "movies" and using the maximal possible number of sensory channels. In complex traumatized children it has proved helpful to instruct them to use the various buttons of the remote control so that they can keep their emotional burden in a median range. In that context, avoiding extremely stressful memories is interpreted as a sign of active self-defense which helps the child to control his/her hyperarousal (constructive avoiding).

Apart from training the child in stabilization techniques, the psychotherapist should explore if the child has any dysfunctional cognitions associated with the trauma (this is true in nearly all cases), such as "It's my fault," "I could/should have prevented it," or "It happened to me because I deserved it. And that is why dreadful things will befall me again and again." These cognitions ("trauma logic") must be addressed in therapy since their concomitant inner tension helps perpetuate trauma and pain symptomatology.

In addition to the standard pain education, we recommend using disorder-specific manuals for trauma education. By means of this education, the child and the parents will learn that generating dysfunctional cognitions is by no means something the child is to blame for, but quite a normal process.

Once the child is stabilized and the family setting provides enough support and safety, it may be adequate to schedule a trauma exposure concurrently with inpatient pain therapy. In addition to classical trauma exposure (e.g., cognitive trauma therapy, narrative exposure, or EMDR), pain provocation may be used for interoceptive stimulus exposure (Sect. 6.4.6) in case of close interoceptive conditioning of trauma and pain stimuli.

Case Report: Miriam (15 Years), CRPS Type I, Left Foot, and PTSD

"Half a year before admission to pain therapy, Miriam had a severe traffic accident in which she and her family came close to death. Every day she recalled the cries, the smell of scorched cables, and some scenes from the hospital. Whenever she saw or heard an ambulance, she experienced a very stressful inner tension. Sitting in a car had become a highly emotional burden for her, so she tried to avoid doing so. Her severe pain due to CRPS resulted in pronounced helplessness and increased her inner tension which itself triggered her bad memories. Experiencing such helplessness frequently reminded Miriam of a stressful event in her childhood (sexual abuse by a stranger). With the help of the "Safe" exercise and mindfulness exercises she was able to be well stabilized. At the same time she practiced active pain coping and followed a stepped plan to treat CRPS, and had a total of 3 trauma exposures (EMDR). This combination resulted in a very successful work-up of the accident. At the end of her stay she was able to sit in a car again, which made her so happy and motivated that she decided to start outpatient psychotherapy, with the focus on trauma therapy, in order to work on the sexual abuse."

Pain provocation is a technique with lower emotional burden (see Sect. 6.4.6 and Chap. 9, Worksheet #18). Children with stressful memories are instructed to focus on both the pain location and the stressful memory. The aim is to enhance self-efficacy and active coping by first increasing and then decreasing both pain intensity and emotional burden (Dobe et al. 2009). The interrelationship between the perception of physical (pain) stimuli and the memory of stressful events may be reduced by this interoceptive stimulus exposure. This type of pain provocation can only be done if the child is both sufficiently stabilized (perhaps with the help of the "Safe Place" or the "Safe"). Thus, the child experiences self-efficacy even if therapeutic trauma exposure is not yet indicated and will have the positive experience of having control over the degree of the emotional load.

After performing pain provocation, children are often surprised at the close relationship between stressful memories and pain stimuli (interoceptive conditioning). This realization again supports the soundness of the education program and makes the patients cooperate with even more motivation. Pain provocation cannot replace trauma therapy in complex traumatized children. It is an additional technique to stabilize the child and can be a good preparation for subsequent trauma-specific therapy.

6.5.3 Passivity and Avoidance: Setting Up a Daily Routine

For various reasons, everyday life for many of the children with chronic pain is characterized by passivity and avoidance. Successful pain therapy is always based on active pain coping in everyday life. A prerequisite of active pain coping is that the child knows what he/she can do. This is by no means trivial, e.g., if the child only has a few friends due to low social competence, hasn't undertaken much for a long period of time, is afflicted by sad or fearful thoughts, and doesn't leave the room due to a dysphoric-petulant atmosphere within the family. Some of these children find it difficult to name any activity they like. They will benefit from making a "list of positive activities" (Chap. 9, Worksheet #15). Other children, however, are that overburdened by organizing their daily routine that even with a structured inpatient life on the ward, they need the strong support of the NET. What does support by the NET look like?

Every morning, the child is handed a piece of paper outlining the schedule of the day. Invariable common activities like the five meals, morning and evening rounds, "beef round," as well as the visiting hour or the rest period in the evening are not listed, but the daily scheduled duties on the ward are included on the sheet. It is the child's responsibility to stick to the schedule exactly. If there are any problems in keeping the schedule, the child is to inform the responsible physician or psychotherapist. If during the course of treatment it becomes obvious that the child has severe problems organizing his/her everyday life, he/she will be told to make a schedule including all variable and invariable appointments. In addition, any active pain coping strategies that could be practiced during the breaks should be noted on the schedule (Chap. 9, Worksheet #15).

In pain therapy one should not tolerate inadequate organization of everyday life. Active pain coping is supported by encouraging the child to strive for autonomy (learn to follow a daily routine) and to take responsibility (organization of the duties on the ward, e.g., organize leisure time activities or common cooking sessions). A good "side effect" is the enhancement of the child's self-esteem; the child will recognize that by working in a structured way, he/she is able to get many more tasks done than expected. The following case report illustrates the implementation of active organization of everyday life as part of inpatient pain therapy.

Case Report: Jana (16 Years), Pain Disorder with Multiple Pain Localizations
After a painful school accident and severe adverse effects of analgesic treatment, Jana increasingly developed pain in all main joints, as well as backache. This started about 4 years before admission to our ward. At times Jana complained about headache, too. After two years her pain had become so severe that she was using a wheelchair for more than a year and was unable to attend school. Due to physiotherapy, she has been able to walk with crutches now for about one year and she is attending a school for the physically handicapped.

Due to her permanent fatigue, Jana usually attends classes while lying down. Several stays in a paediatric rheumatology clinic, invasive pain therapeutic procedures, and the use of various analgesics were so far unsuccessful. Previous therapeutic attempts advocated the application of passive pain coping strategies, and Jana and her family followed the recommendations. Before she fell ill, Jana had been a happy girl. When she was a child she liked to do some sports. She presented at our paediatric outpatient pain clinic following the advice of her paediatrician. At their first outpatient appointment, the ambivalence of Jana and her family towards the demands of an inpatient stay explicitly demanding active pain coping irrespective of the current pain intensity or emotional well-being became evident. During the talk we came to the agreement that Jana should write down her aims for her inpatient stay and declare that she would consent to our therapeutic approach before we would decide on her admittance. Her parents were asked to give their written consent for cooperation. In consideration of Jana's extraordinary impairment, it seemed impossible to us to start with an age-appropriate activity plan from the beginning. Thus, we agreed on gradually increasing activity in her everyday life on the ward. Shortly after Jana and her parents had put our demands into practice, Jana was admitted, walking with crutches and using wrist ortheses. The admission talk was used to explain the treatment plan to Jana and her parents. During that talk it became even more obvious that Jana suffered from comorbid depression and social phobia.

Our Procedure. We agreed jointly on a binding stepped plan. The number of breaks (in which Jana could also lie down) was gradually reduced. Those breaks were operationalized using time-out cards with a value of 30 min each. In consideration of her previously very low activity level (just a few hours a day), we agreed on a total of 6 time-outs of 30 min each during the first step of the treatment plan. Jana was allowed to use these whenever she wanted. Jana had to set up a daily schedule and pick some activities from her "list of positive activities" to practice in her leisure time. In the course of treatment, Jana gradually became more active (attending the clinic's school, participating in sports or pedagogic spare time activities), but at the end of her stay, she still needed three time-out cards a day. Contrary to her fears, active pain coping didn't increase her pain. Though she was frequently fatigued, this helped her fall asleep more easily, and sometimes she woke up in the morning feeling more refreshed than usual. In the course of treatment, the time Jana was allowed to use her crutches was curtailed until she finally only needed the crutches when performing longer activities outside of the ward. Due to her depressive symptoms, Jana needed a lot of encouragement and support from the NET, which she got in the daily evening reflections and by being complimented for every success, small though it might have been.

6.5.4 Anxiety Disorders and Gradual Exposure (Stepped Plans)

"I'll never do it" – Anna (14 years), while planning the last, most difficult step, anxiety hierarchy, with her psychotherapist

Some children don't just suffer a pain disorder but also fears. In some of the children, the fears preceded the pain disease and enhanced the pain chronicity, while other children developed their fears during the course of their pain chronicity. In any case, at the time of first therapeutic contact, the child will present with both a pain and an anxiety disorder that perpetuate and amplify each other. We strongly recommend treating these disorders simultaneously.

6.5.4.1 Integration of the NET

In an *inpatient* pain therapy setting, the close integration of the NET into therapy planning is essential.

How is the therapy of pain and fear best combined in an inpatient setting, integrating the NET in a way that won't confuse or overburden the child?

At the beginning of therapy, there should be an in-depth education session on pain, fears, and their interrelationship. Since both pain and fears tend to become independent, the education on fear is easily combined with that on the vicious cycle of pain. Not only in pain but also with anxiety and fears, important factors are increased body awareness, negative cognitions, and increased muscular tension interpreted as a warning signal. During the education on the vicious cycle of pain (Sect. 6.3.2), the child will learn how pain and fears perpetuate and amplify each other via Black Thoughts, increased body awareness, and muscular tension.

Independent of the type and degree of the fears, these three interventions have proved useful:

1. Most children with fear exhibit low self-confidence and don't take risks. They need encouragement and a sense of achievement to believe in themselves and to face their fears. The *note box* (Sect. 6.5.5) allows this to happen in a structured way. Simply, take a card box with a slot that fits folded notes. The child may make his/her own box, and with some effort some children will create real works of art. The note box is stored in the room of the person in charge within the NET. Each time one of the NET, the physician, or the psychotherapist observes something positive about the child or his/her behavior on the ward (it may also be positive characteristics, a special outer appearance, or a nice habit), they write a note, fold it, and put it into the box. During a daily evening ritual, the box is emptied and the child may read the various notes – alone or, if therapeutically advisable, together with a staff member. At first, most children are very skeptical about this intervention ("You write this only because you are instructed to do so."), but during the course of treatment, they will realize that the notes of different people are often congruent, and they begin to accept them as meaningful and honest. The snippets should be worked within the therapeutic sessions. Children aged 14 years and up often regard a note box as childish. The following intervention might suit them better.

2. Some patients (mostly the older children or adolescents) prefer direct and personal feedback to an anonymous one. To strive for the opportunity to give compliments and express appreciation towards a person is an interaction strategy for this age. The evening reflection only with the child and one member of the NET is a structured form of direct verbal feedback. As with the note box, the various observations and judgments are collected and expressed verbally. The patient is invited to just listen to the feedback and not react to it immediately. In this setting any discussion on how truthful the comments are won't help, and the NET should react to any discussion with a "But that's just the view of him/her" or "Just leave it. He/she just likes that characteristic of you." These interventions may well be continued in an outpatient setting, perhaps by the patient's parents.

3. Biofeedback therapy is an essential module when simultaneously treating pain and anxiety disorders (Sect. 6.4.4). This is also conducted by the NET. As with pain therapy, it is an important experience for the child with an anxiety disorder to understand how his/her body is reacting to fears and how these physical processes may be modified by learned techniques. We use biofeedback therapy before (e.g., when starting a stepped plan) or during (e.g., during a Stress Day) exposure in order to help the patients learn to positively influence their tension and anxiety. Most of the patients are fascinated by the technique, since apart from validating their education (they experience how certain thoughts, memories, or appraisals directly provoke somatic reactions), they find the hope to better control their stressful somatic symptoms on their own.

6.5.4.2 Approaching the Pain Disorder Combined with Specific Fears

If the fears relate to real situations that can be operationalized, it is helpful to use gradual treatment plans. These are practiced together with the responsible caretaker of the NET. First, the child sets up a list of situations with gradually increasing fear together with the psychotherapist (graduated scheme). The list should only include situations that can be managed frequently enough during the stay on the ward or during the Stress Tests. If a situation does not occur during the stay on the ward or during Stress Tests (i.e., fear of class test, fear of a certain person, fear of a certain situation at school or in a club, fear related to a specific family situation), it can be modified in such a way that it triggers a similar anxiety reaction. The following example illustrates our approach using a graduated scheme.

Case Report: Joris (13 Years), Chronic Abdominal Pain and Social Insecurity

Background. On admission, the parents report that Joris is very shy and that he would "take his time to feel comfortable." During his stay on the ward, it quickly became obvious that Joris was not just shy but also suffering distinctive fears (and increased abdominal pain) facing these new social challenges. After being given a comprehensive explanation, he came to understand the relationship between and the mutual amplification of fear and pain. The findings and the diagnostic results were discussed with his parents.

Procedure on the Ward. In the first family talk we presented the procedure indicated to therapeutically treat anxiety (inpatient: graduated scheme, alteration of the dysfunctional fear-perpetuating assumptions, increasing self-esteem; outpatient: psychotherapy presumably necessary) but also outlined the adverse effects of a successful therapy of the anxiety disorder (increased need for autonomy, increased readiness for discussion. For a detailed discussion of this intervention, see Sect. 6.6.4. During the family talk, Joris' parents agreed to the anxiety treatment and accepted the risk of possible adverse effects. Apart from the change of his dysfunctional thoughts (Sect. 6.4.3), Joris, the NET, and his psychotherapist developed the following graduated scheme together:

Step 1: To ask a nurse to hand Joris a sheet of paper.

...

Step 4: To ask a nurse to help him with a certain task.

...

Step 6: To introduce a newly admitted child to his duties on the ward and make himself available as mentor in case of any questions.

...

Step 8: To ask all children aged > 10 years what they like and what they dislike in him and record the answers.

...

Step 10: To present a poster created by him ("That's me" poster) giving all important information on him, his leisure time activities, his strengths, and his weak points and to answer any upcoming questions (total duration, 10 minutes).

At the same time, Joris constructed his "note box" (see Sect. 6.5.4.1). Furthermore, the agreement was that before and after any particularly difficult situation on the ward, the NET will reflect the situation together with Joris and elaborate on suggestions as to how to behave more favorably. With three biofeedback sessions per week, Joris got the opportunity to find the best cognitive or imaginative strategy for the reduction of his anxiety-triggered physical reactions.

The Family's Approach. According to our experience, fears rarely develop without a family model. Joris' family was no different in that regard. During his childhood, his mother had suffered considerable social anxiety. Although his father denied any fears, he denoted himself a "careful person." The parents had the notion that sometimes the environment is dangerous ("You never know what will happen.") and somehow unjust ("Those using their elbows will succeed. All others will have to stand back."). During conflicts they use avoidance strategies (from avoiding any dispute up to using excuses to allow for social withdrawal). They didn't believe that their son could solve any conflict or problem on his own and tried to help him whenever possible. The upbringing of their son was characterized by allowance and missing clear-cut consequences. During the family talks, we had detailed discussions on the anxiety-focused treatment of their son and any advantages or disadvantages of their son's behavior. Finally, the parents agreed not to relieve their son of his commitments, to set up clear rules, and make demands of their son irrespective of his current intensity of pain or anxiety. Furthermore, they were open to doing outpatient psychotherapy in which they would aim to change their own behavior.

Course of Treatment. A couple of months later, Joris' psychotherapist informed us that continuing psychotherapy was no longer necessary. Due to the consistent cooperation of his parents during inpatient therapy, Joris was now much more stable and reported much less anxiety and pain. Both Joris and his parents gradually changed their lives. Twelve months later, Joris had changed, living normally with no pain or abnormal fears. After 24 months, we were informed that Joris planned to go abroad for 1 year.

6.5.4.3 Approaching a Pain Disorder Combined with Panic Attacks

Every now and then, we treat patients with pain disorders and recurrent panic attacks. A panic disorder has a strong negative impact on daily life and quality of life, making normal pain therapy difficult. In children with a panic disorder, one should carefully explore a potential traumatic background. The following approach is suitable in children with a combined pain and panic disorder in whom the panic disorder is less severe, a traumatic background is improbable, and a subsequent outpatient psychotherapeutic treatment is warranted.

The treatment starts with a detailed education on both disorders. Regarding its genesis and maintenance, panic disorder resembles pain disorder more than all other reported comorbidities. Like a pain disorder, panic disorders arise from the spiral of interoceptive perception, its dysfunctional appraisal, and the resulting physiological processes. Unlike pain disorders, the dysfunctional appraisals in panic disorder are of a more existential quality ("I am dying."), resulting in more pronounced fear and physiological processes. Due to the similarities, it is possible to directly transfer some aspects of pain therapy to the treatment of panic disorders. As in the treatment of pain disorders, body-related dysfunctional thoughts are of importance, and often there is a biographical reference that makes the children believe that body signals indicate a life-threatening or even deadly disease (e.g., the father's or the beloved grandmother's heart attack). The dysfunctional thoughts may well be treated together with the dysfunctional thoughts related to pain (Sect. 6.4.3).

Techniques for interoceptive stimulus exposure are successfully used in the treatment of panic disorders. The interoceptive exposure for patients with panic disorders is not very distinct from that for patients with pain disorders (De Peuter et al. 2011). The patients confront themselves with arousal-reactive stimuli that are part of the fear reaction (as in, e.g., perception of the heartbeat). Interoceptive stimuli that do not necessarily increase with fear (as in, for instance, pain or interoceptive sensation with movement) can also play a role. Pain provocation is a variant of interoceptive stimulus exposure (see Sect. 6.4.6). As a first step, these children learn the strategies presented in Sect. 6.4. Next, those with a panic disorder can learn how to reduce their anxiously increased body awareness if they focus on fear-associated signals, instead of concentrating on pain-related bodily sensations. The fear-associated signals can be triggered by intentional hyperventilation or increased body awareness (e.g., focusing on the heartbeat). Some very brave adolescents concentrate simultaneously on their pain and on bodily processes which are connected with the perception of fear. The procedure is otherwise exactly the same as with pain provocation. The fear is then brought back down to the starting point with the help of the techniques described in Sects. 6.4.2 or 6.4.4 or with certain breathing exercises (i.e., intentionally extending expiration in order to interrupt hyperventilation. See also Kuttner 2010).

6.5.4.4 Approaching a Pain Disorder Combined with a Generalized Anxiety Disorder

Children with generalized fears and anxieties benefit the most from a combination of cognitive methods and techniques of fear exposure. Presumably, generalized fears and anxieties are especially perpetuated by mental avoidance techniques. Methods to interrupt or avoid dysfunctional thoughts should be avoided. As a sort of behavioral experiment to verify certain fearful thoughts, it may be helpful to install a graduated scheme focusing on only one of the child's many specific fears. Installation of that scheme can be realized as described for specific fears (see above). The child should be instructed and reinforced by the psychotherapist as well as by the NET to also face other specific scenarios he/she is afraid of during therapy sessions and on the ward.

To this end, observation sheets set up by the child and the NET proved helpful to check and discuss fears concerning the management of common situations on the ward. In addition, a "stamp booklet" can be given to the child, in which he/she collects stamps each time he/she successfully copes with a fear. With those stamps, the child may later "buy" a reward either on the ward or one stipulated by his parents.

6.5.4.5 Integrating the Family System

In order to sustain the reduction in their child's anxiety, the parents must be comprehensively informed about the anxiety disorder early in the course of treatment, as well as the graduated schemes to be integrated into everyday domestic life. In many cases, the parents involuntarily contribute to their child's symptomatology due to their own fears, anxiety disorders, or family burden (i.e., conflict-ridden separation of the parents), for instance, by acting for the child in setting up appointments for him/her and thus helping him/her to avoid a challenging task. If this type of anxiety-perpetuating parental behavior is not stopped, it is extremely difficult for the child to control and reduce his/her fears and the pain. If parents, however, have learned during the education session the necessity of strengthening their child and discovered their own resources, they become invaluable co-therapists, supporting their child in the implementation of graduated schemes or in his courageous behavior in everyday life. Thus, more than one of the involved will benefit from the therapeutic process: the child experiences success in his/her more or less voluntarily handling fears and no longer perceiving his/her parents as helpless but as strong instead, and the parents experience themselves as strong and powerful and able to expect something from their child while simultaneously supporting him/her.

6.5.5   Cognitive Restructuring in the Presence of Comorbid Depressive Symptoms

Many studies have demonstrated an increased comorbidity of chronic pain and depressive symptoms (for a meta-analysis see Pinquart and Shen 2011). Clinically, a depressive symptomatology in children often does not indicate the presence of a depressive episode but is part of an adjustment disorder with depressive reaction, which makes a difference to therapy. Dysfunctional thoughts in children with depressive comorbidity are fundamentally different in some aspects to those of children exclusively suffering a pain disorder.

Examples of Depressive Dysfunctional Thoughts
1. "I'm too stupid to defend myself against the pain."
2. "I'm hardly worth anything."
3. "The whole world is against me."
4. "Why always me? No matter what I do, I will be unlucky anyway."
5. "I hate myself and my body."
6. "Nobody likes me unless I'm tidy and perfect."
7. "I have to be perfect, so that someone will like me."
8. "I'm sure something horrible will happen to me."
9. "I'm so ugly."
10. "I deserve to have pain. It's my own fault."

If depressive symptomatology is suspected, it may be helpful to directly query the patient about his thoughts ("What did you think facing those things?"). The respective topics could be school, friends, oneself, or the family. The psychotherapist may also prompt some thoughts ("Is it possible that sometimes you say to yourself 'I am hardly worth anything,' 'I have to do everything right,' or 'I'm sure something horrible will happen to me'?"). If those thoughts arise more frequently, the psychotherapist should address this in pain therapy. The following example illustrates how to check for perfectionistic thoughts in a child with chronic pain and a slight depressive symptomatology.

Case Report: Jenny (16 Years), Pain Disorder (T = Therapist; C = Child)
T: Hi Jenny. Great that you brought your diary of thoughts with you again. Did you notice something?
C: Yes I did. I notice more and more that I am also having Black Thoughts in other situations. For instance, yesterday morning I was in a bad mood when I had to go to school.
T: Why was that?
C: Well, I overslept and there was no time to put on my makeup. My hair was a mess and I was pressured for time.
T: How did you feel at that moment?
C: I was tense and insecure.
T: What was on your mind?
C: Impossible to go to school looking like that. All the others will laugh at me.
T: What would it mean to you to go to school, your hair being a mess and having no makeup on? What would that tell about your person? (defining the thought to discuss)
C: Well, that I am scruffy and too lazy to take care of myself.

T: What is the worst thing that could happen to you then? (balancing out)

C: The worst thing would be if all the others would point at me and laugh and avoid talking to me the whole day.

T: I understand. And what would be the best case to happen?

C: All this going unnoticed.

T: What do you think will probably happen if you go to school not made up?

C: Well, my friends may wonder and ask if I overslept. But maybe they will think badly of me and won't tell me.

T: How convinced are you about your thought "If I leave not being made up then the others will think I am scruffy and lazy"?

C: About 80 percent.

T: Should we test your thinking?

C: What do you propose?

T: I would like to do an experiment with you. We ponder what you might feel in detail, what could happen if you go to school with your hair being a mess and with no makeup. We do it like scientists: You will perform the experiment and observe if what you fear will happen. (behavioral experiment)

C: Heavens, I will need a lot of courage to do so. I don't dare!

T: Alternatively you could first make a survey on the ward of what people think about people without makeup. Should we plan such a survey?

C: That sounds better. Maybe afterwards I will do the experiment.

Jenny did the survey and found out that nobody thinks a person without makeup scruffy and lazy. Afterwards she dared to show up on the ward without makeup. Nobody was laughing at her, and only a few people noticed the difference. While discussing the experiment with her psychotherapist, she was able to reflect and change her dysfunctional thoughts. This encouraged her to conduct the experiment also in her school at home. That time she was clearly less tense than during the first experiment. Her conclusion was: "People do like me even if I am not always perfect. And anyway, I don't care about those who dislike me." During the course of therapy Jenny's inner tension decreased, making it easier for her to cope with her headache.

Frustrating social experiences (e.g., repeated teasing; devaluation) or interactions (e.g., a difficult family system) play an important role in the development of depressive symptoms. We feel that positive interactions coupled with encouragement and reinforcement should be implemented into daily life on the ward and at home. To this end you can use the following interventions:

6.5.5.1 Note Box

We use this positive feedback technique in children up to the age of 14 years with depressive symptomatology as well as with children with fears (Sect. 6.5.4.1). In these children, it is helpful if they get access to the box at any time to read the positive notes.

6.5.5.2 Positive Evening Reflection

A joint evening reflection of the day between an adolescent with depressive symptoms and the NET can be very helpful (Sect. 6.5.4). Here the patient is asked to name the aspects of the day that in his/her view he/she either did well or experienced in a positive way. The NET adds its own positive observations to this. Besides the positive observations of the adolescent's behavior, explicit positive aspects of his/her personality that were noticed during the day should be reported. This evening reflection should take approximately 5–10 min. The positive evening reflection is extraordinarily loved by the patients. One should not be misled if in the beginning many patients refuse to participate or say very little. That is part of the depressive symptoms, and the adolescents are not usually used to being praised. In the course of the inpatient treatment, the patients start to believe the feedback more and more and can increasingly add their own positive observations. During the Stress Tests (see Sect. 6.6.6) we ask the parents to continue this exercise, so that they also learn to praise and strengthen their children.

6.5.5.3 Success Diary

Alternatively or sometimes even in addition to the positive evening reflection, keeping a diary of success can be arranged, in order that the adolescent becomes more independent of the feedback of others. This way the patients note down autonomously that which they have experienced in a positive way during the day. If fewer than three things per day occur to them, they can get feedback from the NET.

6.5.5.4 Reinforcement Schemes

Especially for children aged less than 12 years it might be helpful to use a reinforcement plan to support newly learned behavior (e.g., distraction during episodes of pain) as well as the use of Colored Thoughts. With this technique, the desired behavior can be rewarded by stamps, for example. Having gained a certain number of entries in the "stamp booklet," the child is allowed to get something he/she desires. Especially if the child does not have much positive time (fun leisure time) with his/her parents, we try to increase that time with the help of a reinforcement scheme (e.g., for a certain number of entries the child can "buy" 30 extra minutes of play time together with his/her mother). Sometimes even older children or adolescents benefit from such a reinforcement scheme. In patients with depressive symptomatology, the use of reinforcement schemes should always be considered.

The successful implementation of cognitive strategies needs much time. In order to avoid any frustration, the patient and his/her parents should be informed in advance that it will take a while until the patient feels the changes and believes in them. Thus, in these children, outpatient psychotherapy is often indicated after the inpatient stay.

6.5.6 Social Insecurity and Dysfunctional Interaction Strategies

Many children with chronic pain have difficulties with social interactions. During the course of their pain disorder, they experience social withdrawal (school, sports club, neighborhood). This may be seen as a consequence of the pain disorder.

Children with chronic pain expect the generally supportive behavior of peers much more often than healthy ones (Forgeron et al. 2011). In most cases their expectations are not fulfilled, they are disappointed and feel misunderstood or hurt and gradually retreat. Pain as the cause for school absence is often regarded as a bad excuse by classmates and teachers. Sometimes the affected children are badly teased and segregated. Finally, during the course of the disease, some children with chronic pain have learned to avoid disliked activities by complaining of pain.

On the other hand, some parents report that their child didn't have many friends, tended to withdraw socially, and had problems coping with peers even before the pain disorder. Presumably, a pain disorder makes it even more difficult for these children to learn age-appropriate social competencies because now they see their pain as the main obstruction to making social contacts, which were associated with fear in the first place.

All this demonstrates that a pain disorder has an unfavorable impact on age-appropriate social development or social competence. If many of these socially incompetent children live together during inpatient pain therapy with its daily structure aiming at active pain coping, social conflicts sometimes are inevitable. To allow for these group dynamic processes on the ward, each week, two group therapy sessions are offered in order to train social competence. Once a week there is a "beef round" where the children may discuss social conflicts and develop or train conflict solving strategies. Since patients at the GPPC are not a cohort but admitted consecutively, it is not possible to offer stepwise social competence training. Instead, current topics are categorized according to the various underlying social problems and the group develops solutions which may be trained doing role plays.

The psychotherapists not involved in that group session get a brief written feedback on relevant behavioral observations. This allows them to continue working on problems or resources in the single therapeutic sessions or family sessions. Often the group therapy sessions inspire the NET to do certain interventions (e.g., to function as mediator in conflicts between adolescents, to arrange an extra appointment for a positive evening reflection, to support certain patients in coping with social conflicts).

There are daily morning as well as evening rounds led by the NET in which the children may express their current mood or well-being (Table 6.1, Sect. 6.2.3). The NET writes down their impressions and hands them over to the next shift or to the physician/psychotherapist. If needed, the following interventions may be requested by the primary psychotherapist:

1. Preliminary discussion and reflection on problematic social situations with the NET. The aim of this intervention is that the NET supports the child to learn to distinguish between favorable and unfavorable social interaction strategies (*favorable*: to ask someone for something in an appropriate way, to enforce a wish in an appropriate way, learning to say "no," to apologize, to broach the issue of someone's disturbing behavior instead of reacting with social retreat; *unfavorable*: avoiding social contacts, lamenting the injustice of others, feeling like a victim).
2. Setting up and implementing a graduated scheme (Sect. 6.5.4) addressing the patient's specific social fears.

6.6   Inpatient Pain Therapy: Module 4 (Integrating the Family System)

"Why did nobody explain that to us before?" – Mr. S. (44 years) after the first family talk

Many parents are not sufficiently informed about the biopsychosocial background of chronic pain and are stuck in their striving for "the one" physical cause of pain. Their understanding of chronic pain is not that different to that of the better part of many medical practitioners. Insufficiently treated pain disorders in children will increase both the degree of impairment of the child's life and the emotional burden of his/her parents (especially his mother), who will be at an increased risk of developing a pain disorder themselves (Lommel et al. 2011).

We feel that it is essential to successful pain therapy to value the parents who are often suspicious or resigned and meet them with understanding. We do not ignore the fact that parental anxiety and affinity for passive coping strategies contributes to the development and perpetuation of their child's pain disorder. However, parents certainly do not do this intentionally. In the light of the complex mutually dependent processes involved, partially intended by society, it would be both unfair and unwise to hold the parents responsible for their child's pain disease, more so as the parents explicitly seek help for their child. We *explicitly* promote the only helpful future-oriented therapeutic attitude: Based on their current knowledge and abilities, parents always strive for the best for their child. Rarely, it becomes evident during the course of treatment that the family's abilities are quite limited due to the mental disorders or somatic diseases of one or even both main attachment figures. Under such conditions, multimodal pain therapy as described in this manual reaches its limits. To the best of our knowledge, therapeutic interventions in children with chronic pain with mentally ill parents have so far not been developed or validated. Fortunately, most family systems are very motivated and able to change their behavior with the ultimate goal of helping their child.

6.6.1   The Admission Talk

At the beginning of inpatient paediatric pain therapy, there is a detailed admission talk scheduled with the patient, his/her family, the physician, psychologist, and paediatric nurse. The aims are as follows:
1. To query previous treatments and their effectiveness:
    (a) Previous diagnostic efforts
    (b) Previous outpatient or inpatient therapy (hospital stays, surgery, invasive pain therapy)
    (c) Previous and current medication (duration of treatment, dose, adverse effects)
2. To query the disease model:
    (a) Of the parents
    (b) Of the child
    (c) Of the patient's relatives.

3. To query any pain modulating factors (strengths; resources; skills of the child or his/her family; other factors that evoke fear, anxiety, fatigue, or desperation)

It is then helpful to summarize again the most important aspects of inpatient pain therapy, previously described during the outpatient appointment at the pain clinic preceding admission (active pain coping irrespective of pain intensity, one therapeutic session with the family per week starting with an education session and then discussion of all aspects relevant to everyday life, three to four single psychotherapeutic sessions a week for the patient, mandatory therapeutic homework, etc.). Based on that information we explore the child's and the parents' aims.

At the end of the admission talk, we construct a family tree including the grandparent generation of the patient, depicting the age, profession, mental disorders, or severe somatic diseases (especially pain disorders) of the family members and the members' interrelationships ("genogram"). The child should help set up the genogram, knowing: "You and your opinion and perception are important." Together with a summary of diagnoses, resources, the most important test results, and a photograph of the patient, the genogram is written on a flip chart. The genogram may later be added to, serving as a memory aid for the team during the multiprofessional ward rounds (Genograms: Assessment and Intervention. McGoldrick et al. (2008)). Figure 6.3 shows an example of a genogram including all essential information. During the ward round, the genogram helps generate important hypotheses with respect to pain perpetuating family structures, as are illustrated by the following examples:

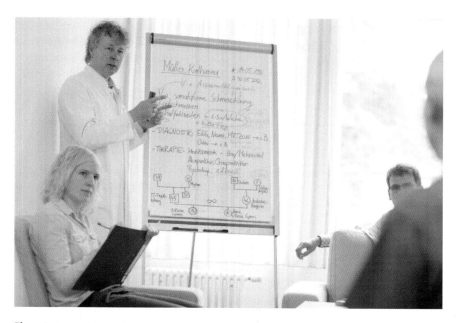

Fig. 6.3 Example genogram

1. All female members of the maternal side of the family suffer pain. What is the significance of this to the child with respect to the disease model or future perspectives?
2. The mother describes the father's family as being very achievement oriented. The father is rarely at home. The genogram shows that there are many relationships in the father's family system that were broken off. What does that mean to the child? Does the child fear that a decrease in performance or an increase in autonomy will result in less approval by his/her father?

Finally, some formalities are settled (e.g., Is the child allowed to leave the ward on his own to visit a store?) and an appointment for the first family talk is set. Only in exceptional cases, for instance, in children with separation anxiety, should the team, the child, and his/her parents agree on a fixed time schedule for telephone talk.

6.6.2 Education, Normalization, Approval, and the Reduction of Guilt

Before the first family talk takes place, some single therapeutic sessions are scheduled. This has several advantages. First, it allows the child to get ahead in knowledge compared to his/her parents. Another advantage is that the child already learns about some basics of pain therapy. In addition, during these single sessions a first identification of pain modulating factors can take place. Finally, this schedule allows us to prepare the family to talk together with the child. The child will decide whether his/her parents need a theoretically or rather a practically oriented education. Which behavioral changes would the child like to see in his parents? Which difficulties will arise from the implementation of certain therapeutic strategies at home? Does the child feel guilty for the family's burden resulting from his/her pain? Does he/she worry about developments, problems, anxiety, or reproaches that have so far not been mentioned?

The first family talk is very important. It is the key to getting the family's compliance with the planned procedure. An insufficiently prepared first family talk may seriously endanger further successful pain therapy. Thus, we recommend investing enough time into the preparation of that talk and collecting essential information on family resources, conflicts, and the family's attitudes towards active as well as passive pain coping strategies. If the child's and his/her parents' disease model is known, the psychotherapist can draw conclusions on which of the Three Thought Traps they might face. The child should be explicitly assured that during the family talk he/she can pipe up anytime in order to correct statements from the NET, the physician or the psychotherapist. We encourage the child to get highly engaged in the family talk and even to explain certain educational topics to his/her parents himself/herself.

After welcoming the family to the first family talk, the session should *start* with a brief summary of the previous course of treatment and the agenda of that talk. Also, the parental efforts and dispensations in order to join this session should explicitly be appreciated. Then the family gets the opportunity to again explain their reasons for proactively deciding on inpatient pain therapy. Don't forget to reinforce the parent's efforts again in this context.

Approval and appreciation of the parents' efforts will be an important basis for the upcoming and sometimes challenging changes in the family system. At the same time, this approach minimizes room for the question of guilt, resulting in a good overall ambience and increased readiness to learn. Most parents expect that previous therapies and psychotherapists will be disparaged and the parents' efforts judged as insufficient or even causal factors of the pain. A (for the parents) surprisingly great appreciation makes them curious and alert, increasing the odds for a successful first family talk before the psychotherapists have even started to convey any educational content. The child should be complimented on his/her motivation to cooperate. Hinting to the parents that "It would be favorable if you as parents would catch up with the knowledge of your child," the education can start.

There are special cases of family systems where one or both of the parents suffer from pain themselves. They may have undergone pain therapy and are familiar with many topics from the education. Usually those parents will be aware of their problems and be motivated for therapy. Nevertheless, some parents with chronic pain are stuck in Thought Trap 2 or 3 (Sect. 4.1), didn't experience any success in their own therapy so far, and thus are skeptical of the biopsychosocial model of chronic pain. If the explicit inclusion of these parents in therapy and the intensified education (described in Sect. 6.3.3) doesn't change their view of chronic pain, sustained success in treatment is nearly impossible.

In such a case one should scrutinize this information to see if the physical and emotional development of the child is endangered (Sect. 6.6.5). It is common in parents who suffer from chronic pain to have difficulties in instructing their child in active pain coping while being in pain themselves. They easily understand the emotional state of their child, but the ability to put oneself in another person's position based on empathy and love means more harm than good for active pain coping. Her child expressing pain or showing pain will remind a pain-diseased mother of her own pain, enhancing her pain perception, and vice versa. Obviously, that has to do with our ability to feel empathy, which presumably is mediated by mirror neurons (Goubert et al. 2005; Singer et al. 2004). The more love a parent feels for his/her child, the greater the empathy will be. Thus, in fact love may hurt. Most affected parents and children can agree with these assumptions. Supposedly, the process outlined here is not directly changeable, but it is our experience that it is of great help to parents suffering from chronic pain and their child if their perception is validated. This makes it easier to implement any interventions and mutual agreements.

At the end of the first family talk, its content is summarized and the parents are asked to write down any questions left in order to discuss them during the next talk. They are advised of the parents' guide "How to stop chronic pain in children: a practical guide" (Dobe and Zernikow 2013). Quite often the parents tell us that it was not until they had read that book, with its many case reports of families in situations comparable to theirs, that they developed some understanding of the biopsychosocial model of the origin and perpetuation of chronic pain. The next family talk is scheduled for 1 week later. Some families need clear arrangements regarding phone contact with the physician or psychotherapist for the time up to the next talk, especially if they tend to catastrophize.

6.6.3 Reducing the Family's Attention Towards Pain and Improving Active Pain Coping

"Mostly I lie down to get a belly rub from my mum." – Jessy (13 years)

One aim of inpatient pain therapy is to help parents support their children in active pain coping and to reduce attention towards pain.

6.6.3.1 Reducing the Family's Attention Towards Pain

Contrary to the assumption that children with pain gain by the increased family attention paid to their pain, most children find it annoying that they are constantly asked about their pain. Not only the child's relatives but also concerned and engaged teachers or members of the child's clique remind the child of his/her pain symptoms by their well-meaning questions. The child, on the other hand, finds it difficult to wall himself/herself off from the questioning. This questioning is a normal behavior and an expression of healthy social relationships in other illnesses. Sometimes children suffer as with time friends and neighbors pull back, school friends don't ask anymore, and social isolation thus arises (Forgeron et al. 2011). In a child with pain, the increased questions lead inevitably to maintaining if not even to aggravation of the pain problem. We have gotten to know a wide range of family attention – from the concerned mother who asks about her child's pain ten times a day, to the father, himself chronically ill with pain, who marks the pain-sensitive areas of his child's back with a felt pen.

No matter who focuses on the child's pain – it will unintentionally amplify the child's pain perception. In order to answer the question "Do you still feel pain?" the child has to set the focus on his/her body and its painful area. In the least favorable case, the child has just been distracted, and the query will confront him/her with the pain again. These queries reflect helplessness. A simple and humorous intervention is the *1 € rule (for the sake of simplicity, we will use the term 1€, but it can easily be adapted to every currency)*.

The 1 € Rule

The education on the interrelationship between parental querying and an increase in pain often does not lead to a behavioral change. Now it's time for the 1 € rule ("bibliotherapy": parents will find information on that method and its background in the parents' advisor "How to stop chronic pain in children: a practical guide" (Dobe and Zernikow 2013)).

In the family talk we agree that whenever a family member asks the child about his/her pain, the respective family member is obliged to immediately give 1 € to the child. Children of every age love this rule. The parents have to understand that the effect of their query now will be that the child primarily thinks of the money gained and not of his pain. So the parents unintentionally asking about the pain causes no further association with pain, since from now on their child will joyfully put out his/her hand. This intervention also emphasizes that asking about the pain induces pain, giving the child some sort of right to claim appropriate compensation ("solatium"). The 1 € rule may be extended at will. There are some parents who want to spare their child, so they take all possibly demanding activities from him (e.g., carrying things for him, tidying up, setting the table). If even comprehensive education does not modify this behavior, a compensation of 2 € for each query or even 5 € should be discussed. In order not to hurt the parents' feelings, we make it clear that introducing that rule is not meant as a criticism of the parents' previous behavior and that in acute pain asking one's child about pain is an absolutely normal and adequate behavior. (In German hospitals pain therapists establish regular postsurgery pain measurements, and the hospitals only get certified if their acute pain patients are regularly assessed for pain). Since nature didn't prepare us for the special case of chronic pain, however, most parents behave as if this is acute pain. Unfortunately, this behavior will contribute to the perpetuation of this type of pain.

Parents often argue that they would like to know how their child is doing. From a therapeutic point of view, it is explicitly desired that parents keep asking the child about his/her well-being, however, not specifically concerning the pain but rather concerning his/her mood. The parents are also invited to express what they perceive about their child's current state. During the long-standing course of a pain disorder, the perception of negative emotions and pain may become closely coupled, and instead of a negative emotion, the child perceives nothing but an increase in pain and is unable to differentiate between the two qualities. Here, parents may help, addressing any negative or positive emotion they notice separately.

The parents should always be instructed to explain the 1 € rule to their relatives and all the child's other attachment figures. The child should be prepared that the odds are that he/she will not make as much money as hoped for, since the parents will usually learn from the intervention quite fast. The record-holder of the last few years, a highly gifted 15-year-old girl, didn't make more than 60 € before her parents completely stopped asking about her pain.

6.6.3.2 Approval and Active Pain Coping

Approval is another option for parents to support their child in active pain coping. Many children with chronic pain have low self-esteem and feel guilty about many of the family's problems. Everyday family life is determined by worries, doctor's visits, and the permanent effort to understand the patient's feelings and state of health. Valuing the child for any active pain coping effort or for other positive behavior is less common. It is important to explicitly highlight this aspect and illustrate it with examples from life on the ward or within the family.

In doing so, we see various parental reactions. While some parents are keen to notice more precisely the achievements of their child, others have difficulties in recognizing positive aspects. For instance, Mrs. G. was very happy to see that her daughter Julia could gradually use her hurting foot more and more, although she still needed crutches. Mrs. H., on the other hand, was bothered that progress in treatment was slow, and she was worried that at such a pace her daughter Mia would need years of convalescence for her foot and might therefore not pass her grade in school this year. In the course of treatment Mia repeatedly showed regression because of lacking motivation and fear of the future. By approving of and complimenting their child, parents are able to provide motivation – but, fueling fears will unmotivate the child. Therefore, we ask the parents to notice and approve of their child's progress, small as it may be, and to meticulously note it down on the Weekend Observation Sheets (Sect. 6.6.6 and Chap. 9, Worksheet #19).

Parents may also be asked to write down their child's progress or positive behavior in a "Success Diary." This intervention takes considerable therapeutic competence because parents are easily offended. Especially parents not used to approving of their child feel guilty and tend to have depressive thoughts and behavior. We don't recommend focusing on that problematic parental behavior; otherwise, treatment resistance will occur easily, counteracting the treatment aim. A psychotherapist focusing on problems is a wrong model for the parents. The majority of patients want their parents to feel good during the family talks (and not "to wear them down," as an adolescent girl called it). A successful family talk in which problems are raised, but laughter and some ease also occur, will motivate both parents and children.

6.6.3.3 Reducing and Preventing Passive Pain Coping

By means of family talks, we try to bring the amount of passive pain coping back to normal. In the past, parents were often told (also by physicians) that they should give their child a break. For them it seems quite normal to go to bed when feeling ill, tired, or exhausted. It is understandable that parents and children make no difference between chronic pain and acute diseases and act accordingly. Rest and passivity – a behavior pattern making sense in an ill or injured child – results in further chronicity in chronic pain. Passive behavior patterns are enhanced by parental worries, and passive pain coping increases pain (Lipani and Walker 2006; Walker et al. 2007; Simons et al. 2008; Dobe et al. 2011; Hechler et al. 2011).

During the family talk, we have to provide the information that especially passive coping strategies (e.g., sleeping, lying down, avoiding movement) will in the long run prevent successful pain therapy. Active pain coping doesn't mean that the patient should permanently be in action – everyone needs a break once in a while. However, the difference between a normal break and rest or pain-related passivity is not obvious to many patients and their parents. A normal break is independent of the presence of pain, while pain-related rest or passivity means avoiding any effort associated with pain.

Passivity and problems in coping with stress and fears contribute to the perpetuation of pain. Most parents, however, are convinced that their child cannot do certain activities anymore due to his/her pain. They erroneously suppose that if pain is reduced, or even stopped, this will automatically lead to normalization of behavior. After long-lasting pain-related school absence and social withdrawal, the child will react with clearly increased physical tension when trying to go to school again.

Generally, negative cognitions will arise ("I don't get it anymore."; "Being in this state, I will never score high on the class test."; "Lara is staring at me, surely she's thinking I intentionally missed school. But she doesn't really know what pain is like."; "Damn, I can't focus mentally anymore."). If the adolescent is not prepared for this situation, there is a huge risk that the pain will be reactivated or increased. Even before starting school again, pain may increase. This phenomenon of learned distress intolerance should be discussed in the family talk *before* doing the first Stress Test. Due to the mechanisms mentioned above, passive therapeutic measures (e.g., massage, acupuncture, homeopathia, pit bags, or cool-pacs) are scientifically proven to have *no* lasting impact on children with pain disorders.

In the following example (Niklas, age 13 years, pain disorder with abdominal pain, during the last semester more than 50 % of school days missed, second family talk, 2 weeks on the ward) the patient's family already understood the education and will now discuss the importance of active pain coping.

Case Report: Niklas (13 Years), Pain Disorder with Abdominal Pain

"Well, Niklas, we explained to you and your parents the origin of chronic abdominal pain and how chronicity happens. What does that mean for you as parents in everyday life? What does it specifically mean now knowing that any type of passive pain coping or avoidance contributes to a further increase in pain? I guess deep in your heart you already know the answer: to do everything despite the pain, even things one doesn't like to do. Obviously you have already tried all this, and I know that severe pain will severely affect you. But, as you already observed on the ward, active coping in everyday life in spite of the pain is awkward but not impossible. You already learned some helpful strategies for how to cope with pain. When you were admitted to the ward, you didn't know those strategies and had to cope with daily life anyway, like all the other patients. And you did it! You can be very proud of yourself! As you notice, it became easier for you each day irrespective of whether or not you used those techniques. Your body got used to that everyday load, and now it is reacting with less distress and less painful muscular tension. Now the task is to use that knowledge, your regained power and the learned techniques in everyday life. Often those strategies will help you better cope with difficult situations in your daily routine. But sometimes – you didn't sleep well and wake up in the morning totally exhausted, wondering how to manage and pass the math exam in such a condition – it may well be that those techniques don't help that much yet. Then it is important to go on in spite of your pain in order to help your pain center learn that pain is not an alarm signal anymore and that it has lost its impact on you, your life and behavior."

"If you succeed in doing so, there is the chance of lasting recovery from your pain disorder. Addressing the parents: It wouldn't be fair to leave that job to your child alone. Your child needs you to be strong parents. Niklas must be able to rely on you to support him with his active pain coping efforts, especially in situations when it is still difficult for him. Do you dare to support Niklas in this? Addressing Niklas: Niklas, are you confident that your parents are able to help you? Addressing the parents: You should understand it doesn't mean that you are bad parents if in such a moment you focus on current worries and your child's pain. Instead you should think about his future. If we succeed in enabling your child to perform more active pain coping on the ward even when he is in severe pain, we are sure you will also succeed."

Now it is time to discuss how far Niklas should go with his efforts *before* he can ask his parents for support. It is helpful to also define the circumstances when the parents should act without the approval of their child. We have had good experiences with changing the domestic systemic context variables before and during particularly problematic interactions. For instance, if it is difficult for the mother, who is suffering from a pain or anxiety disorder herself, to prompt her son to actively cope with his pain during obviously painful episodes, it is a great relief for her if the father feels responsible enough to prompt his child in active pain coping.

6.6.4 Coping with Conflicts Between Autonomy and Dependence

Frequently in outpatient or inpatient pain therapy, it becomes obvious that apart from the pain, there are some open conflicts of autonomy and dependence between the child and his/her parents.

On the one hand, this could mean that the child is striving for more freedom and a voice, i.e., autonomy, against his/her parent's will. This is quite a normal process in human life. It becomes problematic if this conflict is carried out adamantly, resulting in dysfunctional thoughts and muscular hypertension which amplifies pain. This leads to conditioning of family conflicts and increased pain and can culminate in mutual accusations. During these conflicts, many parents do not recognize the child's pain and instead suspect him/her of purposely putting pressure on them. Obviously the child and his/her family suffer in this situation, and it makes successful pain therapy difficult. The child will be worried that successful pain therapy comprising psychological approaches will strengthen his/her parents position that the pain is "mental," "in his/her head," or "imagined."

On the other hand, there will also be developments in the opposite direction. During the course of the pain disorder, the child has spent more time with his/her parents (mostly the mother) and retreated into the secure family environment. Many parents reveal ambiguous feelings indicating they feel unsure how to change to more age-appropriate behaviors – just talking about it is insufficient. For some parents a development towards an increase in parental care and dependency of the child seems pleasing – if there wasn't any pain. In the worst-case scenario, parents and the child are stuck together against the cold and hostile world in which teachers, classmates, physicians, or other people are responsible for the unjust or inappropriate treatment of the child's pain condition. Generally, the child will be lacking motivation to try autonomous behavior and won't undertake anything without the parents.

Irrespective of the specific nature of the conflict, the more the family interaction is dominated by conflict, the more obstructive it will be for success in pain therapy. Regardless of the different positions, seen from a more abstract point of view, the recommended therapeutic approach is quite similar:

1. The first step is to normalize the development of the conflict ("Presumably you all know about families with similar conflicts …") and to find out what was previously undertaken to solve the conflict ("Obviously all of you suffer from this situation. You've probably tried to find a solution. What exactly did you try so far?"). Then the efforts of the family are appreciated ("I can well understand that you are all frustrated. It is quite impressive how you are still willing to cooperate to find a solution in spite of all that mutual hurting in the past. You have explained your conflict quite openly which shows that you are still interested in a solution.").

2. The next step is to identify the family's interaction patterns which have a functional or dysfunctional impact on the family's general well-being and the child's pain. To this end the technique of "circular questioning" is very useful ("Mrs. G., what do you think your child is thinking about the fact that you are seldom complimented by your husband but blamed instead?"). In a next step, techniques aiming at more respectful mutual interactions (e.g., optional time-outs during a discussion which is getting worse) and more autonomous behavior on the part of the child (e.g., giving the child the chance to resolve conflicts on his/her own) should be introduced.

3. Desired behavior is reinforced with a reward meeting the needs of the driving force in the conflict. The reward may be cuddling with the mother after the child has faced a difficult situation on his/her own. Or it might be a reinforcement scheme which provides the desired freedom once housework is done or the child has demonstrated respectful behavior. If each family member is willing to make a compromise, the technique will work and none of the family members will feel outsmarted. The aim of all those interventions is to erase the connection between pain perception and family interaction.

Family conflicts are not the cause of the pain disorder but can contribute much to the pain symptoms in severe cases. The pain is not purely of psychological origin (child) nor caused by wrong upbringing (parents). To avoid polarization in the family talk, we recommend discussing the upcoming family talk in advance. The child is a valuable ally in the family talk if he/she can be sure that the goal is a win-win situation for him/her and his/her parents. Usually the child knows exactly what his/her parents are thinking and how they will react to various interventions. This knowledge should be used to prepare the family talk.

6.6.5   Coping with Stress Factors Within the Family ("The Tip of the Iceberg")

"You were born to help me, not to impose on me" (just one of several things 16-year-old Dana has heard from her mother and experienced as stressful, apart from experiencing physical abuse by her mother).

The family conflicts depicted in Sect. 6.6.4 may make pain therapy difficult but not impossible. The migraine of the single mother that makes it impossible for her to look after her children 4 days a month and the drug abuse of the father with a pain disorder who can still attend regularly are problems that can be solved.

However, for a few children pain is only "the tip of the iceberg," and during the course of therapy, a severely disturbed family interaction becomes obvious. These disturbances may be so severe that the child's well-being is endangered (e.g., severe violence and/or sexual abuse within the family) requiring immediate action (the exact procedures depend on the laws of the respective state). Table 6.4 depicts the gradual procedure we follow.

The classification into five classes of severity reflects just one possibility of facing the different types of extraordinary stress factors within the family. Being an oversimplification, it may still give orientation to set up a preliminary treatment *concept* which may be optimized later. Having no plan and thus being helpless are the main obstacles when establishing suitable support for children and families in need.

On the pain ward, the social worker participates regularly in the ward rounds. With cases of grade 3 or up, he becomes more and more a part of the pain therapy, doing the tasks outlined above (for detailed information on the role of the social worker, see Sects. 6.7.3 and 6.7.4). We feel that with the collaboration of the physician, psychotherapist, social worker, and patient, most affected parents or persons with custody of the child can be motivated to closely cooperate with the staff and the youth welfare institutions.

One technique to get the family's cooperation within a problematic family constellation or with the family's taboo topics is to set up a genogram on a flip chart (Sect. 6.6.1). The genogram is taken into the family talk in order to elucidate striking behavioral patterns repeatedly found in each generation (e.g., on the paternal side, breaking of relationships is only seen with male family members – the (male) patient and his father have increasing verbal conflicts). Sometimes it may be advantageous to use the genogram to introduce topics tabooed by the family without having to explicitly name them (e.g., the alcohol abuse of the father is written down in the genogram. His alcohol abuse is headlined (variant: overwritten) with the bright red letters "TABOO").

Table 6.4 Background and approach dependent on the degree of family burden and danger to the child's wellbeing

Degree of severity	Background	Approach
Grade 1	The family stress factors (e.g. physical or mental disorders of one or both parents; death of a beloved relative; permanent conflict between the couple) result in substantial emotional burden for the child and his parents. But, they are no risk for the further development of the child since everyone involved is ready to work out a solution	Addressing the possibility that the child may feel guilty allows the parents to explain to their child that he/she is not responsible for the family conflicts. The various unfavorable circumstances may be openly outlined and thus are not a taboo. If psychological burden is so high that there is need for further outpatient psychotherapy for the child (or his parents), such a treatment will be initiated
Grade 2	The family stress factors (e.g. conflicts as given in step 1, but also violence; verbally or physically escalating couple conflicts; at least one parent suffering from a severe psychiatric disorder; long-lasting home care of a relative expected to die; brother or sister with a disorder of social behavior and aggressive behavior towards family members) are substantial and generally already resulting in a mental disorder of the child (i.e. adjustment disorder with depressive reaction)	During the family talk all the responsibility is taken off the child. Facing the emotional symptoms, parents or the person having custody agree on co-operation and further efforts in order to avert the imminent risk to the child's development
Grade 3	The stress factors within the family have a severe negative impact on the child and have already resulted in a mental disorder. It turns out that the family resources are insufficient to prevent an imminent risk to the further development of the child	Apart from ongoing outpatient psychotherapy, there is the necessity of family support, or (rarely) inpatient measures of the youth welfare service (Procedure dependent on the laws of the respective state). Parents or the person in custody of the child agree to co-operate
Grade 4	There are severe stressful factors within the family, having resulted in a chronic mental disorder of the child as well as an endangerment of the child's well-being. Often the child is so desperate that he/she has considered committing suicide	Approach is depending on the willingness (and resources) of the parents or the person with custody of the child for co-operation with the ambulatory and transient inpatient support of the youth welfare service and the ambulatory psychotherapist. In most cases there is a fair chance that family stress factors can be reduced so that the child is able to cope with them

(continued)

Table 6.4 (continued)

Degree of severity	Background	Approach
Grade 5	There is the well-founded suspicion of severe domestic violence (physical and/or sexual) or structural or psychological neglect. Hence, the well-being of the child is clearly endangered	If the parents or the person with custody of the child doesn't understand or accept a lasting change or there is a shortage of family resources, the child has to be admitted to an inpatient institution of the youth welfare service as soon as possible (examples: Linda, age 15 years – CRPS type I: continual sexual abuse by her father. When this issue is brought up in a family talk the mother accuses her daughter of lying; Karl, age 14 years – pain disorder with headache, depressive episode: his single mother is unable to look after her child or provide for his basic needs; Yvi, age 17 years – pain disorder with abdominal pain, complex posttraumatic stress disorder due to repeated sexual abuse by different partners of her mother: her mother suffers borderline psychosis, and conflicts with her always escalate to physical violence and mutual destructive insults)

6.6.6   Stress Test and Parent's Observation on the Ward

So far, we have discussed various aspects of including the family within the scope of family talks. Most parents are very interested and increasingly engaged in the implementation of these measures or interventions. But, many difficulties do not become obvious until they try to transfer theory into practice. This is the reason why it is indispensable that *during inpatient therapy* the patient passes two Stress Tests at home, each of 2 or 3 days' duration and including attending class at his/her home school if possible. These Stress Tests are very helpful to figure out the actual family's resources and obstacles to long-term implementation of active pain coping strategies or other measures discussed with the family. For most parents, observations on the ward are another helpful module to learn how to deal with their child.

6.6.6.1 Stress Test
The aim of a Stress Test is to give the child and his/her family the opportunity to examine how well the various techniques can be implemented into the family's everyday life. Thus, it doesn't make sense to start with a Stress Test on the first of the three weekends of the stay. Only the second and third weekends are suitable for a Stress Test. A Stress Test is a regular part of the inpatient pain therapy program and will be omitted only in case of acute risk to the child's well-being or an acute infectious disease within the family. The Stress Test includes attending school at home. A family Stress Test takes 2 days, sometimes 3. If the home is far away from our clinic, the beginning of the Stress Test is scheduled for the same day as the family talk (mostly on Thursday or Friday afternoon), so that the child can go home with the family. The goals for the family are set in detail (e.g., participate in family life irrespective of your back pain, organize meeting up with friends, meet the demands of housework (vacuuming), implement the 1€ rule, practice the techniques, parents should support active pain coping, positive evening discussion with a parent).

The NET records the aims of the Stress Test on the weekend Stress Test sheet (Chap. 9, Worksheet #19). The NET reminds the child and the parents to *separately* document the degree of success at the end of the Stress Test weekend. The reflection discussion on the Stress Test should be very supportive, and the NET will try to get the parents' support. Reprimanding parents is definitely not advisable, as parents are important co-therapists in the implementation of interventions. Since building trust is the NET's responsibility, all NET members need comprehensive training.

The child's estimates of the success of the Stress Test frequently differ from those of the parents. These different views are very helpful for the psychotherapist. The NET should inform the family in advance that these differences are likely to occur. Any ideas or wishes for future work may be recorded in the column "wishes." Finally, the parents are instructed to immediately call the ward if any substantial problems arise in the implementation of the discussed measures (e.g., impossibility of attending school, child is refusing to implement the graduated scheme). Sometimes that phone call helps to avoid the premature interruption of the Stress Test. At the scheduled (or, sometimes, premature) end of the Stress Test, the documentation sheet should be handed to the NET in person. The NET always makes a record of their subjective impressions when the child returns to the ward.

After the Stress Test is finished, the documentation sheet – supplemented by the subjective impressions of the NET and verbal expressions of the child or his parents – is handed over to the physician or psychotherapist in charge. Any modification of the procedure in single sessions and family talks required as a result of the experiences in the Stress Test will be discussed with the patient in upcoming single sessions. Any problems or failures during the Stress Test are an important indicator of obstacles for the long-term implementation of therapeutic interventions and should *never* be neglected.

6.6.6.2 Parent's Observation on the Ward

In case of substantial difficulties in the implementation of active pain coping strategies, an observation of everyday life on the ward for one or both parents may be a very useful addition to the Stress Test. Ideally, such an observation would start at 7:00 a.m. and last until 8:00 p.m. A shorter duration is possible, but should be an exception. The indicated time frame will allow for sufficient opportunities for the parent to observe his/her child in active pain coping on the ward. Observation is especially useful on a child's "Stress Day" (see Sect. 6.4.5.3).

From the medical history, the admission talk, the single appointments, and the previous course of treatment, it is clear in most cases what the aims of observation should be. These are discussed between the NET, physician, and psychotherapist and then edited by the NET and recorded on the observation sheet (Chap. 9, Worksheets #20 and #21). Most often the focus will be on the training of skills and the striving for security in the implementation of active pain coping strategies at home. Often the parents are unsure about what to expect from their child and have feelings of guilt. Often they say, "If I had known what my child could accomplish in spite of the pain, I would have intervened much earlier." Sometimes observation should focus on the modification of dysfunctional interactions between the child and his/her parents. In this case the aims may be to compliment the child, to recognize even small progress, or to implement pleasant shared activities (i.e., spending time together in a relaxation room or playing a game).

At the end of the observation day, the NET and the parent discuss the experiences of the day (Chap. 9, Worksheet #21). This discussion should focus on the degree to which the preset aims were met. The filled-in worksheet is given to the physician or psychotherapist in charge. It will form the basis of the upcoming family talk.

Finally we want to point out a special but rare observation that will not be seen in the agreement of aims: generating hypotheses on the tragic extent of dysfunctional family interaction. Sometimes this is helpful in case youth welfare services are needed after discharge:

1. Mrs. F. is very unkempt when she arrives at 8:00 a.m. to start her observation, as agreed upon. For the following 3 h, she lies on her daughter's bed and is very indignant when asked for collaboration by the NET.
2. Instead of playing with his daughter, Mr. P. prefers to play table tennis with male patients. He shows no interest in stopping until he is summoned by the NET to do so.
3. Even in the artificial environment of inpatient pain therapy and supported by the NET, Mrs. H. is unable to enforce her will on her son. She doesn't stick to the aims jointly agreed to. The child's strong oppositionality is only observed when his mother is with him and not seen in everyday life on the ward.

6.6.7   How the Family Is Advised to Handle Relatives, Friends, and Teachers

Children and their parents report, sometimes with amusement, but more often annoyed or feeling burdened, that they get a lot of advice on how to handle their child's pain. Pain is a universal experience, and everyone has had their own experiences. Unsolicited comments are communicated to the child and the parents, often accompanied by reproaches. The "counselor" expects to be appreciated for his hardly helpful advice! This may provoke interactive distress for the parents or with their child.

Before their admission, the children have usually tried various therapeutic interventions, e.g., acupuncture, homeopathy, osteopathy, diets, massage, physiotherapy, dental corrections, transcranial magnet stimulation, or analgesics.

All advice is based on the assumption that "The child suffers pain because …" This assumption allows for *mono*causality only. These explanations usually stem from one of the Three Thought Traps (see Sect. 4.1). Our parent's guide "How to stop chronic pain in children: a practical guide" (Dobe and Zernikow 2013) presents detailed suggestions for how to get the parents enthusiastic about a view comprising all three dimensions of pain chronicity. This explanation is also understood by relatives, family friends, or teachers. In the following paragraphs, the main ideas of the parent's guide will be presented.

6.6.7.1 How to Handle Relatives and Adult Family Friends?

While abundant well-meant advice is just annoying, it is time for the parents to intervene and protect their child from advice, if relatives talk about their own pain or the child's chronic pain in a catastrophizing way. We recommend that the parents either educate the adviser on chronic pain or, if this seems insufficient, at least temporarily discontinue the discussion or contact. Alternatively, adolescents can be given the consent of their parents to tell the relative or friend of their own wishes and needs.

Example: Asking a Relative or Friend of the Family Not to Question/Inquire About the Pain Anymore

"Up to now we didn't dare to tell you what we are going to tell you now because our child loves you and doesn't want to hurt you. She definitely doesn't want to be questioned about the pain anymore, and she doesn't like to talk about the pain, because this will remind her of it and induce increased pain perception. She decided to undertake an inpatient pain therapy to do something about her pain. I know this will be difficult for you – as it is for us. The physicians asked us to give her 1 € each time you or we still ask about her pain. I hope you will understand. You would do her a great favor. (add the following sentence only if really necessary: If you cannot stop talking about pain, we have discussed that the next step should be to temporarily discontinue your contact with her. But, this is the last thing we want. If you are not willing to stop talking about the pain, however, we will have to take that step to protect our child.)"

Fortunately, most relatives or friends will understand. Rarely some of the relatives (mostly the grandparents) ask to attend the family talk in order to get more information on the background of what they consider a somewhat strange procedure and that their grandchild is so enthusiastic about. If their previous efforts are appreciated, in most cases they are ready to collaborate. Often the "fact sheet for relatives" from the parent's guide "How to stop chronic pain in children: a practical guide" proves helpful to get a better understanding of the issue.

6.6.7.2 How to Handle Teachers?

Most parents of children with chronic pain in need of inpatient pain therapy report having had to argue with their child's teacher about days missed from school. Some parents complain about teachers not trying to understand their child's problems and needs. They often report that their child is exposed to substantial social burden due to the lack of understanding of both teachers and classmates. Those statements should be evaluated carefully. Even if the teacher is acting incorrectly, this normally reflects certain aspects of the child's social behavior. How is the child handling false accusations or wrongful judgments? How does he/she react to teasing? How does he/she behave towards his/her classmates? Does he/she always insist on understanding for his/her problems, or is he/she able to understand his/her peers' or teachers' view (Forgeron et al. 2011)? Most teachers are good at recognizing anxious behavior or avoidance. If during a parent-teacher meeting, a teacher says that in his view the child's headache is an excuse to avoid a class test, then this information should be regarded as valuable. Understandably, with regard to chronic pain, teachers, like most other people, are prone to getting stuck in one of the Thought Traps, especially the First Thought Trap (Logan et al. 2007).

Our experience with schools, their principals, or teachers is more often good than bad. Generally, the teacher's view is helpful: *the child must go to school.* In accordance with most teachers, we don't recommend any type of home schooling, since lessons at home will support a strategy of avoidance and enhance pain. This again will result in social deficits and impair the child's ability to cope with distress and daily hassles.

During the first Stress Test or the first day at school after a (mostly) long school absence, patients typically face the question "What's your disease?" Over the years, we have found a quite simple answer that totally ignores the background of the pain disorder but protects the patient. If there is good reason not to explain the pain disorder in detail to classmates and teachers (as will be in almost all cases), this might be a helpful answer:

> **Example: Explanation of the Pain Disorder to Classmates and Teachers**
> "At last I found a pain clinic that succeeded in diagnosing my disease. The official name is much too complicated to remember, so you just have to know that it is a type of pain-disease. They taught me to how to cope with it. You would help me by not asking about my pain anymore, but approaching me as normally as possible. This would be the very best for me."

That explanation is good for most children. As is the case with relatives, the "fact sheet for teachers" from the parent's guide "How to stop chronic pain in children: a practical guide" has proved helpful. However, it should only be handed over to teachers really interested in the child and his/her pain disorder. In case the teacher asks for a talk with the physician or psychotherapist, one should discuss with the child and his parents *in advance and in detail* what information should be given to the teacher. We proactively offer a talk to the school counselor or the principal in case the school is questioning whether to exclude the child from classes, and the parents see no way of dealing with this themselves.

6.6.8   Pain Therapy in Families with a Migration Background

A person has a migration background (MB) if he/she moved from abroad or was born in this country but at least one of his/her parents is a foreigner. The migration background can have an influence on the expression of pain. According to Ellert et al. (2011), in Germany children with MB report significantly more headache during the last 3 years compared to children without MB. This is in accordance with the results of one other European study on this issue (Bugdayci et al. 2005).

Adults from North American or North European origin seem to express their pain less emphatically than adults from more southern origins (Greenwald 1991). According to our clinical experience, children with MB tend to show their pain more openly. One should accept these differences as culture specific and let the affected families know that they are taken seriously. For therapy planning in general, quality and intensity of pain expression are not that important.

In some families with MB, at least one of the parents has difficulties with the native language or doesn't speak the native language at all. In this case the children often act as interpreters. This is unfavorable for pain therapy aiming at behavioral changes in the family's everyday life. An affected child is not in the best position to translate for his parents, who are often somatically fixated. Furthermore, it's simply not possible for children to translate complex relationships concerning themselves. In rare cases, neither of the parents speaks the native language at all. If only one of the parents speaks the native language a little, there is the risk that the parent will translate only those parts of the discussion to his partner that he/she understands and that fit into his/her view of things. The only professional approach is to ask for a professional interpreter in order to establish some understanding of chronic pain. Apart from its sometimes substantial costs, such an intervention is not without problems. Involving a neutral interpreter might make (mostly) the father feel reproached, his language competence devalued. One should know that it is quite difficult to discuss family conflicts or the child's stressful problems with a stranger, the interpreter, present.

A culturally different distribution of gender roles also means a challenge for pain therapy, for instance, if an adolescent girl opposes the traditional role model, provoking substantial family conflicts. Such a situation is especially difficult since parents are often not ready to discuss those problems or they deny them. Here pain therapy is charged with social problems that cannot always be satisfactorily resolved.

We endeavor to discuss any consequences regarding the patient's life openly. However, a satisfactory solution cannot always be found, but at least some kind of approximation can be attempted. It is good for therapy if continual (pain) psychotherapy following the inpatient treatment can be done by a psychotherapist with the same cultural roots as the family. If the family conflicts are severe, the only solution is to contact the responsible youth welfare service (Sect. 6.6.5).

Many traditional cultures in which the individual's independence of action is subject to a fatalistic or religious interpretation lack an understanding of underlying psychological concepts. In this case it may be helpful to just briefly justify some therapeutic interventions and instead focus on precise instructions for how to do the exercise. It is our experience that irrespective of culture-specific or religious characteristics, lasting changes in family behavior towards active pain coping are more improbable with language barriers between the professional team and the family (lack of understanding) and with families who prefer maintaining their cultural or religious standards over individual well-being (rigidity of thinking).

6.7 Inpatient Pain Therapy: Module 5 (Optional Interventions)

For inpatient pain therapy, we recommend the very close cooperation of the child and his family with selected professions instead of a less intensive cooperation with numerous professions. There is the old saying, "Too many cooks spoil the broth" which is also true in pain therapy. According to their developmental state, children need clear-cut structures and defined contacts, which are reliably accessible. And what is important to the child is also important to his/her parents. Furthermore, therapeutic binding is an unspecific but highly effective tool for successful pain therapy. Our concept of an intensive pain therapy with denominated primary carers meets this requirement. In consequence, other therapeutic options (physiotherapy, social service, body psychotherapy, music or art therapy) are less and exclusively used when indicated. It goes without saying that in musculoskeletal pain, physiotherapy is a crucial treatment modality.

6.7.1 Physiotherapy

Physiotherapy is used whenever advanced chronicity along with avoidance behavior results in impaired functioning or movement. Many of the affected children underwent physiotherapy mostly as a passive procedure, as well as massages, which they enjoyed but were not helpful in the long run. In pain therapy, physiotherapy aims at enhanced active pain coping. The patients should learn exercises they can practice on their own. Not indicated is an increase in the proportion of passive interventions like massage, application of heat, or other solely passive techniques aiming to decrease muscular tension. In the short term, massage is perceived as soothing and has its place in sports medicine or acute local muscular hypertension, miraculously delivering relief. But, massage is not highly effective in chronic muscular hypertension.

Massage also conveys the wrong message, since the primary issue in children with chronic pain is their activation (and decreasing the amount of passive behavior) – "I will do" instead of "You take my pain". This is not the place to describe the various physiotherapeutic techniques and interventions in detail. Instead, we want to focus on the optimization of the cooperation between physiotherapist (independent of his subspecialization), physician, and psychotherapist. We feel the following four aspects are most important:

1. In order to ensure good communication between the physiotherapist and the staff on the ward, the physiotherapist should attend the ward round once a week – at least during the time when his/her patients are discussed. This will allow him/her to get some idea of the underlying biological, psychological, or social aspects of the pain disorder and to better understand the aspects contributing to the development of the impaired functioning and movement. Problems concerning the patient's motivation or sudden regression or progress will be explained in the context of therapy. Any divergent observations of staff and physiotherapist may be directly discussed; the physiotherapist helps the staff understand which movements the child is actually able to do, and to what degree, or which movements are still severely impaired. Together they set up physiotherapeutic exercises that can be practiced on the ward once or several times a day in a graduated scheme.

> **Case Report**
> A boy with CRPS type I in his right foot had to relearn to walk. After having made many small steps of progress, the task was now to set the foot on the ground and to gradually do without the crutches. It was the child's wish to keep one of the crutches for now. But this wish had to be rejected after consultation with the physiotherapist. Rightfully she pointed out that the unilateral weight on the back musculature counteracts the targeted functional improvement.

2. We feel, that it is beneficial to separate professionally led physiotherapy from practice during the daily routine guided by the NET. Stepwise training on the ward simulates life at home quite well, and any motivational problems may be addressed and solved since from everyday attendance the NET knows the child better than the physiotherapist. Frequently the patients talk about fearful or stressful situations especially during times of increased mental tension while practicing their graduated scheme with its inevitable increase in pain. Then it is important for the patient to be emotionally supported by the staff trained in communication and handling of the patient (NET), who will also pass that information onto the physician or psychotherapist in charge.

3. We would like to point out another very important aspect. From their daily work, physiotherapists are used to discussing the background underlying the active exercises. Usually this is alright. *Under no circumstances*, however, should the physiotherapist offer the child monocausal hypotheses to his/her disease, be it blockade, muscular imbalance, muscular tension, trigger points, etc. Most children (and their parents) are stuck in the Second Thought Trap and tearfully tell their parents

about the physiotherapist's "latest discoveries." "The physiotherapist said, such a crooked spine must hurt." Of course, all consulting professions should be cautious with any monocausal model. Any observation made by the physiotherapist is an important contribution to treatment. It should not be directly communicated to the child but to the staff during the ward round in order to discuss its relevance first.

In children with chronic musculoskeletal pain, physiotherapy is an indispensable part of inpatient therapy. The individual benefit of active physiotherapeutic measures embedded into a multimodal treatment program (*not* as a solitary exercise) has been scientifically proven (Ayling Campos et al. 2011). For best treatment success and to ensure a satisfying working environment, both the clear-cut division of the different responsibilities and the establishment of defined communication structures have proved invaluable.

6.7.2 Body Psychotherapy

During inpatient treatment at the GPPC, sometimes we use body psychotherapy techniques. Their indication is primarily with children with traumatic or depressive symptoms next to their pain condition, e.g., experiences with violence or sexual abuse. Before that part of therapy (e.g., Feldenkrais therapy, therapeutic breathing techniques) is started, the aims are discussed with the psychotherapist in charge. Mostly the aim is to let the patient again experience his/her body as a resource. The patient normally rates these exercises as pleasant and helpful. Other methods playfully train the patient's ability to regulate proximity and distance and to nonverbally build a positive image of his body and strengthen his self-confidence.

6.7.3 Art Therapy and Musical Therapy

Art therapy or musical therapy may be indicated sometimes. First of all, both methods are used as supplemental techniques in children that are interested in nonverbal expression. Both methods encourage the children to express themselves with respect to certain issues (family situation, emotions, etc.) by means of different media. The idea is that those methods make it easier for the child to feel and talk about difficult emotional issues and to make them accessible to the child. The instrumental communication during musical therapy allows the child to nonverbally practice listening to other people and follow their play and then to place him/herself, his/her feelings, and personality into focus, leading to an alteration of pacing and leading. Art therapy encourages the child, e.g., by painting his/her pain, e.g., a Pain Fighter or a "Safe Place," to actively engage in pain coping using his/her artistic abilities. The resulting paintings may be used in individual therapies to practice imaginative technique (Sect. 6.4.2).

6.7.4 Social Workers

As with physiotherapy, including a social worker with certain patients is essential. Social workers are engaged in 5–10 % of our inpatient cases (Sect. 6.6.5).

The practical approach of the social worker on the ward, in the family talk, or in the support after discharge is very much dependent on the individual case. For many of the patients, it was very helpful that they were given the opportunity to get accurate information on possible outpatient, day-care, or inpatient options of the youth welfare service meeting the individual's needs. Based on that information, they were able to set up a plan together with their psychotherapist on how to proceed with their treatment. Most parents regard it as supportive if social workers participate in family talks, particularly broaching the issue of the youth welfare service, since they get concrete and reliable answers to their questions. Just making the formal application for help overburdens many of these families, and it is a relief for the child and his/her family to know that there is someone available to support them, not only during but also after their stay on the ward. The social worker may offer support with applications or in responding to a rejection letter. If the child and his/her family give us permission in writing regarding medical confidentiality and the responsible youth welfare service, this will allow us to accelerate the processing of their application, both by phone and by writing a letter. In selected cases the social worker will offer to accompany the child and/or the family to the responsible youth welfare office. Of course either the social worker or the psychotherapist in charge will attend if a first care planning discussion with the youth welfare service is scheduled.

6.7.5   Drug-Based Pain Treatment

This section presents the most often used analgesics, their modes of action, and adverse effects. Their usage should be limited to pain due to inflammation or physical disease proven to be responsive to analgesics (target setting, patient contract).

As part of the evaluation of our inpatient pain therapy program, we analyzed changes in drug use (Hechler et al. 2009) (Table 6.5). On admission, one-third of the 119 patients did not use any analgesic and did not start taking analgesics during therapy. Another third of the patients were on analgesics at the beginning, but discontinued taking drugs. Presumably, in those 39 patients there had never been any indication for analgesics. In the last third of the patients, drug-based analgesia was initiated (mostly in previously undiagnosed migraine) or continued during the inpatient stay because there was a clear indication to do so.

Table 6.5 Drug usage 3 months after discharge from the GPPC

$N=119$	$N\ (\%)$	NSAIDs	Other non-opioids	Triptanes	Opioids	Co-analgesics
No previous analgesic	40 (34)	–	–	–	–	–
Analgesic discontinued	39 (33)	16	18	1	3	1
Analgesic continued	32 (27)	21	2	9	0	0
Analgesic newly started	8 (7)	6	1	1	0	0

NSAID non-steroidal anti-inflammatory drugs

The results of another study comprising 2,249 paediatric pain patients presenting in a 5-year period at our outpatient pain clinic were similar. Ninety percent of the patients had taken analgesics in the past, while 76 % had taken analgesics during the 3 months preceding first presentation. In only 57 % of the patients taking drugs did pain therapists rate drug-based analgesia as indicated and recommend continuation. In other words, *43 % of the patients were on analgesics without any benefit* (Zernikow et al. 2012).

6.7.5.1 Triptans

The chemical structure of triptans is similar to serotonin, and their action is mediated by the activation of serotonin receptors. Triptans are approved for the treatment of migraine and cluster headache. They are used both in adults and children.

Mechanism of Action

Like serotonin, triptans are agonists at both the 5-HT_{1B} and 5-HT_{1D} receptor. Activation of these receptors has two main effects. The blood vessels dilated during a migraine attack constrict, and the secretion of proinflammatory peptides (i.e., substance P, calcitonin gene-related peptide (CGRP)) from CNS neurons is reduced, inhibiting the spreading of pain stimuli along the cortex. Triptans are also agonists at the 5-HT_{1F} receptor. Activation of that receptor reduces the secretion of certain vaso-inactive peptides.

Adverse Effects

Adverse effects of triptans are weakness, dizziness, paresthesia, sensations of warmth or heat, or nausea. Sometimes a transitory increase in arterial blood pressure is observed that is mediated by the activation of $5\text{-HT}_{1B/1D}$ receptors of the cardiovascular system. Seldom reported are dysrhythmia, disturbed blood circulation, or effects on skeletal muscles.

Interactions

If combined with migraine medication based on ergot alkaloids (i.e., ergotamine), there is an increased risk of coronary spasms. Hence, such a combination is contraindicated. Triptans may interact with antidepressants from the selective serotonin reuptake inhibitor family (SNRI) like duloxetine or venlafaxine. Monoamine oxidase inhibitors slow down triptan metabolism.

Under certain circumstances, serotonin may accumulate in the nerve system to a critical level with potentially life-threatening consequences. This serotonin syndrome may present with restlessness, hallucinations, loss of coordination, tachycardia, fluctuating arterial blood pressure, increased body temperature, increased reflexes, nausea, vomiting, or diarrhea.

Contraindications

Triptans must not be used in arterial hypertension or vascular diseases, especially not in coronary artery disease.

6.7.5.2 Opioids

It is still under dispute if opioids should be used only in tumor diseases or also in adults with non-tumor pain, such as backache or joint arthrosis (Stein et al. 2010; Noble et al. 2010). Opioids play only a minor role in multimodal pain therapy of children and adolescents with chronic pain.

Mechanism of Action

The analgesic effect of opioids is mediated via opioid receptors present in high density in the CNS. In the human, endogenous opioid peptides (encephalines and endorphins) can activate those receptors and inhibit nociceptive afferences. Morphine and other exogenous opioid analgesics also bind to those receptors, mimicking the effect of endogenous opioids. The analgesic effect of opioids is mediated by several mechanisms:

1. Dampening of the limbic system reduces affective pain processing, and the patient perceives the pain as less threatening.
2. Activation of descending pain-inhibiting tracts.
3. Inhibition of the conduction of ascending nociceptive signals at the spinal level.

Opioid receptors are categorized into several subclasses. The opioid's pattern of receptor activation explains the individual profile of effect and adverse effect.

The μ_1-receptor is exclusively found presynaptically. Its activation results in a decrease of Ca++ influx into the cell and a reduced release of neurotransmitters responsible for pain signal conduction. Thus, activation of the μ_1-receptor has a predominantly analgesic effect.

The μ_2-receptor is mainly found postsynaptically. Its activation results in an increased probability that K+ channels will open with subsequent hyperpolarization. Activation of the μ_2 receptor leads to decreased pCO_2 reactivity and may lead to respiratory depression. Since there are intestinal μ_2 receptors, their activation leads to a prolonged intestinal passage, increasing the risk of constipation.

Adverse Effects

Activation of the μ-receptor reduces propulsive peristalsis and may result in gastro-intestinal disturbances like delayed emptying of the stomach, nausea, vomiting, or constipation. Sometimes bladder emptying dysfunction or urinary retention is observed, as are heat sensations and lowering of the seizure threshold. Gradual respiratory depression is already seen in normal analgesic doses. If the opioid dose is increased too fast and not titrated to the pain score, there is the risk of disturbed vigilance up to somnolence, coma, or death. If the opioid dose is titrated to actual pain and effect, the body will adapt to even the highest doses.

Due to adaptation, some opioids require regular dose escalation (this is especially the case with synthetic opioids used in intensive care). There is no adaptation with regard to the adverse effects of constipation. Since opioids are also psychotomimetic (reducing anxiety, etc.), opioid therapy may result in opioid addiction, especially if fast-acting preparations are used (immediate release droplets, fast intravenous injection, etc.) since the fast flooding in the CNS has strong psychoto-mimetic (adverse) effects. The risk for addiction is reduced with slow release preparations, due to their delay in effect. Physical dependency is *always* observed in opioid therapy, since the body habituates itself to external opioids and will react with symptoms of withdrawal if the opioid is suddenly stopped. Any opioid therapy lasting more than a week must be tapered.

Contraindications
Contraindications and interactions of the various opioids are not necessarily identical (for details, see the individual drug sheet). Due to their risk of addiction, most of the opioids are subject to regulatory restrictions on their availability and accessibility that differ from country to country. Patients with a history of addiction are especially endangered.

6.7.5.3 Nonsteroidal Anti-inflammatory Drugs (NSAIDs)
Mechanism of Action
Nonsteroidal anti-inflammatory drugs like ibuprofen quite unselectively inhibit the enzymes cyclooxygenase I and II which results in an inhibition of prostaglandin synthesis. Prostaglandins as mediators of inflammation are involved in the generation of pain signals. Those mechanisms explain why nonsteroidal anti-inflammatory drugs exert analgesic, antiphlogistic, and antipyretic effects. Due to its antiphlogistic activity, ibuprofen is the drug of choice to begin with.

Adverse Effects
The unspecific inhibition of prostaglandin synthesis results in an altered composition of the protective mucus layer of the stomach's mucous membrane and in impaired platelet aggregation which explains the ulcerations and bleeding from the mucous membrane seen especially after prolonged use of those drugs. Since ibuprofen impairs renal perfusion, renal insufficiency is a contraindication for this drug. A number of adverse effects which are not all mediated by inhibition of cyclooxygenases are only seen after treatment for 1 week or longer. If given for only 3 days or less or just once as in migraine, NSAIDs are very well tolerated.

6.7.5.4 Gabapentin
In the treatment of neuropathic pain, apart from the local application of lidocaine (e.g., Versatis®, not suitable for all skin areas), other drugs are used that originally were developed for the treatment of epilepsy. Both gabapentin and pregabalin act by regulating calcium channels.

Indications
Gabapentin is used to treat neuropathic pain as observed with post-herpetic neuralgia where pain persists for up to several months with the herpetic exanthema having already vanished.

Gabapentin is also used in the treatment of neuropathic pain in diabetic polyneuropathy and that of phantom pain.

Mechanism of Action

In impaired peripheral nerves, the calcium channels become increasingly dysregulated, resulting in spontaneous depolarization of the affected fiber. Important in the context of pain therapy are the membrane stabilizing features of gabapentin with concomitant inhibition of calcium channels. Gabapentin also inhibits the glutamate-mediated signal transmission.

Adverse Effects

The most frequent adverse effects are tiredness, dizziness, headache, nausea, vomiting, increase in bodyweight, nervousness, insomnia, ataxia, nystagmus, paresthesia, or altered appetite. The blood smear may be altered with leuco- or thrombocytopenia, and there are mental symptoms that may arise such as anxiety, depression, hallucinations, thought disorder, or amentia.

Interactions

The simultaneous intake of antacids based on calcium or magnesium may influence the bioavailability of gabapentin.

6.7.5.5 Pregabalin

Pregabalin shows less interaction with other drugs than gabapentin, which makes pregabalin more suitable for a combination therapy.

Mechanism of Action

In the CNS, pregabalin binds to a subunit of voltage-dependent calcium channels, restricting the influx of calcium ions into the neuronal endings, thus normalizing the secretion of noradrenaline and substance P. Therefore, pregabalin is used both as an anticonvulsant and in the treatment of neuropathic pain.

Adverse Effects

The most frequent adverse effects, especially at the beginning of treatment, are dizziness, tiredness, drowsiness, and lack of concentration. Blurred vision, double image, disturbance of equilibrium, nausea, and vomiting are also observed, and occasionally reported are muscle cramps, dysrhythmia, weakness, or falls.

6.7.5.6 Amitriptyline

Amitriptyline is approved for the treatment of depression and for long-term analgesia in chronic pain. Due to its proved effectiveness in the prophylaxis of adult migraine, amitriptyline is used with this indication. In children and adolescents, it proved *ineffective* for prophylaxis.

Mechanism of Action

In the CNS, amitriptyline unselectively inhibits monoamine reuptake from the synaptic gap into the presynaptic neuron, leading to an increased neurotransmitter concentration (serotonin and noradrenaline) in the synaptic gap.

Adverse Effects

The most frequent adverse effects of amitriptyline are neurologic (i.e., headache, dizziness, tremor, drowsiness), cardiovascular (i.e., palpitation, tachycardia, orthostatic hypotonia), gastrointestinal (i.e., dry mouth, constipation, nausea), increase in bodyweight, blurred vision/disturbed accommodation, or increased sweating. Other central nervous adverse effects are paresthesia, ataxia, or tiredness. The most frequent mental disturbances seen under amitriptyline are amentia and a lack of concentration. Finally, ECG alterations like AV block or other conduction disorders were observed.

Interactions

The combination of amitriptyline and MAO inhibitors may lead to the life-threatening serotonin syndrome. If amitriptyline is used in conjunction with drugs affecting QT-time (i.e., macrolides), there is a risk of prolonged QT-time with dysrhythmia, torsades de pointes, or sinus tachycardia.

6.8 Inpatient Pain Therapy: Module 6 (Planning the Time After Discharge)

At the end of the patient's stay, it is the physician's or primary psychotherapist's responsibility to set up a treatment plan together with the patient and parents for the time after discharge. This plan is based on the previous course of treatment. With a complex mental or psychosocial stress situation, we recommend already discussing that plan in the middle of the stay in order to allow the child to grapple with his own aims and wishes regarding that time.

6.8.1 Relapse Prevention

At the end of his/her stay, the child points out which intervention was helpful, which one he/she would like to continue, and if there is need for family support for the further implementation of the learned interventions. Since the discharge talk with the whole family is scheduled after the last single therapeutic session, the psychotherapist discusses family interventions with the child, which from the child's point of view might help avoid a relapse (e.g., the child's wish for a special psychotherapeutic pain treatment of his/her parent with a pain disorder). In addition to the discussion of the treatment plan (Sect. 6.8.2), the following three interventions proved helpful for relapse prophylaxis:

1. Again, the child and his/her family are explicitly referred to the fact, already taught in our education sessions, that a pain disorder means increased pain sensitization, which implies that the child will have a higher risk of experiencing more pain during a common cold or injury than those without a pain disorder. Due to the patient's medical history, distinct pain sensitization and concomitant fatigue are to be expected during the months following discharge. *Increased pain perception*, e.g., *when attending school again, should never result in a relapse to passive pain coping strategies.* Anticipating any hypothetical increase in

symptomatology in conjunction with a detailed action plan will help the child and his/her family to master the time after discharge.

2. Many children are very exhausted from the incessant burden during the previous years and seem to be more prone to infections. After discharge from the ward, it is possible that these children are more prone to catching viral infections. Of course fever is a somatic alarm signal demanding rest and perhaps a visit to the child's physician. If indicated and prescribed by the physician, analgesics are allowed during those infections. A feverish infection will often lead to a combination of severe pain, pronounced passivity, and exhaustion. This carries the increased risk of reactivating former behavioral patterns. Already in the discharge talk, the parents are told that after the second day without fever, all regular activities should be performed *irrespective* of pain intensity or exhaustion. If this agreement is not followed (generally, 2 days absent from school allowed if fever has disappeared), the parents will call the GPPC and an appointment in the outpatient clinic will be made in order to support the family in the implementation of what was learned on the ward.

3. It should be decided which member of the family will contact our outpatient pain clinic and for which specific problems. The threshold for calling the clinic should be set high to make it clear that not every difficulty arising from everyday life automatically has to result in a plea for professional help.

6.8.2   Therapy Plan

During the discharge talk, we determine *who* is responsible *for what, when, and where* regarding the implementation of therapeutic techniques at home or elsewhere. This information is recorded in the patient's chart as well as in the discharge letter. We also record which strategies the child has chosen to implement until the outpatient appointment is scheduled 3 months after discharge and to what degree the parents will participate in the implementation of active measures. In the discharge talk we frequently have to point out that the parents have the difficult task of doing *nothing* (besides promoting active coping and encouraging their child) since they can't do anything. Naturally this is more difficult for them than actively doing something for their child's relief. Thus, we compliment the parents for already having tried to abstain from action and ask them to be forgiving of themselves if they did not succeed. At the GPPC the child's primary psychotherapist is always present when the patient returns for follow-up.

6.8.3   Special Case: Readmission

In some cases after discharge, the patient may relapse. When this occurs it is necessary to openly discuss the possible reasons in order to evaluate whether a second inpatient treatment might contribute to a solution.

Before readmission, it is essential to have the outpatient appointment together with the patient, his/her parents, and the primary psychotherapist of the former inpatient stay, since that psychotherapist is most familiar with the relevant intrapsychic and interpersonal issues. Together we explore if readmission is necessary and if it makes sense. If the answer to both questions is "yes," the aims for the following stay should be negotiated and fixed during that appointment. We strongly recommend *not* just adopting the aims from the former stay. Instead, one should focus on the factors that hindered the implementation of the learned techniques at home or that allowed for reactivation of the pain disease. This means that during the second stay one should focus more on those features of the child that hampered his/her development to more autonomy, or on a more intense training of coping with the daily hassles or distress, irrespective of the actual pain intensity. Since readmission usually means more intense psychotherapeutic interventions, a second stay will be even more demanding than the first one. This should be made clear in advance.

Sometimes the child or his/her parents are ambivalent with respect to readmission. Then we advise them to "apply" for readmission, writing down their aims of therapy and how much effort they are willing to invest. Depending on the patient's age we expect detailed information. Such an approach seems hard, but it is our experience that clarifying those questions before readmission is essential to making the stay a success.

Case Report: Maren (17 Years), Pain Disease with Headache, Light Depressive Episode

At an outpatient appointment 12 months after discharge from inpatient pain therapy, Maren and her parents reported that her pain and mood had very much deteriorated again. Since the time on the ward "had been very good for Maren," Maren and her parents asked for readmission. Maren was currently suffering a light depressive episode which presented as a joylessness, loss of motivation, and difficulties in falling asleep. During the outpatient appointment, Maren expressed the view that she would like "to see us again." But, since she couldn't imagine any reason why there was a relapse, she was unable to say how the aims set during last pain therapy should be modified so that she could sustain her improvement (or success). So we asked both Maren and her parents to write down their modified aims of therapy as well as their speculations about the factors perpetuating Maren's negative mood and pain and mail them to us before we could make any decision. While the parents were doing their homework, Maren wrote the following letter.

Maren's Letter

"I can't tell you what exactly contributed to my impairment in the last few weeks. I wish I could relearn how to better cope with my pain, and how to get more self-confidence, as I did during my last stay. Maybe some new techniques to handle my problems. For the time afterwards – after my second stay at the clinic – I wish to be able to practice the learned techniques and to better manage my problems."

We rated this letter as insufficient. Maren seemed to have problems precisely naming the various factors contributing to her current situation and her relapse. Hence, we decided to pose our questions more precisely in a letter to Maren.

Our Letter to Maren in Response

"Dear Maren, many thanks for your letter. To better prepare your readmission, we need more precise information. The problem is that we can't just do the same things as last time. Since you answered our questions the best you could, we decided on posing more precise questions. We beg your pardon that we didn't already do so during our last appointment. So please answer the following questions and send us back the answers in writing:

  1) At the moment, what makes you feel sad when thinking of friends?
  2) At the moment, what makes you feel sad when thinking of school?
  3) At the moment, what makes you feel sad when thinking of your pain?
  4) At the moment, what makes you feel sad when thinking of your mother?
  5) At the moment, what makes you feel sad when thinking of your father?
  6) At the moment, what makes you feel sad when thinking of your future?
  7) At the moment, what makes you feel sad when thinking of yourself?
  8) How well do you generally cope with distress?
  9) How many stress-days will you need on the ward?
10) Let's leave the pain out. What do you think you still have to learn to lead a happier life in future?

  Finally, a very specific request: Will you and your parents please organize outpatient psychotherapy? As we did the last time, we will focus on doing the first steps towards active pain and distress coping. We are sure you will be able to do those steps on the ward. But, 3 weeks is not enough time to learn to stabilize your mood on your own forever. Usually after discharge, ambulatory support is needed for a while. There is still some time left until we see you again. So take the time you need to answer our questions."

One week later, we received a nice and much longer letter from Maren with all the required answers that enabled us to better prepare the second inpatient stay. Following is a small segment of the letter:

"It makes me sad that I often have the feeling that I will soon lose my friends because I'm not good enough for therm. …The way I behave, I think I bother them and they soon won't want to have anything more to do with me. At school I'm always asked to say something, but I don't dare because I think I'll just answer wrongly. …I feel sad and unmotivated because of my continuing headaches. That's why I'm often afraid that I'm disappointing my parents and can't achieve what they want of me."

We have found it very important early on to be as clear as possible about how much active cooperation is required from the child and his/her family. Especially in children with a more passive attitude and/or depressive symptomatology, you will discover the resources but also the disease-perpetuating negative factors still present in the child and the family system that will be discovered when proceeding as outlined.

In some very rare cases, it may make sense to schedule a date for readmission at the time of discharge. Between discharge and readmission, there should also be an outpatient appointment 4–6 weeks after discharge. Prescheduling these appointments is a source of security for the child and his/her family, especially for children with distinct rare pain disorders (i.e., CRPS type I and II), or an extreme degree of chronicity, together with substantial psychosocial stress factors present. To minimize the risk that those patients get too closely attached to the ward, we indicate to the patient that this will be a unique intervention to consolidate the treatment effect in order to find a trade-off between the four aspects outlined in the following paragraphs:

1. Rightfully so, the health insurance will insist on an outpatient treatment when inpatient pain therapy isn't indicated anymore.
2. Between the two inpatient treatments, both the child and his/her family have the chance to discover which individual factors are helpful or dysfunctional during the absence of the therapy which provided a highly structured life. This will enable them to better substantiate any wishes on how to proceed with outpatient treatment. It is essential to communicate this strategy in advance with the family. Nevertheless, in spite of many doubts ("Can we stand it?"; "Isn't it too early now?"; "Shouldn't we have waited another fortnight before discharging our daughter?") for the families described above, it is a relief to have a second inpatient treatment already scheduled at discharge. This gives the child and his/her family the opportunity to try out the long-term implementation of the learned measures at home without pressure. If the parents are not successful in implementing the learned inpatient measures at home with their child, there is the danger with CRPS of a permanent impairment of the affected body part, be it hand or foot. On the other hand a planned readmission offers psychosocially highly burdened families at escalation level 1–3 (Sect. 6.6.5) and who are very skeptical of youth social services outpatient measures, the possibility of first trying out the interventions themselves.
3. When chronicity persists, sometimes the families request an extension of the inpatient treatment course, since it is "so good" for the child, so that any treatment success can be "stabilized." Certainly, in some children it seems reasonable to extend their stay by a couple of days (e.g., to allow them to pass another Stress Test). We feel that any additional extension is useless and will not be a solution in the long run. Apart from supporting the child in his/her tendency to avoid the exposure to everyday life in the family or at school, a prolonged inpatient stay is counterproductive since we want to avoid the possibility that the child will feel safer in the institution than at home. Such a development would be also detrimental to the patients, and, if fearful, they might intensify their complaints in order to postpone the day of discharge.
4. Some pain disorders are progressive, for example, CRPS, and require inpatient readmission after a short interval if in the course of outpatient treatment, a

renewed deterioration occurs. In order to allow the child and his/her family enough leeway to use individual resources in case of difficulties arising during the subsequent outpatient treatment course (and not want readmission as soon as the first problems arise), an ethically sound trade-off is to aim for readmission 8–10 weeks after discharge, in case of relapsing symptoms.

6.9   Therapy of Pain Disorders in Children and Adolescents: Conclusion

At a time of limited human resources and a shift to technical medicine, the inpatient pain therapy program of the GPPC with its personnel-intensive multimodal approach focusing on the child and his/her family may seem to be a relic from the past. However, it is exactly these human approaches that make the program so successful.

References

Asmundson GJ, Norton PJ, Nortöon GR (1999) Beyond pain: the role of fear and avoidance in chronicity. Clin Psychol Rev 19(1):97–119

Asmundson GJ, Coons MJ, Taylor S, Katz J (2002) PTSD and the experience of pain: research and clinical implications of shared vulnerability and mutual maintenance models. Can J Psychiatry 47(10):930–937

Asmundson GJ, Noel M, Petter M, Parkerson HA (2012) Pediatric fear-avoidance model of chronic pain: foundation, application and future directions. Pain Res Manag 17(6):397–405

Ayling Campos A, Amaria K, Campbell F, McGrath PA (2011) Clinical impact and evidence base for physiotherapy in treating childhood chronic pain. Physiother Can 63(1):21–33

Bailey KM, Carleton RN, Vlaeyen JW, Asmundson GJ (2010) Treatments addressing pain-related fear and anxiety in patients with chronic musculoskeletal pain: a preliminary review. Cogn Behav Ther 39(1):46–63

Barsky AJ, Wyshak G, Klerman GL (1990) The somatosensory amplification scale and its relationship to hypochondriasis. J Psychiatr Res 24:323–334

Bugdayci R, Ozge A, Sasmaz T, Kurt AO, Kaleagasi H, Karakelle A et al (2005) Prevalence and factors affecting headache in Turkish schoolchildren. Pediatr Int 47(3):316–322

Craske MG, Wolitzky-Taylor KB, Labus J, Wu S, Frese M, Mayer EA et al (2011) A cognitive-behavioral treatment for irritable bowel syndrome using interoceptive exposure to visceral sensations. Behav Res Ther 49(6–7):413–421

Crombez G, Bijttebier P, Eccleston C, Mascagni T, Mertens G, Goubert L et al (2003) The child version of the pain catastrophizing scale (PCS-C): a preliminary validation. Pain 104(3):639–646

Crombez G, Van Damme S, Eccleston C (2005) Hypervigilance to pain: an experimental and clinical analysis. Pain 116(1–2):4–7

Crombez G, Eccleston C, Van Damme S, Vlaeyen JW, Karoly P (2012) Fear-avoidance model of chronic pain: the next generation. Clin J Pain 28(6):475–483

De Peuter S, Van Diest I, Vansteenwegen D, Van den Bergh O, Vlaeyen JW (2011) Understanding fear of pain in chronic pain: interoceptive fear conditioning as a novel approach. Eur J Pain 15(9):889–894

Dobe M, Zernikow B (2013) How to stop chronic pain in children: a practical guide. Carl-Auer-Verlag, Heidelberg

Dobe M, Hechler T, Zernikow B (2009) The pain provocation technique as an adjunctive treatment module for children and adolescents with chronic disabling pain: a case report. J Child Adolesc Trauma 2(4):297–307

Dobe M, Hechler T, Behlert J, Kosfelder J, Zernikow B (2011) Pain therapy with children and adolescents severely disabled due to chronic pain: long-term outcome after inpatient pain therapy. Schmerz 25(4):411–422

Domschke K, Stevens S, Pfleiderer B, Gerlach AL (2010) Interoceptive sensitivity in anxiety and anxiety disorders: an overview and integration of neurobiological findings. Clin Psychol Rev 30:1–11

Eccleston C, Crombez G, Aldrich S, Stannard C (1997) Attention and somatic awareness in chronic pain. Pain 72(1–2):209–215

Eccleston C, Crombez G (2007) Worry and chronic pain: a misdirected problem solving model. Pain 132(3):233–236

Eccleston C, Malleson P (2003) Managing chronic pain in children and adolescents. We need to address the embarrassing lack of data for this common problem. BMJ 326(7404):1408–1409

Ellert U, Ravens-Sieberer U, Erhart M, Kurth BM (2011) Determinants of agreement between self-reported and parent-assessed quality of life for children in Germany-results of the German Health Interview and Examination Survey for Children and Adolescents (KiGGS). Health Qual Life Outcomes 9:102

Feinstein AB, Forman EM, Masuda A, Cohen LL, Herbert JD, Moorthy LN et al (2011) Pain intensity, psychological inflexibility, and acceptance of pain as predictors of functioning in adolescents with juvenile idiopathic arthritis: a preliminary investigation. J Clin Psychol Med Settings 18(3):291–298

Flink IK, Nicholas MK, Boersma K, Linton SJ (2009) Reducing the threat value of chronic pain: a preliminary replicated single-case study of interoceptive exposure versus distraction in six individuals with chronic back pain. Behav Res Ther 47(8):721–728

Forgeron PA, McGrath P, Stevens B, Evans J, Dick B, Finley GA et al (2011) Social information processing in adolescents with chronic pain: my friends don't really understand me. Pain 152(12):2773–2780

Goubert L, Craig KD, Vervoort T, Morley S, Sullivan MJ, de Williams AC et al (2005) Facing others in pain: the effects of empathy. Pain 118(3):285–288

Goubert L, Eccleston C, Vervoort T, Jordan A, Crombez G (2006) Parental catastrophizing about their child's pain. The parent version of the Pain Catastrophizing Scale (PCS-P): a preliminary validation. Pain 123(3):254–263

Greenwald HP (1991) Interethnic differences in pain perception. Pain 44(2):157–163

Gregory RJ, Manring J, Berry SL (2000) Pain location and psychological characteristics of patients with chronic pain. Psychosomatics 41(3):216–220

Haggard P, Wolpert DM (2005) Disorders of body scheme. In: Freund HJ, Jeannerod M, Hallett M, Liguarda R (eds) Higher-order motor disorders. Oxford University Press, Oxford

Hechler T, Dobe M, Kosfelder J, Damschen U, Hübner B, Blankenburg M et al (2009) Effectiveness of a three-week multimodal inpatient pain treatment for adolescents suffering from chronic pain: statistical and clinical significance. Clin J Pain 25(2):156–166

Hechler T, Dobe M, Damschen U, Schroeder S, Kosfelder J, Zernikow B (2010) The pain provocation technique for adolescents with chronic pain: preliminary evidence for its effectiveness. Pain Med 11(6):297–310

Hechler T, Vervoort T, Hamann M, Tietze AL, Vocks S, Goubert L et al (2011) Parental catastrophizing about their child's chronic pain: are mothers and fathers different? Eur J Pain 15(5):515. e1–515.e9

Hermann C, Hohmeister J, Demirakça S, Zohsel K, Flor H (2006) Long-term alteration of pain sensitivity in school-aged children with early pain experiences. Pain 125(3):278–285

Hohmeister J, Kroll A, Wollgarten-Hadamek I, Zohsel K, Demirakça S, Flor H et al (2010) Cerebral processing of pain in school-aged children with neonatal nociceptive input: an exploratory fMRI study. Pain 150(2):257–267

Katzer A, Oberfeld D, Hiller W, Gerlach AL, Witthöft M (2012) Tactile perceptual processes and their relationship to somatoform disorders. J Abnorm Psychol 121:530–543

Kuttner L (1997) Mind-body methods of pain management. Child Adolesc Psychiatr Clin North Am 6:783–796

Kuttner L (2010) A child in pain. What health professionals can do to help. Crown-House, Bethel

Kuttner L, Culbert T (2003) Hypnosis, biofeedback, and self-regulation skills for children in pain. In: Breivik H, Campbell W, Eccleston C (eds) Clinical pain management: practical applications and procedures. Arnold, London

Labbé EE (1995) Treatment of childhood migraine with autogenic training and skin temperature biofeedback: a component analysis. Headache 35(1):10–13

Leeuw M, Goossens ME, van Breukelen GJ, de Jong JR, Heuts PH, Smeets RJ et al (2008) Exposure in vivo versus operant graded activity in chronic low back pain patients: results of a randomized controlled trial. Pain 138(1):192–207

Liedl A, Müller J, Morina N, Karl A, Denke C, Knaevelsrud C (2011) Physical activity within a CBT intervention improves coping with pain in traumatized refugees: results of a randomized controlled design. Pain Med 12:234–245

Lipani TA, Walker LS (2006) Children's appraisal and coping with pain: relation to maternal ratings of worry and restriction in family activities. J Pediatr Psychol 31(7):667–673

Logan DE, Catanese SP, Coakley RM, Scharff L (2007) Chronic pain in the classroom: teachers' attributions about the causes of chronic pain. J Sch Health 77(5):248–256

Lommel K, Bandyopadhyay A, Martin C, Kapoor S, Crofford L (2011) A pilot study of a combined intervention for management of juvenile primary fibromyalgia symptoms in adolescents in an inpatient psychiatric unit. Int J Adolesc Med Health 23(3):193–197

Martin AL, McGrath PA, Brown SC, Katz J (2007) Anxiety sensitivity, fear of pain and pain-related disability in children and adolescents with chronic pain. Pain Res Manag 12(4):267–272

McGoldrick M, Gerson R, Petry S (2008) Genograms: assessment and intervention, 3rd edn. W.W. Norton & Company, New York

Meulders A, Vansteenwegen D, Vlaeyen JW (2011) The acquisition of fear of movement-related pain and associative learning: a novel pain-relevant human fear conditioning paradigm. Pain 152(11):2460–2469

Noble M, Treadwell JR, Tregear SJ, Coates VH, Wiffen PJ, Akafomo C et al (2010) Long-term opioid management for chronic noncancer pain. Cochrane Database Syst Rev (1):CD006605

Pagé MG, Stinson J, Campbell F, Isaac L, Katz J (2013) Identification of pain-related psychological risk factors for the development and maintenance of pediatric chronic postsurgical pain. J Pain Res 6:167–180. doi:10.2147/JPR.S40846. Epub 2013 Mar 5

Palermo TM, Eccleston C, Lewandowski AS, Williams AC, Morley S (2010) Randomized controlled trials of psychological therapies for management of chronic pain in children and adolescents: an updated meta-analytic review. Pain 148(3):387–397

Pinquart M, Shen Y (2011) Depressive symptoms in children and adolescents with chronic physical illness: an updated meta-analysis. J Pediatr Psychol 36(4):375–384

Reddemann L (2005) Imagination as healing power. Klett-Cotta, Stuttgart

Reinecke H, Sorgatz H, German Society for the Study of Pain (DGSS) (2009) S3 guideline LONTS. Long-term administration of opioids for non-tumor pain. Schmerz 23(5):440–447

Rief W, Barsky AJ (2005) Psychobiological perspectives on somatoform disorders. Psychoneuroendocrinology 30(10):996–1002

Rief W, Broadbent E (2007) Explaining medically unexplained symptoms-models and mechanisms. Clin Psychol Rev 27(7):821–841

Sansone RA, Pole M, Dakroub H, Butler M (2006) Childhood trauma, borderline personality symptomatology, and psychophysiological and pain disorders in adulthood. Psychosomatics 47(2):158–162

Schlarb AA, Stavemann HH (2011) Einführung in die KVT mit Kindern und Jugendlichen: Grundlagen und Methodik. Beltz PVU, Weinheim

Scholz OB, Ott R, Sarnoch H (2001) Proprioception in somatoform disorders. Behav Res Ther 39:1429–1438

Seemann H, Schultis J, Englert B (2002) Children with headache. Klett-Cotta, Stuttgart

Seng JS, Graham-Bermann SA, Clark MK, McCarthy AM, Ronis DL (2005) Posttraumatic stress disorder and physical comorbidity among female children and adolescents: results from service-use data. Pediatric 116(6):e767–e776

Sherry DD, Wallace CA, Kelley C, Kidder M, Sapp L (1999) Short- and long-term outcomes of children with complex regional pain syndrome type I treated with exercise therapy. Clin J Pain 15(3):218–223

Simons LE, Claar RL, Logan DL (2008) Chronic pain in adolescence: parental responses, adolescent coping, and their impact on adolescent's pain behaviors. J Pediatr Psychol 33(8): 894–904

Simons LE, Sieberg CB, Kaczynski KJ (2011) Measuring parent beliefs about child acceptance of pain: a preliminary validation of the Chronic Pain Acceptance Questionnaire, parent report. Pain 152(10):2294–3000

Singer T, Seymour B, O'Doherty J, Kaube H, Dolan RJ, Frith CD (2004) Empathy for pain involves the affective but not sensory components of pain. Science 303(5661):1157–1162

Stallard P (2005) A clinician's guide to think good feel good: the use of CBT with children and young people. Wiley, Chichester

Stein C, Reinecke H, Sorgatz H (2010) Opioid use in chronic noncancer pain: guidelines revisited. Curr Opin Anaesthesiol 23:598–601

Sullivan MJ, Martel MO, Tripp DA, Savard A, Crombez G (2006) Catastrophic thinking and heightened perception of pain in others. Pain 123(1–2):37–44

Trautmann E, Lackschewitz H, Kroner-Herwig B (2006) Psychological treatment of recurrent headache in children and adolescents – a meta-analysis. Cephalalgia 26(12):1411–1426

Turk DC, Wilson HD (2010) Fear of pain as a prognostic factor in chronic pain: conceptual models, assessment, and treatment implications. Curr Pain Headache Rep 14(2):88–95

van der Kolk BA, Courtois CA (2005) Editorial comments: complex developmental trauma. J Trauma Stress 18(5):385–388

Vlaeyen JW, Linton SJ (2000) Fear-avoidance and its consequences in chronic musculoskeletal pain: a state of the art. Pain 85(3):317–332

Vlaeyen JW, Linton SJ (2012) Fear-avoidance model of chronic musculoskeletal pain: 12 years on. Pain 153(6):1144–1147

Wald J, Taylor S, Chiri LR, Sica C (2010) Posttraumatic stress disorder and chronic pain arising from motor vehicle accidents: efficacy of interoceptive exposure plus trauma-related exposure therapy. Cogn Behav Ther 39:104–113

Walker LS, Smith CA, Garber J, Claar RL (2007) Appraisal and coping with daily stressors by pediatric patients with chronic abdominal pain. J Pediatr Psychol 32(2):206–216

Wallace DP, Harbeck-Weber C, Whiteside SP, Harrison TE (2011) Adolescent acceptance of pain: confirmatory factor analysis and further validation of the chronic pain acceptance questionnaire, adolescent version. J Pain 12(5):591–599

Watt MC, Stewart SH, Lefaivre MJ, Uman LS (2006) A brief cognitive-behavioral approach to reducing anxiety sensitivity decreases pain-related anxiety. Cogn Behav Ther 35:248–256

Weydert JA, Ball TM, Davis MF (2003) Systematic review of treatments for recurrent abdominal pain. Pediatric 111(1):e1–e11

Wicksell RK, Melin L, Olsson GL (2007) Exposure and acceptance in the rehabilitation of adolescents with idiopathic chronic pain – a pilot study. Eur J Pain 11(3):267–274

Wicksell RK, Melin L, Lekander M, Olsson GL (2009) Evaluating the effectiveness of exposure and acceptance strategies to improve functioning and quality of life in longstanding pediatric pain – A randomized controlled trial. Pain 141(3):248–257

Wicksell RK, Olsson GL, Hayes SC (2011) Mediators of change in acceptance and commitment therapy for pediatric chronic pain. Pain 152(12):2792–2801

Witthöft M, Basfeld C, Steinhoff M, Gerlach AL (2012) Can't suppress this feeling: automatic negative evaluations of somatosensory stimuli are related to the experience of somatic symptom distress. Emotion 12:640–649

Young Casey C, Greenberg MA, Nicassio PM, Harpin RE, Hubbard D (2008) Transition from acute to chronic pain and disability: a model including cognitive, affective, and trauma factors. Pain 134(1–2):69–79

Zernikow B, Wager J, Hechler T, Hasan C, Rohr U, Dobe M et al (2012) Characteristics of highly impaired children with severe chronic pain: a 5-year retrospective study on 2,249 pediatric pain patients. BMC Pediatr 12(1):54

Michael Dobe and Boris Zernikow

Contents

M. Dobe (✉)
German Paediatric Pain Centre (GPPC),
Children's and Adolescents' Hospital, Witten/Herdecke University,
Dr.-Friedrich-Steiner Street 5, Datteln 45711, Germany
e-mail: m.dobe@kinderklinik-datteln.de

B. Zernikow
German Paediatric Pain Centre (GPPC),
Children's and Adolescents' Hospital, Witten/Herdecke University,
Dr.-Friedrich-Steiner Street 5, Datteln 45711, Germany

Chair Children's Pain Therapy and Paediatric Palliative Care
Witten/Herdecke University, School of Medicine,
Datteln 45711, Germany
e-mail: b.zernikow@deutsches-kinderschmerzzentrum.de

M. Dobe, B. Zernikow (eds.),
Practical Treatment Options for Chronic Pain in Children and Adolescents,
DOI 10.1007/978-3-642-37816-4_7, © Springer-Verlag Berlin Heidelberg 2013

Abstract

The main goal of this chapter is to present general treatment aspects of children suffering both a pain disorder and a mental disorder. We pinpoint the specifics for paediatric pain therapy in children with a pain disorder and concomitant depressive symptomatology, anxiety disorder, trauma disorder, or adjustment disorder. We furthermore discuss the specific therapeutic needs of children who are accused of school truancy or who actually have learning disabilities or intellectual giftedness. Finally, we discuss children with chronic pain also suffering a severe somatic disease or living in highly burdening family systems.

This chapter will provide information on general aspects of the simultaneous treatment of pain, anxiety, depression, or trauma that may be implemented in both outpatient and inpatient therapy. We will discuss some specifics for the treatment of children being accused of *school truancy* or who are diagnosed with learning disabilities or intellectual giftedness. Finally, we will discuss treatment in children suffering a severe somatic disease or living in highly burdening family systems.

7.1 Specifics of Pain Therapy in Children with an Anxiety Disorder

The following case report depicts the close relationship between a pain disorder and an anxiety disorder.

Case Report: Lea (10 years) (Pain Disorder and Anxiety Disorder)

Lea has always been a clingy child, anxious in new and unknown situations. When she started kindergarten, she already had difficulty separating from her mother. She frequently wept when her mother dropped her off at the kindergarten. Sometimes she complained about abdominal pain in the morning. However, the pain didn't last long. When she had gotten used to the kindergarten, she was a reserved but very popular child. The symptoms did not reemerge until she started primary school. But also then, symptoms vanished again after a couple of months. According to Lea's mother, Lea's empathetic class teacher had been a big help in this process.

Lea was shocked when she found out her class teacher had to quit due to a severe illness. Lea developed a severe gastroenteritis along with high fever, nausea, vomiting, gastric spasms, and diarrhea. After her symptoms had diminished, Lea frequently reported abdominal pain over a period of weeks. The pain ceased after a recreational autumn vacation. Resuming school, the abdominal pain reoccurred and became more frequent and more intense. Lea has now been suffering constant daily pain for about half a year. The new class teacher has repeatedly stated her doubts and incomprehension concerning the situation; she openly assumed educational issues to be the problem behind the pain. Since Lea's spasm-like pain peaks occur suddenly and unexpectedly, even after school, Lea has been refraining from her former leisure time activity (horseback riding) and has withdrawn from most of her friends, fearing that her mother might not be beside her during pain peaks.

The desperate parents ordered many investigations which didn't yield any significant result. Frustrated from all these attempts to explain the disease ("psychosomatic"; "functional disorder"), they turned towards alternative therapies. Lea underwent homeopathy and acupuncture. The parents were told that Lea had a lactose malabsorption. Her nutritional intake was changed to a lactose-free diet. While homeopathy and acupuncture were unsuccessful, the frequency of abdominal spasms decreased somewhat while she was on the diet, which caused her mother to focus even more on dietary therapies. During the first contact with our clinic, Lea reported permanent abdominal pain with an intensity of 7 (NRS 0–10). She had been absent from school for 2 months and was supported and taken care of by her mother all day. Apart from the fear of pain, she admitted fear of her class teacher who, as she said, was "so mean" to her. Both parents reported being exhausted and helpless.

The case report shows that Lea had already suffered slight separation anxiety and fear of unknown situations in early childhood. In these situations abdominal pain was presumably mainly a reaction to mental stress. At first, Lea and her family managed to cope with the situation, but then a sequence of events brought forward both a pain disorder and a childhood anxiety disorder.

7.1.1 Pain-Related Versus Non-Pain-Related Fears

When treating children with pain disorders and increased anxiety, it is important to distinguish between pain-related and non-pain-related fears. In pain disorders, even pronounced pain-related fears (e.g., fear of an internal injury in case of severe pain, fear of increasingly painful movement, or fear of an underlying disease) are common and by no means signs of a separate anxiety disorder. The treatment of these fears is an implicit part of pain therapy in children with chronic pain. Children suffering an anxiety disorder and complaining of their pain as part of their anxiety symptomatology usually suffer little pain-related fear. Their pain will rapidly decrease as soon as the fearful situation is over or can be avoided. Thus, it is not that difficult to differentiate anxiety disorder from combined pain-anxiety disorders.

7.1.2 Anxiety and Pain: Which One Should Be Treated First?

If a child has chronic pain and fears not related to this pain, the latter (e.g., fear arising before a test, with separation, with social demands) have to be explicitly addressed during treatment. Otherwise, anxiety-induced muscular tension will perpetuate the pain. In anxiety therapy, gradual exposure is usually indicated, and this needs a separate and detailed education session. Gradual exposure requires a lot of time and will often result in transient pain amplification due to the concomitant increase in muscular tension. Hence, a child should be taught relaxation techniques *before* doing gradual exposure.

In the case report described above, Lea is suffering permanent abdominal pain apart from the increased pain in stressful situations. In the morning and in the evening, she needs a hot water bag. Her mother worries a lot about a possible somatic cause and has already arranged several diagnostic appointments and therapies (e.g., lactose-free diet). As presented in the case report, the child's history does not always give a clear-cut time sequence of events (e.g., pronounced avoidance behavior first, then increased abdominal pain). In Lea's case, diagnoses are most probably a pain disorder and a childhood anxiety disorder with fear of separation. Which one of these diagnoses is assigned as the main one is less important for therapy.

For pain therapy this means that part of the education should focus on the mutual perpetuation of pain and fears. In the beginning of pain therapy, pain-therapeutic techniques focusing on emotional stabilization (e.g., imaginative techniques like "Safe Place") are used. Having experienced a first success with these techniques, it is time to increasingly focus on the patient's fears (first, gradual exposure and then pain provocation). In childhood and adolescence, an anxiety disorder is rarely an isolated disorder within the family system. The family talks serve to identify perpetuating factors and parental fears, to illustrate that the child is not the only one with symptoms, and to identify the origin of the other family member's fear. During the family talk, it is helpful to ask the following question to the child: "Who do you believe understands your fears best?" or to the parents: "Meanwhile, much is known about the origin of fears in childhood. It is undisputed that an interplay between genetic, biological, and family factors like model learning is important in the manifestation of fears. Which one of you is best able to understand your child's worries due to his/her own (biographical) experiences?"

Unfortunately, the course of therapy as suggested above cannot always be followed. If in Lea's case she reported additional pain peaks (up to score 10, NRS) before or during a situation of separation, apart from her constant abdominal pain, those pain peaks would presumably reflect a childhood anxiety disorder with fear of separation (nevertheless, the pain is real since the increased inner tension *in fact* may trigger painful intestinal spasms). Since primarily addressing the abdominal pain in this case would most probably not be effective in itself, treatment for Lea would also have to include the aspects described in the next chapter.

7.1.3 Special Case: Emotional Disturbance in Childhood with Fear of Separation

A childhood anxiety disorder with fear of separation requires special treatment. Since the inpatient setting implies a separation, this aspect needs to be worked on first. In our experience, four agreements and interventions can be helpful:

1. Due to their pain-related worries and heavy burden, parents and their child can usually be reached in a talk before they are actually separated. In that talk we address the worries and burden that contributed to their decision for inpatient pain therapy. We address their love for their child that underlies the fear of separation, and we agree on scheduled daily times for visits or phone calls (in childhood, separation anxiety often results from an ambivalent fear-perpetuating interaction of at least one of the parents and thus is not solely a disorder of the child). Then we discuss how to cope with separation anxiety. In order to not prolong the parents' and the child's suffering unnecessarily, a member of the NET may support the child during the good-byes, which are confined to a certain duration (e.g., taking the child into one's arms while he/she is kissing his/her parents and then a "good-bye" and the scene is over). Such a time limit should be addressed in advance in order not to shock the child and his/her parents. Finally, the parents are allowed to call the NET to find out how their child is doing after the separation (by the way, the child usually does quite well. The shorter the good-bye scene, the faster the child will show normal behavior on the ward).

2. To some children, it is beneficial if their performance during separation is coupled with a reinforcement plan (that only makes sense if there is a suitable reward).

3. Motivation for therapy may be increased if good cooperation in pain therapy is rewarded by means of a reinforcement plan with longer visiting hours or longer-lasting visits at home (Stress Tests; see Sect. 6.6.6). If such a plan is arranged and the child has experienced that his/her parents actually will separate from him/her (rendering parental behavior predictable), we find that during the course of inpatient therapy, separation anxiety plays only a minor role in most cases. The outlined procedure will only work if the parents understand its background, explain it to their child, *and adhere to the agreements.* By no means should this task be accomplished by the therapist, physician, or NET. It is *essential* for the child to recognize that the responsibility for this action is *with his/her parents.*

4. One should try to avoid sending the child to his/her room "to calm down" after a separation. In most cases that will be counterproductive since the child will be lacking adequate strategies to regulate his/her emotions before, during, or after the separation; otherwise he/she would apply them. Instead, the child should be actively distracted by a member of the NET and be included in some other forms of distraction (e.g., group activity). This will make the child feel taken seriously with all his/her worries and fears, and with that support he/she will learn faster to cope with those worries and fears on his/her own.

The boundaries between a pain disorder and an anxiety disorder can be blurred. Chronic pain is not just a minor symptom of an anxiety disorder. It has to be addressed during therapy to underline its seriousness. In a child with separation anxiety, it suffices to explain to him/her during the education session (Sects. 6.3.2 and 6.3.3), as follows:

"Of course your pain is real. Nobody imagines pain or longs for it. Since you often get your pain in situations very awkward and stressful to you (e.g., separation from your parents), it fortunately doesn't indicate inflammation within your body. While being in extreme distress, your body gets tense which naturally results in pain. It would be odd if it didn't. Since your pain is so closely connected to fear or distress, analgesics won't help. Pain can only be resolved when you distract yourself in such a situation or when you don't experience the stress or the fear anymore."

Taking the child's fear or pain seriously to some therapists erroneously means devotion to the child and giving him/her a secondary gain from illness. We believe this is a substantial mistake. Such an approach will rather jeopardize the course of therapy since the child will feel devalued and not taken seriously with all his/her aims and wishes. As a result, he/she will boycott or interrupt therapy or the compliance will become insufficient. From our viewpoint, this "resistance" is understandable and should be regarded as a warning signal requiring fundamental changes in the therapeutic interaction or therapy plan.

7.2 Pain Therapy in Children with Depressive Symptomatology

A pain disorder is accompanied by depressive symptomatology in many cases (for a meta-analysis, see Pinquart and Shen 2011). What does this mean for therapy? In order to answer that question, one has to clarify first what the origin of the depressive symptoms may be:

1. Do they reflect grief after having lost a beloved attachment figure (e.g., the grandmother)?
2. Do they arise from low self-esteem and the experience of failure (or the lack of success)?
3. Does the patient report on generalized negative thoughts regarding herself/himself, his/her surroundings, or his/her future (*cognitive triad*)?
4. Are the symptoms dependent on certain situations (e.g., symptoms arising when being reminded of something)?

5. Does the patient gradually withdraw from both his/her family and his/her peers, or does he/she have a normal social life?
6. Does the child have problems falling asleep or staying asleep?

It makes a substantial difference whether a child suffers a pain disorder for years and irrespective of that has had sad thoughts concerning the deceased grandmother for half a year or whether he/she has lost faith in him/herself due to massive teasing combined with numerous devaluations in the family environment. In Sects. 6.4 and 6.5, we discussed some interventions to act on depressive symptoms. In this section, we describe attitudes and general approaches towards children with a concomitant depressive episode or an adjustment disorder with a depressive reaction. The example case reports of "Svetlana" and "Mike" serve to illustrate the different approaches.

Case Report: Svetlana (15 years) (Pain Disorder and Depressive Episode)
Together with her mother, Svetlana, a very fine girl, presents at our outpatient clinic with constant severe headache (score 9/10, NRS 0–11) for the last 3 years. Numerous medical investigations yielded no pathological result. Svetlana reports that apart from the constant pain, once in a while she also experiences pain peaks (10/10 NRS) with concomitantly increased nausea, vertigo, and increased sensitivity to noise and light. Several types of migraine medication have been prescribed without effect. In the course of the talk, however, it becomes obvious that on at least 5 days a week Svetlana has been taking an analgesic (most often ibuprofen, sometimes paracetamol or acetyl-salicylic acid). The respective doses and intake patterns remain uncertain. Meanwhile, Svetlana is missing school 1 day a week and is withdrawing from her family and friends, spending much time alone in her room. Every now and then Svetlana meets her friends, but this has no significant impact on her headache. In addition, her mother is worried about her daughter's casual intentional cutting of her arms with a knife. This started after Svetlana was bullied in school. Meanwhile, the bullying was supposedly clarified in school and had stopped. Svetlana's mother presumes the cause of Svetlana's social withdrawal and self-harm is either that she has problems she doesn't want to discuss with her or that she is seeking attention "although everything is revolving around her." While her mother is either heaping reproaches on her daughter or addressing her readiness to open her heart, Svetlana denies her mother's reproaches, at times being dysphoric and irritable, then depressed again, and then keeping silent. Due to her symptomatology and clinical relevant scores on the depression inventory (Sect. 3.3), Svetlana is queried for any suicidal intentions which she credibly denies. But she says that she is not interested in most things and has previously thought about not living anymore. Svetlana's mother reacts huffily and reproachfully to her daughter's statement, since at home everything "is perfectly fine." The mother tells us that due to her numerous symptoms, Svetlana has started with outpatient psychotherapy which has not so far led to any positive change.

Svetlana told us at the beginning of pain therapy that she suffered from her mother's permanent devaluations, that her father was an alcoholic, and that she was badly bullied at school. She reported being beaten by her parents (especially her mother) during her childhood, and this is still the case once in a while. She didn't tell the outpatient psychotherapist since she didn't know if she could trust her. On the cognitive level, she reported general dysfunctional cognitions with respect to herself, her surroundings, and her future. Generally, her situation was hard to bear, and she was tense most of the time. She reported that cutting herself would improve her well-being for a couple of hours. This was the reason why she regularly cut herself before meeting her friends. Basically her mood was sad, but she still had the capacity to act. She didn't know which was more burdensome to her, the pain or the sadness. Her belief was that it would be easier to reduce the pain than the sadness, and that "would be a first step."

7.2.1 Modified Education for Depressive Symptomatology

During the education, we explained at length to Svetlana the vicious cycle of pain, also using neurobiological charts, the origin of chronic pain, and the impact of negative emotions. According to Svetlana, her pain was making her sad, and increasing sadness would amplify her pain. She would perceive her pain more intensely while being passive, or alone, or unable to get the necessary distance from her negative thoughts (which was mostly the case). She was very interested in the neurobiological charts and very relieved to know that there was "proof" that her pain was not imagined (as her mother was blaming her for) but real. She was very astonished that pain inhibition is a predefined basic cerebral function. Based on her education, we agreed to first set up a proof that both pain perception and negative thoughts can be interrupted for a couple of hours. To this end, distraction techniques (chaos ABC with permanently altered themes or Distraction-ABC using lines of poems) were used. It turned out that Svetlana was very amenable to figurative imaging. Based on that ability, she created two very different Safe Places (one for use in public, the other in privacy). With their help she succeeded in influencing her general mood. Biofeedback helped her verify the effectiveness of the various techniques. During the following six single therapeutic sessions, she was working on her negative basic beliefs, collecting arguments for or against her negative basic assumptions (for details, see Sect. 6.5.5), as well as working on training verbal interaction strategies for contact with her mother. Like many children with depressive symptomatology, Svetlana was able to reflect her own thoughts and behavior. Due to the support during her stay on the ward, she succeeded in significantly influencing her mood for the better; she was able to notice this change herself. It turned out that the severe pain attacks were due to internal or external tension, and thus the presence of an additional migraine could be excluded (and an analgesic therapy with potentially severe side effects was unnecessary indeed).

7.2.2   Adapting the Daily Routine for Patients with Depressive Symptomatology

According to the approach outlined in Sect. 7.2.1, Svetlana set up a structured plan for her daily activities together with the NET and a "list of pleasant activities" (Sect. 6.5.3 and Chap. 9, Worksheet #15). In the evening, Svetlana had a 10-min talk with her contact person from the NET (evening reflection). The NET member gave her feedback on her behavior, her personality, or special skills and abilities observed during the day. In addition, several times during therapy Svetlana's task was to query her peers and the therapeutic team about what they liked about her and to record their answers. Those records were integrated into the individual therapeutic work with Svetlana.

7.2.3   Working with the Family in Patients with Depressive Symptomatology

Using examples from everyday life, it was demonstrated in the family talks that there was an interrelationship between pain perception, depressive thoughts, and internal tension. Against Svetlana's expectations, her parents actively cooperated, and they repeatedly expressed their deep concern about their daughter's future.

The primary issue of the following family talks was appreciating the parents' various efforts to educate their daughter. From our experience, especially in family systems such as the one described for Svetlana, it is important to highlight and compliment the parents' good intentions irrespective of any obvious dysfunctional patterns of family interaction (note: this is true as long as there is honest motivation to cooperate and any acute endangerment of the child's well-being is absent).

As mentioned before, also in this case a humorous approach has proven helpful to increase the parents' motivation to cooperate. After having reflected their biography, the parents were able to admit to their daughter that they unintentionally contributed to her problems. Svetlana had described her mother as hard and adamant. Contrary to Svetlana's expectations, her mother burst into tears during one talk. On this basis they came to binding agreements regarding the further course of psychotherapy. At the end of her stay on the ward, Svetlana was able to decrease her pain up to 3 scores and to better control her dysfunctional thoughts. During the Stress Tests, Svetlana's mother tried to praise her daughter and not to interrupt her when she was talking. After having signed a release of the obligation of confidentiality, the background and course of the disease were discussed with the outpatient psychotherapist, allowing a seamless continuation of the therapeutic process. Motivated by the positive experiences from the inpatient stay, outpatient psychotherapy was successful because now Svetlana had learned to open herself towards her therapist.

Svetlana's case illustrates how a simultaneous approach to pain disorder and depressive symptomatology may be helpful even if in the framework of pain therapy most probably not all factors relevant for the symptomatology can be determined.

7.2.4 Adjustment Disorder: Coping with Grief and Death

The case of Mike illustrates our approach in a case of a very sad onetime experience (e.g., the death of a beloved one) being the trigger of depressive symptomatology.

Case Report: Mike (12 years) (Pain Disorder and Adjustment Disorder)

Twelve-year-old Mike is quite a content and calm boy. According to him and his mother, he had a happy, though unremarkable, childhood. Due to his above-average power of comprehension, he passed primary school without any problems. Also the change to high school was uncomplicated. Every now and then he would suffer migraine which presumably was inherited from his mother (and by his mother from *her* mother). An analgesic (ibuprofen 400 mg) taken early in the course of the episode would help, and migraine was never an issue with him. Because both parents were employed, he often visited his grandparents living in the neighborhood. He did a lot, especially with his grandfather, whom he loved passionately. Unfortunately, 1½ years ago, after having played together with Mike all day, his grandfather suddenly and unexpectedly died at home, supposedly due to stroke. From that moment everything went downhill for Mike and his family. Only a few weeks after the grandfather's death, his father lost his job because of the economic crisis and had to reestablish himself professionally. Five months later, his mother suffered disc prolapse, "presumably due to all that stress," and had to attend a rehabilitation clinic for 4 weeks. Mike changed from a fun-loving boy to a secluded, depressed, and contemplative boy who hardly went out. Apart from constant headache, Mike also often complained about very severe headache attacks. During those headache attacks, his migraine medication would not help anymore. It was no longer possible to attend school because Mike was not able to get out of bed in the morning, weeping due to pain. Due to the extremely high number of days missed in school, it was not possible to grade him, and passing to the next class was in doubt. His parents seemed very exhausted and desperate. They told us that they didn't know how to go on and that they were at the end of their rope.

On the background of a very well-treated migraine (without aura), after the very stressful loss of a beloved one, Mike developed both a pain disorder and an adjustment disorder with a depressive reaction. The high family burden is obvious. When we explored the case history, it was unclear how much Mike's mother was burdened by the mourning process and therefore failing as a support for Mike. How should Mike's history modify the necessary inpatient pain therapy?

Contrary to what could be assumed and in accordance with our experience, the implications for treatment are minor. A "standard" pain therapy in a child with pain disorder with an underlying migraine is not much different to that in a child with additional adjustment disorder after loss of a beloved one. The basic therapeutic strategies as educated for use in "standard" pain therapy are also suitable to coping with grief. Active pain coping in everyday life, better differentiation between migraine and pain disorder, and much resource-oriented reinforcement are of value for a sad child as well. Especially in the treatment of mourning children, one should consider the following thoughts:

1. During the *first* education session, using the vicious cycle of pain, the therapist should carve out the close relationship between severe pain and sad Black Thoughts: "Many children report that Black Thoughts regarding pain (such as "Why me?") provoke other Black Thoughts or stressful memories that cause the situation to deteriorate further. Does that make sense to you? Do you know this from your own experience? How much does the pain have to score to automatically result in stressful memories or thoughts?" (In Mike's case, "…do you then think about your grandfather?")

2. Frequently, feelings of guilt or the wish to tell something really important to the deceased play a role. Be cautious with that. Children appreciate when the therapist reflects their mood and thoughts in an appreciative and normalizing way. Any therapeutic options (e.g., to accompany the child in his/her process of grief, for instance, jointly writing a farewell letter to be laid down at the grave or talking about thoughts and feelings of guilt) should be cautiously offered to communicate to the child that the therapist respects the needs, but also the boundaries.

3. The interventions should be examined to determine which one is most helpful in reducing stressful memories in the evening – at the time when "everything comes to rest" and the probability of stressful memories increases. If the child tells us he/she is sufficiently stabilized, pain provocation (Sect. 6.4.6) is a suitable technique to simultaneously reduce fear of pain and stressful memories conditioned with most severe pain. The affected children report that after frequent application of pain provocation, the stressful memories are now "far away" and even the most severe pain would more and more seldom trigger stressful memories. They have successfully faced their memories and pain, resulting in increased self-efficiency.

4. All these aspects should be addressed at length in the family talks. Usually, sadness in at least one of the parents is a factor maintaining the adjustment disorder. Just expressing that assumption while the child is listening may validate the child's perception and may therefore be very helpful. The child's choice not to talk "about that" with his/her parents to protect them from their own feelings is normalized. Then we jointly ponder which steps the mother or the father could take in order to work on their own grief or sadness. Finally, we emphasize that the parent's own efforts will relieve the child by relieving his/her worries concerning the parent(s).

7.3 Pain Therapy in Children with Trauma Disorder and Pain Disorder

On the one hand, traumatized children frequently suffer chronic pain (Seng et al. 2005). On the other hand, a substantial proportion of children and adults with chronic pain suffer symptoms of posttraumatic stress disorder (PTSD), other trauma disorders, or an adjustment disorder (Seng et al. 2005; Sharp and Harvey 2001; Asmundson et al. 2002). The significantly increased comorbidity of chronic pain and symptoms of PTSD was emphasized even 10 years ago (e.g. Sharp and Harvey 2001; Asmundson et al. 2002). Asmundson et al. (2002) hypothesized that anxiety sensitivity (see also Sect. 6.4.6) is of importance for the perpetuation of both traumatic symptoms and pain disorder. In line with this hypothesis, Wald and Taylor (2007) were able to show that harmless physiological activation, such as sports, could trigger stressful intrusions in about 60 % of adult patients with PTSD. They supposed that the perception of physiological activation triggers traumatic memories because high physiological activation was closely associated with the traumatic situation (interoceptive conditioning). It is still unclear, though, to what extent either the premorbid anxiety sensitivity or the maladaptive interoception as a result of traumatization (or both) could better explain the results of the study (see also Sect. 6.4.6 for a more detailed definition of the concepts). Anxiety sensitivity, on the other hand, is closely connected with fear of pain in children suffering from chronic pain (Martin et al. 2007). Meulders et al. (2011) confirm that fear of pain can also be conditioned by the perception of muscle tension. It can be assumed that anxiety sensitivity is closely connected with increased maladaptive interoception in children with chronic pain (see Fig. 6.2 in Sect. 6.4.6). Thus, if there is an additional pain disorder in traumatized children, increased body awareness (see Sect. 6.4.6) may enable mutual conditioning (Asmundson et al. 2002; Liedl et al. 2011; Dobe et al. 2009). Hence, there is a necessity to develop new therapies covering both diagnoses. The meaning of these associations for the clinical context is illustrated in Wiebke's case (see below).

Case Report: Wiebke (13 years) (Pain Disorder and PTSD)
Wiebke presented at our outpatient clinic accompanied by her mother with the diagnoses of juvenile fibromyalgia syndrome and a moderate depressive episode. She scored high on the depression and anxiety questionnaires (T-values: depression=68; general anxiety=80), and she rarely attended school due to her pain. Several inpatient therapies focusing on "rheuma therapy" were successful only for as long as Wiebke was in the clinic. As a consequence, drug therapy escalated. When Wiebke presented at our clinic, she was on two different antidepressants and an oral retarded opioid. Despite substantial adverse effects (excessive weight gain, lack of concentration, constipation), there were no positive drug effects at all. The treating physicians and therapists offensively questioned the presence of pain as well as Wiebke's motivation for treatment. This led to a worsening of the conflict-ridden relationship between Wiebke and her mother. The neat, friendly, and sociable girl seemed hopeless when we first met her. She didn't believe in a change for the better in her life. But a friend had told her about the GPPC, her very positive view of it, and the possibility of inpatient pain treatment. With respect to Wiebke's severe emotional burden (depression and anxiety), we told her our assumption that she

was suffering not only pain but was also impaired from other stressful life events. Wiebke was astonished at first but confirmed our assumption that there were very stressful memories. She asked curiously how we would suggest proceeding in inpatient therapy. After giving an extended overview of our work with a focus on single therapeutic sessions, Wiebke agreed to our conditions for inpatient treatment.

During her treatment on the ward, we were able to identify several critical and two traumatic life events (witnessing severe domestic violence by her biological father, sexual abuse by a stranger). Regarding the sexual abuse, the criteria for PTSD were fulfilled. In the past, interoceptive conditioning resulted in mutual conditioning of pain and trauma factors. Since Wiebke had so far not been told about these mechanisms and associations, she didn't dare to talk about those issues. Following inpatient therapy, we tapered the medication, monitored by several follow-up visits. One part of the therapy was family therapeutic interventions. One year after finishing inpatient treatment, Wiebke was off medication, free of constant pain, attending numerous social activities, and regularly attending school. She told us that her emotional burden was steadily decreasing due to successful psychotherapy. Both her mother and her stepfather were still sticking to the arrangements made during the stay on the ward, and the dysphoric-irritated family mood had normalized.

In children with PTSD, the very high emotional burden and decreased ability to regulate one's emotions are problematic for pain therapy. A further important factor is the fact that the previous passive pain coping behavior of the affected child was some kind of problem-solving strategy (avoidance) in the coping with stressful memories. Active pain coping would take away an effective short-term problem-solving strategy, resulting in an increased emotional burden which very well could become critical in a child with an impaired ability to regulate his/her emotions. As the case report shows, children with PTSD or other trauma disorders don't generally report those life events if not specifically queried about them, and their parents don't like to talk about stressful family conflicts. Thus, there are the risks of missing a diagnosis and an escalation of medical and drug therapy, as seen in Wiebke.

7.3.1 Coping with an Increased Need for Control and Security

Children like Wiebke learned during their life to have only a small impact on things happening to them or their body. Their experience was that many people are malevolent, not respecting a person's basic needs. This makes the child cautious and suspicious in his/her interactions. In addition, most of these children report that they fear becoming "mad" due to the long-standing emotional overburdening by their chronic pain, intrusive memories, reduced stress tolerance, lack of concentration, or other dysfunctional cognitive thoughts. It is understandable if at first these children behave in a reserved or distrustful way towards the team, their psychotherapist, and any new information. In patients with an exaggerated need for control, it may be advisable to make the therapeutic attitude and any therapeutic decision very transparent. In addition, we ask the child to scrutinize the therapist, all information given, and the communication within the team and to give feedback on any discrepancy.

With traumatized children, we discuss all steps and therapeutic interventions extensively *in advance*. The child should understand the reason why the intervention is done. Such an approach is very time-consuming and requires good communication within the therapeutic team.

We advise against inpatient therapy of traumatized children with chronic pain in an institution where the therapeutic approach of the nurses or physicians on the ward is not predictable (e.g., team conflicts, no clear-cut assignment of responsibilities), since lacking predictability will cause the patient to experience loss of control. The patient would try to get control by means of his/her behavior (e.g., avoidance, refusal). His/her increased physiologic activation as a consequence of loss of control would result in adverse somatic symptoms which themselves are experienced as making the patient insecure and will often lead to more frequent consultation with the physician. All this increases the risk of a split of perception within the team (e.g., "She is seeking attention" vs. "It's her emotional burden") being more damaging/detrimental than beneficial to the patient.

7.3.2 Adaptation of the Education

During the course of treatment, one should try to find out if certain traumatic contents are triggered by a certain type of pain, and vice versa. Ask for a description of the respective context (e.g., domestic surroundings). The education should address the dysregulation of the limbic system due to traumatization and the permanently reduced ability to cope with stressors.

Supplementary Pain Education in the Traumatized Child
As a consequence of one or several traumatizing events, a cerebral emergency mechanism is triggered in order to prevent you from having to go through that horrible event a second time. You will become more watchful, scanning your environment for any sign that *it* could happen a second time. Your experience has been so stressful/traumatizing that you were overburdened with the task of processing the event, and you grew scared stiff. Later your memories reemerge, especially when you try to rest. Those memories are called "intrusions" or "flashbacks." A main feature of them is their liveliness and intensity; this makes it difficult to distinguish them from reality.

As a consequence, you are unable to relax because the stressful memories may reemerge any time. Falling asleep or staying asleep may become difficult. Frequently, nightmares emerge. And after not having slept well, you will wake up tired in the morning. Some children have experienced such horrible things that their only way of dealing with them is that their brain dissipates the memory into small packages in such a way that they can only remember one package at a time or only certain packages or that the flashback is confined to the visual or auditory sensory channel. It becomes quite bewildering if certain people or actions imbued with aspects associated with the trauma (e.g., a certain haircut, voice, threatening gesture) trigger a flashback confined to purely somatic perception (e.g., severe pain, intense heartbeat, extreme dizziness, other sudden physiological reaction) though the child may not understand why this happens at that very moment. In most cases, this will contribute to the child's feelings of insecurity.

The permanently anxiously increased tension combined with sleeping problems results in a dysregulation of the stress system and thus gradually reduced ability to cope with daily hassles. In the end, the patient is severely impaired in concentration. Regarding emotions, wide swings of mood will be observed or feelings of emptiness and numbness. Sometimes this happens in fast sequence. The patient is pondering "why?" and tries to cope with the event. Many affected children come to the conclusion that it was their fault or that they are doomed to horrible experiences. This is not "standard" logic but trauma logic arising from the desperate attempt to make sense of what happened in order to keep a minimum of control. However, the price is high, since this mostly leads to substantial self-devaluation. The patient starts to hate himself for not having done anything to prevent the event. Depending on the exact type of trauma, a feeling of shame may arise which makes it difficult to verbally address what happened.

The symptoms described result in permanent tension and fear, leading to an increase in pain frequency. Many patients start to withdraw from social activities because they feel exhausted. Finally, dysregulation of the stress system impairs the immune response of the body, the patient is ill more often, and the risk of minor inflammatory illnesses increases. Due to the increased body awareness caused by the trauma, the patient perceives these body signals as very differentiated and intense. In this way, the concern that something is wrong with the body and him/herself arises. In case of any acute painful event (e.g., accident, severe flu, common cold, migraine attack, or relapse of a rheumatic disease), the probability of entering the vicious cycle of pain and that acute pain converting to chronic pain is high.

Complex traumatized children (e.g., children with a yearlong history of neglect and/or witnessing or experiencing physical violence and/or sexual abuse) need an even more specifically adapted and detailed education as well as specific consideration of their basic interactional needs. In these children, it makes sense to choose a physician or psychotherapist especially trained in trauma therapy.

Chronic pain that suddenly sets in after a traffic accident is a special case. In most of these cases, we expect at least some traumatic aspects of the accident to be of importance regarding the chronicity of the pain. With respect to the education, it is especially important to address the point that the experience of pain often triggers the memory of the accident, and vice versa. As mentioned above, the memory of the accident is often fragmented, requiring meticulous inquiry as to what exactly happened during that accident.

Having explained the interrelationships, it is essential to repeatedly and empathetically normalize the patient's experience and perception in therapy. For many children it is beneficial to learn to better anticipate their somatic symptoms since this means better control and security. The child is encouraged to pose any question (even repeatedly) about any somatic symptom experienced which triggers a feeling of insecurity. In addition, the child's homework is to record a few times a day which situations his/her body reacts in a certain way to, depending on his/her appraisal (ABC model according to A. Ellis, Sect. 6.4.3).

7.3.3 Specifics Concerning Active Pain Coping

For many children with a combined pain and trauma disorder, passive pain coping represents a kind of trauma avoidance and thus problem-solving or coping strategy (as already described, increased physiological activation, for instance, within the framework of a stepped plan for active pain coping, can trigger traumatic memories). Thus, increased active pain coping may result in an increased emotional burden resulting in ambivalent motivation for therapy. If the suspicion of such a connection is present, it is important to value it and to normalize the reasons for these connections as well as the resulting ambivalent motivation for therapy. If this is done, the therapist may refer to the education session and the prediction of ambivalence in order to normalize the child's feelings and behavior. If the interrelationship between active pain coping and a consequent increase in trauma-associated emotional burden is not addressed, this should be made up for at the first sign of ambivalent therapy motivation. Otherwise, there is the risk of splitting the team in the inpatient setting because the child's behavior allows for several different and contradictory interpretations. In an outpatient setting, a situation like this would most likely make the child interrupt therapy.

Apart from normalizing and appreciating their previous efforts, it should be made clear to the child and his/her parents that passive pain coping will increase both pain and trauma symptomatology in the long run. After having normalized the patient in acute ambivalent therapy motivation, we usually discuss the following aspects with the patient:

"Which way do you want to go? The way of passivity and avoidance made your life the way it is now and prompted you to decide for an inpatient therapy. Do you want to continue in this way? Or would you prefer to change to active coping strategies?"

At this point, it is worthwhile once more explicitly addressing the seemingly simple and understandable solutions like somatic fixation, drug medication, and in some cases alcohol, where one doesn't have to leave the course of passivity and avoidance.

"It would be great if there were a pill available that would just wipe everything out, wouldn't it? This is what we all wish for once in a while. The question is, what can you do now to make yourself feel better? How can we support you?"

For the parents, it is also important to develop an understanding of these inter-relationships. This is the only way to enable them to expect active pain coping from their child. With this issue most parents are as ambivalent as their child. Some parents fear that their child will do worse if they apply educational consequences. The child knows about that ambivalence and will take advantage of it when planning his/her behavior. Some parents feel pity and don't want to expect "even more" of their child. Anyway, parental education should make it clear that only increased active pain coping in everyday life and in school gives the therapy a chance for success.

7.3.4 Coping with "Side Scenes" and Dissociative Symptoms

In the jargon the expression "side scenes" implies something negative and is used in conjunction with a devaluating view of the patient's motivation. Some children with low motivation for therapy try to avoid or prevent certain situations by presenting with somatic or behavior-related symptoms. Mostly, however, the presence of "side scenes" is an indicator of substantial insecurity and overburdening of the child. If children don't dare to ask questions or to criticize out of shame or social insecurity, they try another way to get answers to their questions, for instance, by presenting more somatic symptoms.

In this respect a self-critical attitude while talking to the child will pay off, which does not mean that the therapist should give up basic positions (e.g., aiming at active pain coping in the daily routine). But it may be advisable to take an increased somatic concern of the child seriously and let him/her talk to the doctor about his worries for 10 min a day. Or the therapist explicitly asks the patient for critical feedback and alternative solutions to the situation experienced by him/her as critical. Usually such an approach will result in a reduction in the number of "side scenes." If these measures are ineffective, presumably an approach as outlined in Sect. 7.3.5 is necessary.

If, nevertheless, the child is considerably overburdened with inpatient pain therapy, he/she might show dissociative symptoms presenting as psychogenic syncope, sudden loss of vision, deafness, muscular weakness, or pareses. Transitorily impaired vigilance, somnolence, derealization, or depersonalization is observed as well as (seldom) seizures. Primarily it is complex traumatized children presenting with these symptoms.

Those symptoms are liable to severely hinder inpatient pain therapy or make it even impossible (this is different with outpatient psychotherapy). Regarding the decision whether to continue inpatient pain therapy despite the presence of those symptoms, it is crucial how far from awareness the dissociations are. Regarding the dysregulation of the stress system, we recommend normalizing the symptomatology by talking to the child:

"You have experienced so much in the past, and you survived. So far you haven't had the opportunity to perorate with all those stressful experiences and make "it" end. Hence, your brain and your body are still in emergency mode, which might mean that your brain is protecting you from further overburdening by switching off your awareness for a while. This is harmless; nothing will be damaged in your brain. And you definitely aren't mad."

While doing so, the therapist should state his/her concerns about the child's well-being (e.g., in case of psychogenic syncope: "You feel life can't go on like this. Your brain is protecting you from overburdening, but this way it is impossible for you to learn how to cope with distress, problems, or memories more appropriately, and in the long run leading a normal life becomes impossible").

If the exploration of the symptomatology shows that the child is able to at least have a presentiment of the context triggering dissociative symptomatology (or of trigger memories or external triggers) and is motivated to learn to better influence symptomatology, it is appropriate to continue with inpatient therapy, keeping the dissociative symptoms in focus. Otherwise, having excluded acute endangerment of the child's well-being within the family system, inpatient therapy in a paediatric psychiatric institution focusing on dissociative and trauma disorders is the better choice (Sect. 7.3.5).

If the family wishes to continue inpatient therapy, limiting the dissociative symptoms is of primary concern. If this is the case, some interventions deriving from ego state therapy (according to Watkins and Watkins 1997) in conjunction with interventions transferring the responsibility for the emergence of the symptoms to the child ("weather forecast," see below) have proven helpful. We use interventions in which the child writes, paints, or tinkers with his/her perceivable personality features. More hidden parts of the personality (or ego states) like "the inner child" or self-destructive and destructive personality parts should also be written, painted, or tinkered with. Optionally the ego states may be marked with a name and/or a symbol. In the next step (and if the child wants to), it is helpful to highlight the specific role of the different ego states in coping with stressful or traumatic life events in the child's biography. This should also be done explicitly with destructive ego states (e.g., the patient's parts as offender). Then the various ego states are supported to jointly decide how to proceed (e.g., to implement certain therapeutic interventions). For a deeper understanding of that approach and its theoretical background, we advise a specific trauma-therapeutic training. We advise such an approach only if the child agrees to participate in outpatient psychotherapy after having finished his/her inpatient stay or if outpatient therapy is already arranged.

It makes sense to accompany interventions deriving from ego state therapy with interventions such as "weather forecast." Since during exploration of the child some dissociative symptoms close to awareness have become evident, it is important for the control of dissociative symptoms to have the child learn to predict the emergence of his/her symptoms. Practicing "weather forecast," the child is queried each morning for the probability and frequency of the dissociative symptoms to appear that day. Interestingly this intervention often results in a quick resolution of dissociative symptoms, and the child quickly recognizes the interdependencies.

For some children (e.g., those with psychogenic pareses), it is helpful to gradually learn, via gradual exposure, to reduce their dissociative symptoms. Gradual exposure in children with dissociative symptoms is principally the same as outlined elsewhere (Sects. 6.4.5 and 6.5.4).

7.3.5 Contraindications for Inpatient Pain Therapy of Traumatized Children

Children with active and severe emotional instability with self-injuring and/or aggressive behavior do not fulfill the criteria for inpatient pain therapy. To some of the children, it might make sense – after having them extensively educated during the primary outpatient talk about the requirements (no self-injury, no aggressive behavior, sticking to the ward rules, regularly doing therapeutic homework – otherwise immediate interruption of therapy) – to contractually demand their agreement and evaluate their motivation in a written letter (see Sect. 6.8.3). Actually, some of our older patients with a beginning borderline personality disorder could be admitted to inpatient pain therapy and kept to the rules so therapy was conducted regularly. *Traumatization with concomitant ongoing drug abuse and severe dissocial or dissociative symptoms is an absolute contraindication for our type of inpatient pain therapy.*

In case any doubt about the eligibility of a patient arises during the first outpatient appointment, we generally recommend performing a detailed and written motivation check. This will allow the child to become aware of his/her ideas and what he/she is ready to invest. At the same time we protect the child from otherwise inevitable disappointment. In all other cases, outpatient or inpatient therapy focusing on the dissociative or traumatic symptoms is preferable to inpatient pain therapy.

To summarize, in the treatment of children with both a pain and a trauma disorder, an adapted education focusing on processes of interoceptive conditioning and aiming at normalization of physical symptoms and interrelationships is a prerequisite for successful therapy. Thus, treating only the pain or trauma symptomatology is useless. For these patients, predictability of interventions is very important. This and the possibility of close interprofessional cooperation with all its necessary arrangements on short notice can be guaranteed only by an inpatient treatment program. Any suddenly arising emotional or somatic symptoms should trigger self-critical evaluation by the therapist, a detailed exploration of the symptomatology, and intensified education. If after having done so it is still impossible to confine the symptoms, one should critically evaluate the indication for participation in the treatment program and envisage a transfer to a better-suited institution. In the light of the variability and complexity of traumatic or dissociative symptoms demanding special knowledge, we recommend that at least one member of the therapeutic team be certified in trauma therapy.

7.4 Pain Therapy in Children Suspected of School Truancy

Some parents report that the school, the psychiatrist, the psychotherapist, the responsible paediatrician, or the general practitioner often suspects school truancy in children with chronic pain and absenteeism from school. The child is accused of lacking motivation, lacking readiness to perform, idleness, and laziness. The pain is regarded as an excuse.

7.4.1 Myth and Reality

Many children with chronic pain act insecure in their interactions with teachers or classmates. They cannot deal with their daily hassles and show social withdrawal. However, to construct school truancy from this is inadequate and does not capture the impact of their disorder. Another argument against assumed school truancy is that after successful inpatient pain therapy even in the long run, these children don't show abnormal absenteeism from school (Eccleston and Malleson 2003; Hechler et al. 2009; Dobe et al. 2011; Hirschfeld et al. 2013). Interestingly, a reduced number of days missed from school is seen in children even without significant pain reduction. These results support the hypothesis that children miss school due to pain, and not due to school aversion. The proportion of children with primary school aversion or truancy in our clinical population is lower than 5 %.

7.4.2 Specifics in Pain Therapy

In a child with high pain-related school absence, pain therapy should focus on the improvement of his/her ability to cope with daily hassles and distress. The Stress Day (see Sect. 6.4.5.3), active pain coping irrespective of pain intensity, or scheduling the day is of special importance. In many cases, even 2 Stress Days during the inpatient stay are advisable since it often does not become obvious before the first Stress Day which specific coping abilities in everyday life should be addressed during the further course of treatment.

Finally, we would like to mention three other aspects relevant for the treatment of children with high school absence:

1. Children with extensive absenteeism from school should *not* be admitted for therapy just before school holidays. During holidays, the daily routine on the ward is different, with fewer commitments. Among other things, this is because the patient does not have to attend the clinic's school. During holidays it is impossible to schedule Stress Tests with attendance at the home school. But in these children the Stress Test at school is of special importance, allowing for targeted therapy planning.
    (a) Is the patient motivated due to his/her knowledge and newly learned abilities and is he/she attending school on his/her own?
    (b) How do the parents cope with their child's school problems after a total of two family talks and one extensive education session on active pain coping in everyday life?

(c) How do the teachers and the classmates react to the patient who in some cases did not or only sporadically attended school for months? Quite often the patient has to bear the teacher's mocking comments, which later must be therapeutically addressed.

(d) In case of increased pain: when exactly is it observed? Is it already there in the evening before the school visit is scheduled? Or does it emerge at night, in the morning, on the way to school, at school, or even after school has finished?

(e) How does the patient cope with his/her pain?

(f) Do the learned techniques and strategies work?

2. The therapist should discuss with the child and his/her parents the signs signaling that the child is refusing school irrespective of pain and that it is not primarily the pain disorder with its concomitant absenteeism from school. Children refusing school will quickly learn to use the learned strategies to influence their pain on the ward. In their family surroundings, they still have these abilities but they use them primarily outside the time scheduled for school, so that they still do not attend school. Some of these children will suddenly exhibit altered symptomatology, e.g., tiredness, exhaustion, or a prolonged flu. It quickly becomes obvious that the family's structures are unable – or sometimes unwilling – to implement the therapeutic arrangements. If this is the case, one must inform the child welfare office with its outpatient or institutional inpatient therapeutic programs. Often these children have to be moved to alternative accommodation, and this is not seldom at the parents' request because they are at the end of their rope.

3. The possibility of the presence of trauma-associated disturbance or PTSD, or permanent bullying at school, should be examined. In one of our patients where we discussed school truancy, it finally turned out that the child had been repeatedly sexually abused at school and was getting death threats from the offender in person, by phone, and via the Internet. In another case, a boy was attacked by a group of adolescents from another school on his way home and threatened with death if he talked to his parents. Most (but unfortunately not all) children will report such experiences in the talks if they are informed about the therapeutic team's confidentiality.

7.5 Pain Therapy in Children with Learning Disabilities or Intellectual Giftedness

If the patient's intelligence is out of the normal range, the pain-therapeutic approach has to be adapted.

7.5.1 The Child with a Chronic Disorder and Learning Disabilities

In children with learning disabilities, the education program should be modified as follows:

1. The lessons teaching theoretical knowledge or techniques are shortened. Each educational appointment is confined to just *one* topic.

2. Many affected children know by intuition that it is harder for them to grasp complex interrelationships as quickly as their peers. This will evoke shame and insecurity with regard to theoretical content. Some of the children try to hide their weakness by not asking much or pretending that they did comprehend everything. But a basic understanding of the biopsychosocial model is necessary for pain therapy. Hence, it is very important to prompt these children to cooperate honestly. We've had good results when the therapist has humorously and self-ironically communicated any assumed insecurity or difficulty in understanding by the child as a sign of the therapist's lack of didactic capabilities. It may be worthwhile to try the following approach to check the child's comprehension: "Sorry, I just lost my thread. Could you please help me to resume the last topic by telling me what you have learned so far?"

3. Finally, we recommend asking the child to summarize the content of the crucial education sessions the way he/she understood the topic. If the child is able to write, this should also be done in children with learning disabilities. It is advisable to add "in your own words," "just as you understood the education," "in keywords," or "as you like."

7.5.2 Children with Chronic Pain and Intellectual Giftedness

A highly gifted child needs a lot of input and needs to be challenged. Often a highly gifted child judges an education that is below his/her competence level as an insult and doesn't feel taken seriously.

But even a highly gifted child often missing school cannot know the missed subject matter. In addition, some highly gifted children tend to overrate their cognitive capabilities, which is their weak point, and similar to their peers with learning disabilities, their feelings are easily hurt. One has to carefully balance out the demands on the child. Three conclusions are important for the educational process:

1. A highly gifted child needs more exercises or homework than other children.

2. A highly gifted child seems to love to scrutinize any existing structure. Yes, this could be very annoying. But this also gives the therapist the chance to modify preexisting therapeutic methods and interventions for the better. One way could be to give the child some tasks and then ask him/her to check the methods or interventions for any flaws and to make any suggestions for improvement.

3. As with any child, the therapeutic process should be made as transparent as possible. The various options and interventions in the current as well as future therapeutic process should be addressed *early*. This will increase the amount of information to be exchanged, sometimes significantly stretching the appointments. But at the end of therapy, many of our patients explicitly tell us that they always feel taken seriously and integrated into the therapeutic process by this very approach and are able to retain control over treatment.

7.6   Pain Therapy in a Child with a Burdening Underlying Disease

"Pain is always there. It is the worst if I sit in my wheelchair for too long." – Christina (17 years), pain disorder and spina bifida

Children with a severe underlying somatic disease (e.g., spina bifida, multiple sclerosis, epidermolysis bullosa dystrophica, Ehlers-Danlos syndrome, juvenile poly- or oligoarthitis, celiac disease, or Crohn's disease) are prone to developing a pain disorder. For most professional helpers (physicians, psychologists), this is difficult to understand. They see the primary disease and they know that it is often combined with pain. Severe pain in juvenile idiopathic arthritis, for example, indicates an inflammatory relapse and is regarded as an important diagnostic marker. A pain disorder is present and has to be diagnosed if the patient reports a high pain score, shows typical pain behavior, and is emotionally impaired, without the somatic disease being strongly active (see Chap. 3 for diagnosis criteria). At the time the patient presents at the paediatric outpatient pain clinic, drug therapy has in many cases already been escalated (glucocorticosteroids, biologicals, anti-inflammatory drugs) without any additional therapeutic effect. Such a constellation, with the disease activity not explaining the pain score and pain-related impairment, hints at the presence of a pain disorder. In most cases pain-modulating psychosocial factors can be explored. To diagnose a pain disorder on top of an "obvious" severe somatic disease is difficult not only for somatically focused physicians but also for psychologists not familiar with the biopsychosocial model. Paediatric patients suffering from a severe organic disease as well as from a pain disorder need a multiprofessional therapeutic team with intact interprofessional communication.

Because there are a lot of potentially painful severe somatic diseases, we will confine our discussion to some important general pain-therapeutic principles.

7.6.1   Adaptation of Education

Many children suffering a severe underlying somatic disease have gotten used to medical examinations and clinic stays over the years. Over and over the child has been queried by his parents for symptoms of his underlying disease. Dependent on his/her specific diagnosis, the child will depend more on parental support than on his/her peers. A significant part of his/her leisure time is sacrificed to disease-related matters. What does that mean for education?

1. *First,* these children and their parents are accustomed to both a very somatic approach and somatically oriented disease models. Due to their proximity to at least one parent, these children rely very much on this parent for judgment of their physical symptoms, much more so than is age appropriate. The increased somatic focus and worries could make education extremely difficult. This, however, is *normal* and *appropriate* considering the underlying disease. With the background of emotional or physical burden of any severe underlying somatic disease, the therapist should examine the individual suffering experiences and recognize the

resources used for dealing with the disease. This is crucial for establishing a good working atmosphere within the therapeutic relationship. For most affected children, it is a challenge to join pain therapy, leaving familiar diagnostics or medication behind. That aspect is important to the child, but even more important when working with the parents. There is a high risk that at least one of the parents suffers depressive symptoms facing such nearly unbearable experiences. If there was ever a life-threatening event related to the child's underlying disease, one should bear in mind that the patient, the parents, or siblings might suffer PTSD. All those aspects should be considered in the family talk, which is best done by querying for current sources of strength, worries, and the degree of exhaustion. In so doing, the therapist will quickly gain an overview of the current burden and resources of the family. If the parents feel taken seriously with their coping strategies, they usually agree to readjust their behavior as best they can.

2. *Second,* the complexity of the biological problem requires one to address during the education session the point that the ability to inhibit pain is "already part of the brain." Due to the family's background in these cases, we choose a somatically oriented education program. It may be helpful to use metaphors such as "analgesics of the brain" or "integrated pain-inhibition system," meaning that the ability to distract ourselves from pain is intrinsic to the brain. Such a system may prove to be lifesaving in case of danger (e.g., fighting a tiger in the Stone Age) or just beneficial (today: going to work or pursuing one's hobby in spite of injury). Thus, mental or social aspects of pain don't contradict physical ones but use the same biological systems that can also cause disease (Eippert et al. 2009). The child and his/her parents will be keen to know why pain inhibition doesn't work properly anymore. Before coming to the details, one should summarize the essentials.

"The more I focus on my body, the more I worry; the more I choose to be passive and take a rest when pain emerges, the more cerebral pain inhibition is switched off. (Break.) This is one of the main reasons why in many children suffering a severe painful disease, the risk of experiencing a chronic impairment in addition to their acute pain increases with time. Let me explain this to you in more detail (now follow Sect. 6.3.3)."

3. *Third,* it is important to meticulously distinguish between acute pain (e.g., due to a relapse in rheumatic disease) and chronic pain. With this differentiated education, we aim to instruct the patients to a more differentiated body awareness and judgment. In the long run, this is the only way to allow them to distinguish pain signals indicating acute disease from those due to pain sensitization. This is a challenge to pain therapy. We will address it in detail in Sect. 7.6.3.

7.6.2 Striving for Independence and Autonomy with an Underlying Somatic Disease

The older the child, the more he/she wants to follow his/her own path, enforce his/her own will, and use his/her own problem-solving strategies. As a consequence of this striving, conflicts will arise. This is a normal part of adolescence.

For many children with a severe underlying somatic disease, it is difficult to go their own way. In the presence of further stress factors, especially in puberty, severe conflicts between the child and the family will emerge, making coping with the disease and pain therapy much more difficult. This will be illustrated by the next case report.

Case Report: Jürgen (15 years) (Pain Disorder and Ehlers-Danlos Syndrome)
For many years Jürgen has been medically treated due to various complications of his underlying disease. The last treatment was surgical stabilization of his spine. Afterwards, Jürgen was able to cover short distances without a wheelchair again. In spite of this success, his family has been at the end of their rope for some time now. Because of the increased nursing efforts, the many visits to the doctor, and Jürgen's various surgeries, his mother feels burned out. She always says, "I can't see the horizon!" During the last couple of years, Jürgen hasn't learned to look after himself. Being extraordinarily intelligent, he attends senior high school supported by an integration assistant. However, social contacts outside of school are rare because Jürgen's family lives in the countryside, and Jürgen would need transportation for every contact. Being severely handicapped, Jürgen cannot walk longer distances without his wheelchair. After school, Jürgen is often frustrated; this has been going on for several years already. According to his mother, this is due to Jürgen's lack of ability to proactively make social contacts. She has always tried to help him with his social deficits, but that is something he doesn't want to talk about. There are continuous conflicts between Jürgen and the rest of the family instead, as all family members agree. Meanwhile, Jürgen refuses to practice his essential physiotherapeutic exercises or to proactively work on an improvement of his situation. He would prefer to sit in his wheelchair and let someone push him. This is, however, causing his physical symptoms to deteriorate. Now the parents are too exhausted to enforce their will. As his mother told us, resignation is spreading all over the family. Hence, the contact between Jürgen and his family is restricted to a minimum. Jürgen retreats to his room more and more. With his exaggerated and worrying body awareness, he focuses on numerous somatic processes and has been repeatedly admitted into an inpatient clinic for diagnostics of indistinct complaints. The interrelationship between the frequency and intensity of his complaints and absenteeism from school is obvious to the family.

These conflicts are not necessarily that severe. This example illustrates how increasing parental exhaustion, learned passivity, medically indicated increased body awareness, physical disability, low social competence, resulting mental problems, and difficulties in school merge to a vicious cycle in which no way out is obvious.

Certainly there is no patent remedy. On the contrary, especially in the family talks with the physician or the psychotherapist, substantial skills in family therapy as well as knowledge of systemic relationships are needed in order to create the prerequisites for successful therapy. In such a situation, the first step is to address the parents' burden and exhaustion and to appreciate their efforts during the long course of the disease. The next step is to check if any family member still believes in a change for the better. Then the family members should briefly record their contribution to an improvement of the situation. In case the family members are no longer confident in finding a solution and are not able to draw an alternative solution for the family, we address the solution of boarding schools or other types of accommodation outside the family.

Certainly such a family talk is emotionally quite stressful. But it will make obvious the resources present or those lacking. Having made it clear that there is confidentiality, don't forget to ask the child in a single session the same questions. With Jürgen it became obvious that a boarding school would be the best possible trade-off. The reader should be aware that any solution based on accommodation outside of the family can usually only be put into practice together with the respective child welfare office. With the widespread municipal shortage of money, it takes a good argument to get a municipal subsidy for external accommodation. During the family talks, the therapist should try to convince the family to ask for the clinic's social worker's support to set up the respective application.

7.6.3 "Double-Entry Accounting": Oath and Blessing of Body Awareness

Due to the unpredictable course of most severe underlying somatic diseases, it is medically important for the children to pay attention to certain physical symptoms that indicate a relapse or increased disease activity. This is a matter of survival. But the increased body attention is the largest obstacle for successful pain therapy. Given the great variety of somatic disorders or complications, each patient has to find his/her own way to manage body awareness according to his/her own and his/her family's resources and accompanying stress factors.

A successful way will provide the answers to the following six questions:
1. Did I understand that I can influence pain perception?
2. How can I distinguish disease-related acute pain from chronic pain?
3. To what degree am I ready to work actively and autonomously to improve my pain and my situation?
4. Which strategies can I use for acute or chronic pain?
5. How can I contribute to the de-escalation of family problems?
6. What is the plan for after my stay on the ward (or after therapy has finished)? What can I contribute to making my success last? Where do I need support? Who will support me?

7.6.4   Considering Painful Medical Procedures

It goes without saying that chronically diseased children – as any child – should be supported in their coping with painful medical procedures. Unfortunately, adolescents often are treated in hospitals for adults where they and their parents are confronted with phrases such as "This doesn't hurt. Don't make such a fuss" or "The way your child is acting, there must be another underlying problem."

For an overview of especially helpful strategies, we refer the reader to the extensive literature on this subject (e.g., Kuttner and Culbert 2003; Kuttner 2010; Kohen and Olness 1993). Besides various hypnotherapeutic as well as imaginative strategies, classic cognitive distraction strategies are helpful (e.g., strategies from Sects. 6.4.1, 6.4.2, and 6.4.3). Besides these techniques, children should have time within the framework of a stepped plan to get used to the medical situation. Painful medical procedures, especially those not sufficiently supported, will contribute to an aggravation of a pain disorder because they provoke helplessness and fear and often trigger any preexisting traumatic memories, both resulting in increased tension. Quite often children report that they experience medical procedures as so severe that symptoms similar to PTSD arise, including flashbacks of procedures perceived as especially horrible. For pain chronicity, this is devastating.

In order to render the necessary medical procedures as gentle as possible, the therapist, the NET, and the child should jointly set up a stepped plan (gradual exposure) with the last step being the very procedure perceived as especially stressful (e.g., lumbar puncture). According to the model of systematic desensitization, the steps preceding the last one should gradually make the child familiar with the medical procedure, thus reducing anxiety. Simultaneously, the child learns hypnotherapeutic and/or imagery and/or distraction techniques (depending on the child's resources). Finally, a detailed plan should be set up to schedule the step at which the child should practice which special technique.

7.6.5   Coping with Pain and Future Perspectives

Treated adequately, most children with a pain disorder will face quite a normal life with all its common challenges, which seem to be unconquerable for many healthy adolescents. Children with a severe underlying somatic disease resulting in permanent handicap (e.g., spina bifida) or advancing impairment of quality of life (e.g., multiple sclerosis) are facing a much bigger challenge: typically they perceive fear, insecurity, resignation, or despair. In some children, such an emotional challenge is more than they can handle with their coping strategies. As a consequence, they may develop dysfunctional coping strategies regarding their thinking and acting, which should better be diagnosed as an adjustment disorder. Apart from the dysfunctional judgment of somatic processes, catastrophizing thoughts about future perspectives are common. Thus, this leads to an increase in internal and external tension and therefore contributes to pain amplification and chronicity.

The patient's task is to develop an attitude of acceptance towards the underlying disease. The targets for therapy and life should match the possibilities. This is often of significance not only to the patient but also to his/her parents. At the beginning of pain therapy, the Three Letters (Sect. 6.4.3; Chap. 9, Worksheet #17) and projective questionnaires (Sect. 3.3.3) are well suited to gaining an overview of the state of acceptance of the disease. Also from these, the therapist will get information about the resources currently available. This gives an idea of how to best support the patient with his/her disease coping. Sometimes an increased acceptance of the disease and a more realistic future perspective contribute to successful pain therapy, due to the concomitant emotional relief and improved ability to substantially regulate the patient's stress and emotions.

7.7 Contraindications for Pain Therapy

Contraindications of paediatric pain therapy have not so far been investigated. We feel that one should be cautious with the usage of pain-therapeutic methods in anorexia nervosa or in the presence of psychotic symptoms.

7.7.1 Children with a Pain Disorder and Concomitant Anorexia Nervosa

In our past experience, pain therapy as described in this manual was not successful in children with not yet sufficiently treated concomitant anorexia nervosa, even if bodyweight had stabilized for some time. Extremely increased body awareness and distorted body perception are two of the main symptoms of anorexia nervosa, and are nearly inaccessible to pain therapy while concomitant anorexia nervosa is not sufficiently treated, while increasing pain perception. A sufficient and successful treatment of anorexia nervosa seems to be a prerequisite for successful pain therapy.

7.7.2 Children with a Pain Disorder and Psychotic Symptoms

Generally, it is presumably possible that children with chronic pain and concomitant psychotic symptoms will benefit from some pain-therapeutic methods in an inpatient psychiatric setting. Psychotic disorders may be accompanied by disturbed attention, vigilance, or thinking. Additionally, there may be unpredictable fears along with very high mental and muscular tension. Thus, we urge not using imaginative techniques or relaxation (e.g., autogenic training, PMR). It goes without saying that these methods are absolutely contraindicated during an active episode of psychosis. During inpatient psychiatric therapy, however, a very experienced psychotherapist familiar with children suffering from psychotic symptoms might apply more simple variants of distraction techniques or acceptance-based techniques to improve the patient's situation.

References

Asmundson GJ, Coons MJ, Taylor S, Katz J (2002) PTSD and the experience of pain: research and clinical implications of shared vulnerability and mutual maintenance models. Can J Psychiatry 47(10):930–937

Dobe M, Hechler T, Zernikow B (2009) The pain provocation technique as an adjunctive treatment module for children and adolescents with chronic disabling pain: a case report. J Child Adolesc Trauma 2(4):297–307

Dobe M, Hechler T, Behlert J, Kosfelder J, Zernikow B (2011) Pain therapy with children and adolescents severely disabled due to chronic pain: long-term outcome after inpatient pain therapy. Schmerz 25(4):411–422

Eccleston C, Malleson P (2003) Managing chronic pain in children and adolescents. We need to address the embarrassing lack of data for this common problem. BMJ 326(7404):1408–1409

Eippert F, Finsterbusch J, Bingel U, Büchel C (2009) Direct evidence for spinal cord involvement in placebo analgesia. Science 326(5951):404

Goubert L, Craig KD, Vervoort T, Morley S, Sullivan MJ, de C Williams AC et al (2005) Facing others in pain: the effects of empathy. Pain 118(3):285–288

Hechler T, Dobe M, Kosfelder J, Damschen U, Hübner B, Blankenburg M et al (2009) Effectiveness of a three-week multimodal inpatient pain treatment for adolescents suffering from chronic pain: statistical and clinical significance. Clin J Pain 25(2):156–166

Hirschfeld G, Hechler T, Dobe M, Wager J, von Lützau P, Blankenburg M et al (2013) Maintaining lasting improvements: one-year follow-up of children with severe chronic pain undergoing multimodal inpatient treatment. J Pediatr Psychol 38(2):224–236

Kohen DP, Olness K (1993) Hypnotherapy with children. In: Rhue JW, Lynn SJ, Kirsch I (eds) Handbook of clinical hypnosis. American Psychological Association, Washington, DC, p xxv

Kuttner L (2010) A child in pain. What health professionals can do to help. Crown-House, Bethel

Kuttner L, Culbert T (2003) Hypnosis, biofeedback, and self-regulation skills for children in pain. In: Breivik H, Campbell W, Eccleston C (eds) Clinical pain management: practical applications and procedures. Arnold, London

Liedl A, Müller J, Morina N, Karl A, Denke C, Knaevelsrud C (2011) Physical activity within a CBT intervention improves coping with pain in traumatized refugees: results of a randomized controlled design. Pain Med 12:234–245

Martin AL, McGrath PA, Brown SC, Katz J (2007) Anxiety sensitivity, fear of pain and pain-related disability in children and adolescents with chronic pain. Pain Res Manag 12(4):267–272

Meulders A, Vansteenwegen D, Vlaeyen JW (2011) The acquisition of fear of movement-related pain and associative learning: a novel pain-relevant human fear conditioning paradigm. Pain 152(11):2460–2469

Pinquart M, Shen Y (2011) Depressive symptoms in children and adolescents with chronic physical illness: an updated meta-analysis. J Pediatr Psychol 36(4):375–384

Seng JS, Graham-Bermann SA, Clark MK, McCarthy AM, Ronis DL (2005) Posttraumatic stress disorder and physical comorbidity among female children and adolescents: results from service-use data. Pediatrics 116(6):e767–e776

Sharp TJ, Harvey AG (2001) Chronic pain and posttraumatic stress disorder: mutual maintenance? Clin Psychol Rev 21:857–877

Wald J, Taylor S (2007) Efficacy of interoceptive exposure therapy combined with trauma-related exposure therapy for posttraumatic stress disorder: a pilot study. J Anxiety Disord 21(8):1050–1060

Watkins J, Watkins H (1997) Ego states – theory and therapy. W W Norton & Co Ltd., New York

Is It All Worthwhile? – Effectiveness of Intensive Interdisciplinary Pain Treatment

8

Tanja Hechler, Michael Dobe, and Boris Zernikow

Contents

T. Hechler • M. Dobe (✉)
German Paediatric Pain Centre (GPPC),
Children's and Adolescents' Hospital, Witten/Herdecke University,
Dr.-Friedrich-Steiner Street 5, Datteln 45711, Germany
e-mail: m.dobe@kinderklinik-datteln.de

B. Zernikow
German Paediatric Pain Centre (GPPC),
Children's and Adolescents' Hospital, Witten/Herdecke University,
Dr.-Friedrich-Steiner Street 5, Datteln 45711, Germany

Chair Children's Pain Therapy and Paediatric Palliative Care,
Witten/Herdecke University, School of Medicine,
Datteln 45711, Germany
e-mail: b.zernikow@deutsches-kinderschmerzzentrum.de

M. Dobe, B. Zernikow (eds.),
Practical Treatment Options for Chronic Pain in Children and Adolescents,
DOI 10.1007/978-3-642-37816-4_8, © Springer-Verlag Berlin Heidelberg 2013

Abstract

This chapter addresses three topics: First, the evidence for the effectiveness of intensive interdisciplinary pain programs is summarized. Data was gathered from eight studies which report positive short-term treatment results, especially for decreases in pain-related disability and absence from school. Long-term effectiveness was shown in one study with 67 % of the children maintaining positive changes over a 12-month period. Second, characteristics of children in need of intensive interdisciplinary pain treatment are summarized. While grading systems for paediatric chronic pain are scarce, preliminary evidence for the utility of the Chronic Pain Grading System (CPG) of von Korff et al. (Pain 50(2):133–149, 1992) for children is presented. At present, clinicians mainly rely on clinically evolved criteria for treatment allocation, though these have not yet been evaluated. Third, research on process variables which modulate treatment response is presented. There is clearly a paucity of research in this area. The few existing studies demonstrate sex differences in treatment response, the importance of changes in pain coping, psychological flexibility, willingness to change, and adherence to the treatment regimen for treatment response. Future research is warranted to provide evidence for the effectiveness through randomized-controlled trials, to provide validated grading systems for paediatric chronic pain for treatment allocation, and to investigate the specific impact of process variables on treatment outcome.

8.1 Introduction

Intensive interdisciplinary pain treatment is advocated as the treatment of choice for children who are severely affected by their chronic pain condition (Zernikow et al. 2012). In this chapter, we follow the definition of an intensive interdisciplinary pain program set out by the German Pain Society (Arnold et al. 2009) defined as treatment provided by a minimum of three health-care disciplines including medical, psychological, and physical therapy which are provided concurrently. There are two forms of intensive interdisciplinary pain treatment: an inpatient-based approach (Dobe et al. 2006; Hechler et al. 2009) and a day-hospital approach (Eccleston et al. 2003; Logan et al. 2012), which share similarities in therapeutic interventions and program philosophy. These programs address underlying pain mechanisms, adapt pain medication, treat specific symptoms such as emotional distress, and teach active coping skills (Hechler et al. 2010c; Maynard et al. 2009). The advantage of the intensive interdisciplinary pain treatment is that professionals from several disciplines can see the child daily in various situations, thus allowing a systematic change in pain-related disability and distress to be achieved (Maynard et al. 2009). Given the high intensity of treatment and the involvement of several specialists, intensive interdisciplinary pain treatment is expensive. It is therefore worth knowing how effective these intensive interdisciplinary pain treatments are in reducing the severity of pain and pain-related disability. In this chapter, we address three questions: Chap. 8.2 provides an overview of existing studies into the effectiveness of the treatment. Chapter 8.3 discusses for whom this treatment may be warranted. Chapter 8.4 reviews knowledge on potential process variables modulating treatment response.

8.2   Evidence for the Effectiveness of Intensive Interdisciplinary Pain Treatment in Children with Chronic Pain

How effective intensive interdisciplinary pain treatment is for children is difficult to determine for two reasons: First, these programs and their evaluation are still scarce worldwide (Hechler et al. 2010b) even though their number is rising with yet only nine publications (five of which are from the German research group of the German Paediatric Pain Centre) (Dobe et al. 2006, 2011; Eccleston et al. 2003; Hechler et al. 2009, 2010a: Hirschfeld et al. 2013; Logan et al. 2012; Maynard et al. 2009; Palermo and Scher 2001). In comparison, there are more than a hundred nonrandomized studies in adults (Guzman et al. 2002). In addition, the few programs are diverse in terms of interventions provided (exercise therapy (Sherry et al. 1999) compared to multimodal interventions (Eccleston et al. 2003)).

Here we present an overview of existing effectiveness studies (Table 8.1). We included studies on treatment programs in accordance with the definition of an intensive interdisciplinary pain program provided previously. We were able to identify eight studies presented by five research groups from the USA, Great Britain, Sweden, and Germany.

Table 8.1 Studies into the effectiveness of intensive interdisciplinary pain treatment for children with chronic pain

Study	Treatment follow-up (FO)	Sample description: diagnosis, age	Outcome measures	Statistical analysis	Pain	Disability	School absence	Emotional distress
Palermo and Scher (2001)	Inpatient-based intensive interdisciplinary treatment 3 weeks FO: 6 months	Case study of a girl with somatoform pain disorder 11 years	Anxiety depression Functional disability Health-related quality of life	Descriptives of changes after 6 months	No information	→	→	No information
Eccleston et al. (2003)	Day-hospital program of interdisciplinary cognitive behavior therapy 3 weeks Post-treatment FO: 3 months	N = 57 adolescents with various pain conditions (72 % girls) N = 57 parents Age: 11–17 years	Pain intensity Anxiety Catastrophic thinking Disability Somatic awareness Depression School attendance	T-test for repeated measure Confidence interval	No change	→	→	No change
Maynard et al. (2009)	Inpatient-based intensive interdisciplinary pain program FO: 3 months	N = 41 (73 % girls) with various pain conditions	Retrospective chart review School attendance Sleep Functional status	Descriptive statistics; T-tests for dependent samples; Wilcoxon signed-rank test for dependent samples	No information	→	→	No information

Logan et al. (2012)	Day-hospital approach of intensive interdisciplinary pain therapy including CBT, physiotherapy and occupational therapy FO: Discharge and follow-up (2–24 months)	Longitudinal case series N = 56 adolescents with CRPS spectrum conditions (89.3 % girls) Age: 8–18 years	Pain Functional disability School functioning Anxiety Depression Lower Extremity Function Scale Canadian Occupational Performance Measure	Paired t tests, Wilcoxon signed rank tests; repeated measures analysis of variances	→	→	→	→	→
Hechler et al. (Dobe et al. 2006, 2011; Hechler et al. 2009, 2010a; Zernikow et al. (2012); Hirschfeld et al. 2013)	Inpatient-based intensive interdisciplinary pain program; CBT-based FO: 3 and 12 months	N = 200 (60 % girls) children and adolescents with severe chronic pain and various pain conditions Age: 9.9–18.3 years	Pain intensity Pain-related disability School absence Emotional distress	ANOVA for repeated measures Clinical significance of achieved changes according to Jacobson and Truax (1991) McNemar tests to determine maintenance of achieved improvement status	→	→	→	→	→

8.2.1   Design

The majority of the studies included children with various pain conditions (7/8). The age range was comparable across studies, ranging between 9 and 18 years. All studies included more girls than boys (60–89 % girls). Primary outcome variables included pain intensity in 6/8 studies, pain-related disability (8/8), school absence (8/8), and emotional distress (6/8). Two studies reported on posttreatment results; 4/8 studies reported on short-term effectiveness (ranging between 3 and 6 months). One study investigated long-term effectiveness (≥12 months).

8.2.2   Short-Term Effectiveness

Statistically reductions in pain intensity were reported by 6/8 studies. Two studies also reported clinically significant changes. All studies reported significant decreases in pain-related disability and school absence following intensive interdisciplinary pain treatment. Significant reductions in emotional distress were reported by 5/8 studies. Two studies reported also clinically significant reductions. In addition, Hechler et al. (2009) defined an overall improvement status by use of the construct of clinical significance (Jacobson and Truax 1991). Patients were classified as showing overall improvement if they did not show deterioration in any pain-related variable (i.e., in pain intensity, pain-related disability, and school absence) and had clinically significant improvements in one or both disability-related variables (pain-related disability or school absence). All other patients were classified as showing no overall improvement. Of their sample, 55 % were assigned to the group with overall improvement 3 months following treatment.

In summary, all studies provide evidence of the short-term effectiveness of intensive interdisciplinary pain treatment.

8.2.3   Long-Term Effectiveness

The research group of the German Paediatric Pain Centre (Dobe et al. 2011; Hirschfeld et al. 2013) investigated the long-term effectiveness of the intensive interdisciplinary pain program with two research questions: First, what was the degree of change in primary outcome variables 12 months following treatment? Second, how stable were the achieved treatment effects over two assessment periods, i.e., 3- and 12-month follow-up (Hirschfeld et al. 2013)? They defined the following groups based on overall improvement status at 3- and 12-month follow-up: (1) "stable long-term improvers" (improved on both assessments), (2) "short-term improvers" (improved at 3-month follow-up only), (3) "long-term improvers" (improved at 12-month follow-up only), and (4) "children with unsuccessful treatment results" (not improved at either follow-up). They found that participants showed statistically significant reductions in all variables 12 months after treatment, such that they reported less pain, disability, and fewer school absences. Over the two time points, 53 (46 %) of the adolescents were "stable long-term improvers," 16 (14 %) were "long-term improvers," 22 (19 %) were "short-term improvers," and 25 (22 %) had an "unsuccessful treatment outcome."

To sum up, children with chronic pain are able to maintain accomplished positive changes 12 months following treatment. Approximately 50 % recover quickly (after 3 months) and are able to maintain this status long term. Another 14 % take longer to improve but maintain this status as well. Approximately 20 % deteriorate over time, and another 20 % do not (yet) benefit from the intervention.

8.2.4   Limitations

There are some methodological problems of the existing studies ranging from a heterogeneous definition of core endpoints (Maynard et al. 2009; McGrath et al. 2008) and, most importantly, a lack of control groups and randomization (Eccleston et al. 2003; Hechler et al. 2009; Maynard et al. 2009; Sherry et al. 1999). There are only five randomized controlled trials (RCT) available yet (Hechler 2011; Lanzi et al. 2007; Lee et al. 2002; Lommel et al. 2011; Wicksell et al. 2009) – compared to 12 RCTs in adult samples (Guzman et al. 2002). Four of the five RCTs, however, did not provide intensive interdisciplinary pain treatment as defined previously.

8.2.5   Evidence from a Randomized Controlled Trial

In the study by Hechler (2011), adolescents (aged 9–17 years) were randomly assigned to either immediate referral (fast track sample) or a 3-week waiting list (best practice sample). Assessments were made before treatment and 3 weeks following randomization, after the intervention group had completed the treatment. Main outcomes were pain intensity, pain-related disability, and school absence; trial compliance was considered as a secondary endpoint. Over a 19-month recruitment period, 120 adolescents were recruited and 1:1 randomized. Nine children of the intervention group discontinued treatment. Only the intervention group showed locally significant changes in all three core parameters. More children in the intervention group compared to the best practice group showed clinically significant changes in pain-related disability (22 % versus 6 %) and school absence (36 % versus 11 %). This pattern was not found for pain intensity. Significantly more children in the intervention group showed overall improvement (54 % compared to 16 %; Fisher $p < .001$; 95 % CI for incidence difference: 19–(.57 %). The study provides evidence that inpatient-based intensive interdisciplinary pain treatment improves pain-related disability and school absence in paediatric chronic pain patients.

8.3   Who Should Be Admitted?

Children and adolescents with chronic pain differ with regard to their pain intensity, pain-related disability, and school absence as well as emotional distress. These differences in the severity of the chronic pain problem have an important impact on the kind of treatment that may be required. For example, a child with high pain intensity but low pain-related disability and school absence may not necessarily be admitted to an inpatient-based treatment setting. The question of how the severity of the chronic pain problem should be graded in children is still unanswered. Which factors should be taken into account when assigning children to different degrees of treatment intensity?

In Germany, we refer children who display unsatisfactory treatment results in primary care to our inpatient-based treatment (see also Chap. 5 for a more detailed description). In addition, all patients meet the following criteria for inpatient admission in accordance to the medical service of the health-care insurances (Hechler et al. 2009):

1. No malignant disease
2. Patient and parent compliance with inpatient treatment

In addition, at least three of the following five criteria have to be met to be admitted to the inpatient unit:

1. Pain duration ≥6 months
2. Average pain intensity of ≥5 over the preceding 7 days (Numeric Rating Scale: NRS 0–10)
3. Pain peaks (pain intensity ≥8) occurring at least twice a week
4. At least 5 days absent from school within the preceding 4 weeks
5. Severe pain-related disability as assessed by the Paediatric Pain Disability Index (P-PDI) (Hübner et al. 2009) with scores ≥36/60 (Dobe et al. 2006)

Unfortunately, the specificity and sensitivity of these criteria have not yet been investigated.

While there are assessment tools to grade chronic pain in adults, such as the severity grading system of Von Korff et al. (1992), the Chronic Pain Grading (CPG) adaptation of such a system for children and adolescents with chronic pain is scarce. In the CPG, pain severity is calculated based on an algorithm including pain intensity, disability days, and an overall judgment of pain-related disability.

Huguet and Miro (2008) applied the CPG to a sample of school children. They found that 37 % of their sample had chronic pain, but only 5 % reported chronic pain that was classified as moderate or severe. They further showed that increasing pain severity was associated with decreased quality of life, increasing visits to a doctor, and medication usage. A limitation of this study is the low number of children assigned to the higher CPGs; only 4 % ($n=22$) were experiencing moderate and only 1 % ($n=6$) high chronic pain severity.

Vowles et al. (2009) developed another severity grading system for adolescents, including psychological variables based on the Bath Adolescent Pain Questionnaire (BAPQ; Eccleston et al. 2005). It comprises four distinct groups differing in daily functioning, emotional functioning, family functioning, and development. While those results are promising with regard to a potential grading system for children and adolescents, the findings are hampered by the fact that they are based on children with musculoskeletal pain only and are specifically developed for the BAPQ, which is so far only available in English. Furthermore, the clinical applicability of this measure is limited due to the use of a rather complex algorithm for group assignment. Even though conducted in a clinical sample, this study did not test the utility of the measure for treatment assignment.

To sum up, previous studies that either tried to apply the CPG to paediatric samples or develop novel grading systems provided neither a comprehensive valid assessment nor a test of its usefulness as a measure of outcomes or its prognostic utility for treatment assignment.

The research group of the German Paediatric Pain Centre (Wager et al. 2013) has recently investigated the application of the CPG to a large sample of adolescents with chronic pain admitted to a tertiary clinic. Results indicate that most adolescents were assigned to the three higher severity grades. Higher CPG assignment was associated with more pain locations, higher pain frequency, longer pain duration, extensive use of health care, and more depressive symptoms. Adolescents with a high CPG received recommendations for inpatient treatment more often; however, the prognostic utility for therapy recommendation was low. Sensitivity to change was assessed via reassessment at follow-up for a subsample of 490 adolescents. The majority of adolescents improved to a less severe CPG; changes were more common in the high severity range.

To summarize, a standard assessment tool to grade paediatric chronic pain and enable assignment to different treatment intensities is not yet available. Clinicians therefore rely on clinically developed assignment procedures which have not yet been critically evaluated. There is clearly a need for research in this area. The following research questions may be addressed: first, to investigate and evaluate comprehensive grading systems for paediatric chronic pain; second, to determine their clinical and prognostic utility for treatment decisions; and third, to compare the effectiveness of different treatment intensities for patient groups assigned by varying severity of the chronic pain condition.

8.4   Process Variables and Their Effects on Treatment Response

Intensive interdisciplinary pain treatments aim to achieve reductions in the child's pain-related disability, school absence, and psychological distress (Eccleston et al. 2006; Hechler et al. 2009; Simons et al. 2010). The importance of decreases in reported pain ratings is critically discussed, given study results that pain in itself does not explain the extent of pain-related disability (Wicksell et al. 2009). It is therefore argued that, in contrast to pain reduction per se, the child's ability to act effectively in the presence of pain and distress constitutes a key factor for improvement in accordance to acceptance and commitment therapy (ACT) (Hayes et al. 1999). We have previously reported on the effectiveness of the programs in accomplishing these treatment goals, i.e., the effect of treatment on outcome measures (see Table 8.1).

Here, we address the question of which process variables might moderate or mediate treatment response. Analyses of these variables provide knowledge of the treatment's impact on a process (e.g., changes in coping) and that process' effect on the treatment outcome. For example, cognitive behavioral therapy (CBT) aims to increase the self-management of pain and to accomplish decreases in pain-related disability and pain intensity. Differences in pain coping (active versus passive) may be particularly relevant to understanding improvements in pain-related disability (Hechler et al. 2010c).

There is still a paucity of research on associated factors of treatment response in paediatric pain research (Wicksell et al. 2011). To the best of our knowledge, there are to date five studies addressing this issue. We subdivided their results with regard to the factors they investigated. These ranged from sociodemographic factors (do boys respond better than girls?) (Hechler et al. 2010a) to psychological factors inherent in the child or parents (such as changes in pain coping) (Hechler et al. 2010c) and adherence to the treatment regimen (Simons et al. 2010).

8.4.1 Sociodemographic Factors Associated with Treatment Response

Hechler et al. (2010a) investigated differences in treatment response between boys and girls and between children and adolescents. In their study, with 33 children (aged 7–10 years) and 167 adolescents (aged 11–18 years) including 60 % girls, they found that boys displayed better treatment responses than girls at 12-month follow-up. Specifically, girls reported higher pain intensity and higher school absence than boys 12 months following treatment. They also maintained higher use of analgesics over the study period compared to boys. The authors suggest two potential reasons for these differences: (a) girls' pain experience and pain behavior and (b) parental reactions towards pain. Girls may have benefited less from the program with less reduction in pain intensity. This may lead to pain expressions and pain-related behavior which may trigger parental reactions towards pain. Parents are typically responsible for delivering analgesics to the child. Hence, girls' parents may still focus on a medical model of chronic pain leading to higher use of analgesics.

8.4.2 Factors Inherent in the Child and Parents

8.4.2.1 Maladaptive Pain Coping
Multidimensional models of chronic pain such as the psychobiological perspective emphasize the role of pain-related coping strategies to the experience of pain as well as to the development and maintenance of pain-related disability (Hermann et al. 2007; Novy et al. 1995). Accordingly, intensive interdisciplinary pain programs with a CBT-approach focus on changes in pain-related coping strategies during treatment to impact on core outcomes such as pain and disability. Few studies,

however, have explored changes in coping with pain over treatment and how these changes are associated with treatment response. Hechler et al. (2010c) investigated changes in coping with pain and their association to treatment response in 167 adolescents (aged 11–18 years). They found significant decreases in maladaptive coping strategies such as passive pain coping (such as the inability to change or improve the pain experience) and seeking social support (such as relying on others when in pain). Their regression model including changes in coping with pain and sex was able to explain 28 % of variance in changes in pain ratings and 34 % of variance in changes in pain-related disability. Decreases in maladaptive coping were significantly associated with positive treatment response. In addition, boys and girls differed with regard to these associations. Specifically, the interaction between sex and changes in seeking social support emerged as a significant predictor. Analyses revealed that a reduction in seeking social support was only related to a reduction in pain intensity in girls. To summarize, changes in maladaptive coping have been shown to be associated with positive treatment response. For girls, strategies for reducing seeking social support may be especially important to achieving decreases in pain ratings.

8.4.2.2 Willingness to Self-Manage Pain

The majority of interdisciplinary pain programs emphasize the child's self-management in that children are expected to participate actively in treatment and take over responsibility for their pain management (Simons et al. 2010). This philosophy often requires a profound change in the child's and parents' attitudes. Logan et al. (2012) recently investigated changes in readiness to change of the child and parents after intensive interdisciplinary pain treatment and associations of these changes with treatment response. They included 157 children with primarily neuropathic or musculoskeletal pain (aged 10–18 years). Results suggest a significant change in readiness to change in both children and parents (from precontemplation to activation) following treatment. In addition, these changes were positively associated with decreases in functional disability, depression, and fear of pain.

8.4.2.3 Psychological Flexibility

In contrast to CBT approaches, ACT for children with chronic pain aims to increase the child's ability to experience difficult emotions, thoughts, or pain sensations without avoidance behavior (Wicksell et al. 2009, 2011). Symptom reduction (i.e., pain reduction) is therefore not the primary treatment goal but rather to increase functioning in the presence of pain. It is assumed that increases in psychological flexibility, i.e., the capacity to engage in value-oriented behaviors while in the presence of potentially interfering pain and distress, mediate treatment outcome in ACT interventions. Wicksell et al. (2009) recently demonstrated in a group of 32 children with various pain conditions significant improvements in the group of children randomized to ACT. Significant differences were seen in pain impairment beliefs, pain interference, health-related quality of life, kinesiophobia, depression, and pain intensity when comparing the ACT group to a group receiving multidisciplinary pain treatment with amitriptyline. Multidisciplinary pain treatment was performed by a psychiatrist, a child psychologist, a physiotherapist, and a pain physician in an outpatient setting. Interventions included education on the pain problem, discussions of physical activity, relaxation and imagery techniques, physiotherapy sessions, contacts with the school, and goal setting. Over a 10-month period, children were seen for on average ten sessions, equally divided by the physician, physiotherapist, and psychiatrist/psychologist (Wicksell et al. 2009). Amitriptyline was administered over a 10-month period.

Wicksell et al. (2011) also showed that in the ACT group variables related to psychological flexibility (pain impairment beliefs and pain reactivity) mediated treatment response, while variables related to symptom reduction (pain intensity, catastrophizing) did not mediate treatment response. This confirms the importance of psychological flexibility as a process variable on treatment response.

8.4.3   Adherence to the Treatment Regimen

Adherence is usually defined as the extent to which a patient's behavior coincides with medical or health advice. Given that the intensive interdisciplinary pain programs require self-management of pain, and given that the child and the parents are often required to engage in multiple interventions (psychological interventions, changes in use of analgesics, physiotherapy), it is important to investigate adherence to these complex treatment regimens and its association to treatment response (Simons et al. 2010). In a sample of 57 adolescents with primarily musculoskeletal pain, Simons et al. (2010) found that adherence to multidisciplinary recommendations ranged from 50 to 100 %, with the highest level of adherence to physical therapy. They also found significant associations between adherence and treatment response. Specifically, adherence to psychological recommendations was associated with improvements in functioning and decreases in visits to medical doctors.

Conclusions

In the words of Eccleston et al. (2006), the skies are brightening with regard to evidence for the effectiveness of intensive interdisciplinary pain programs. These programs are on the rise worldwide. The summary of the eight existing studies showed significant and clinically relevant reductions – short term and long term – in primary outcome measures such as pain intensity, pain-related disability, and school absence. This is of importance given that children in need of intensive treatment are seriously affected in their lives and that their conditions are at risk of chronicity into adulthood (Zernikow et al. 2012). Potential factors in positive treatment response are changes in coping with pain, psychological flexibility, willingness to change, and adherence to the treatment regimen. Notwithstanding these positive developments, there remain important topics to be addressed in future research: First, evidence for effectiveness needs to be confirmed in appropriate study designs such as RCTs. Second, a grading system for paediatric chronic pain is warranted to enable treatment allocation in clinical practice. Third, the individual contribution of factors modulating treatment response is yet unknown. For example, do changes in pain coping and psychological flexibility exert similar effects on changes in outcome measures? How important for treatment response are changes in pain-specific emotions such as fear of pain? These future studies will provide important knowledge of mechanisms of change warranted for treatment conceptualization.

References

Arnold B, Brinkschmidt T, Casser HR, Gralow I, Irnich D, Klimczyk K, Müller G, Nagel B, Pfingsten M, Schiltenwolf M (2009) Multimodal pain therapy: principles and indications. Schmerz 23(2):112–120

Dobe M, Damschen U, Reiffer-Wiesel B, Sauer C, Zernikow B (2006) Multimodal inpatient pain treatment in children – results of a three-week program. Schmerz 20(1):51–60

Dobe M, Hechler T, Behlert J, Kosfelder J, Zernikow B (2011) Pain therapy with children and adolescents severely disabled due to chronic pain – long-term outcome after inpatient pain therapy. Schmerz 25(4):411–422

Eccleston C, Malleson P, Clinch J, Connell H, Sourbut C (2003) Chronic pain in adolescents: evaluation of a programme of interdisciplinary cognitive behaviour therapy. Arch Dis Child 88(10):881–885

Eccleston C, Jordan A, McCracken LM, Sleed M, Connell H, Clinch J (2005) The Bath Adolescent Pain Questionnaire (BAPQ): development and preliminary psychometric evaluation of an instrument to assess the impact of chronic pain on adolescents. Pain 118(1–2):263–270

Eccleston C, Connell H, Carmichael N (2006) Residential treatment settings for adolescent chronic pain management: rationale, development, and evidence. In: Finley A, McGrath PJ, Chambers CT (eds) Bringing pain relief to children: treatment approaches. Human Press, Totowa

Guzman J, Esmail R, Karjalainen K, Malmivaara A, Irvin E, Bombardier C (2002) Multidisciplinary bio-psycho-social rehabilitation for chronic low-back pain. Cochrane Database Syst Rev 1:CD000963

Hayes SC, Strosahl KD, Wilson KG (1999) Acceptance and commitment therapy: an experiential approach to behavior change. Guilford Press, New York

Hechler T (2011) Is multimodal treatment effective for children? – Problems and solutions for clinical trials for children with chronic pain. Conference proceeding. Der Schmerz 25(1)

Hechler T, Denecke H, Hünseler C, Schroeder S, Zernikow B (2009) Pain assessment. In: Zernikow B (ed) Pain therapy for children and adolescents. Springer, Heidelberg/Berlin

Hechler T, Blankenburg M, Dobe M, Kosfelder J, Hübner B, Zernikow B (2010a) Effectiveness of a multimodal inpatient treatment for pediatric chronic pain: a comparison between children and adolescents. Eur J Pain 14(1):e1–e9

Hechler T, Dobe M, Zernikow B (2010b) Commentary: a worldwide call for multimodal inpatient treatment for children and adolescents suffering from chronic pain and pain-related disability. J Pediatr Psychol 35(2):138–140

Hechler T, Kosfelder J, Vocks S, Mönninger T, Blankenburg M, Dobe M, Gerlach AL, Denecke H, Zernikow B (2010c) Changes in pain-related coping strategies and their importance for treatment outcome following multimodal inpatient treatment: does sex matter? J Pain 11(5):472–483

Hermann C, Hohmeister J, Zohsel K, Ebinger F, Flor H (2007) The assessment of pain coping and pain-related cognitions in children and adolescents: current methods and further development. J Pain 8(10):802–813

Hirschfeld G, Hechler T, Dobe M, Wager J, von Lützau P, Blankenburg M, Kosfelder J, Zernikow B (2013) Maintaining lasting improvements: one-year follow-up of children with severe chronic pain undergoing multimodal inpatient treatment. J Pediatr Psychol 38(2):224–236

Hübner B, Hechler T, Dobe M, Damschen U, Kosfelder J, Denecke H, Schroeder S, Zernikow B (2009) Pain-related disability in adolescents suffering from chronic pain: preliminary examination of the Pediatric Pain Disability Index (P-PDI). Schmerz 23(1):20–32

Huguet A, Miro J (2008) The severity of chronic paediatric pain: an epidemiological study. J Pain 9(3):226–236

Jacobson NS, Truax P (1991) Clinical significance: a statistical approach to defining meaningful change in psychotherapy research. J Consult Clin Psychol 59(1):12–19

Lanzi G, D'Arrigo S, Termine C, Rossi M, Ferrari-Ginevra O, Mongelli A, Millul A, Beghi E (2007) The effectiveness of hospitalization in the treatment of paediatric idiopathic headache patients. Psychopathology 40(1):1–7

Lee BH, Scharff L, Sethna NF, McCarthy CF, Scott-Sutherland J, Shea AM, Sullivan P, Meier P, Zurakowski D, Masek BJ, Berde CB (2002) Physical therapy and cognitive-behavioral treatment for complex regional pain syndromes. J Pediatr 141(1):135–140

Logan DE, Carpino EA, Chiang G, Condon M, Firn E, Gaughan VJ, Hogan M, Leslie DS, Olson K, Sager S (2012) A day-hospital approach to treatment of pediatric complex regional pain syndrome: initial functional outcomes. Clin J Pain 28(9):766–774

Lommel K, Bandyopadhyay A, Martin C, Kapoor S, Crofford L (2011) A pilot study of a combined intervention for management of juvenile primary fibromyalgia symptoms in adolescents in an inpatient psychiatric unit. Int J Adolesc Med Health 23(3):193–197

Maynard CS, Amari A, Wieczorek B, Christensen JR, Slifer KJ (2009) Interdisciplinary behavioral rehabilitation of pediatric pain-associated disability: retrospective review of an inpatient treatment protocol. J Pediatr Psychol 35(2):128–137

McGrath PJ, Walco GA, Turk DC, Dworkin RH, Brown MT, Davidson K, Eccleston C, Finley AG, Goldschneider K, Haverkos L, Hertz S, Ljungman G, Palermo T, Rappaport BA, Rhodes T, Schechter N, Scott J, Sethna NF, Svensson OK, Stinson J, von Baeyer CL, Walker L, Weisman S, White RE, Zajicek A, Zeltzer L (2008) Core outcome domains and measures for pediatric acute and chronic/recurrent pain clinical trials: PedIMMPACT recommendations. J Pain 9(9):771–783

Novy DM, Nelson DV, Francis DJ, Turk DC (1995) Perspectives of chronic pain: an evaluative comparison of restrictive and comprehensive models. Psychol Bull 118:238–247

Palermo TM, Scher MS (2001) Treatment of functional impairment in severe somatoform pain disorder: a case example. J Pediatr Psychol 26(7):429–434

Sherry DD, Wallace CA, Kelley C, Kidder M, Sapp L (1999) Short- and long-term outcomes of children with complex regional pain syndrome type I treated with exercise therapy. Clin J Pain 15(3):218–223

Simons LE, Logan DE, Chastain L, Cerullo M (2010) Engagement in multidisciplinary interventions for pediatric chronic pain: parental expectations, barriers, and child outcomes. Clin J Pain 26(4):291–299

Von Korff M, Ormel J, Keefe FJ, Dworkin SF (1992) Grading the severity of pain. Pain 50(2):133–149

Vowles KE, Jordan A, Eccleston C (2009) Toward a taxonomy of adolescents with chronic pain: exploratory and discriminant analyses of the Bath Adolescent Pain Questionnaire. Eur J Pain 14(2):214–221

Wager J, Hechler T, Darlington AS, Hirschfeld G, Vocks S, Zernikow B (2013) Classifying the severity of paediatric chronic pain - an application of the chronic pain grading. Eur J Pain. doi:10.1002/j.1532-2149.2013.00314.x. [Epub ahead of print]

Wicksell RK, Melin L, Lekander M, Olsson GL (2009) Evaluating the effectiveness of exposure and acceptance strategies to improve functioning and quality of life in longstanding pediatric pain – a randomized controlled trial. Pain 141(3):248–257

Wicksell RK, Olsson GL, Hayes SC (2011) Mediators of change in acceptance and commitment therapy for pediatric chronic pain. Pain 152(12):2792–2801

Zernikow B, Wager J, Hechler T, Hasan C, Rohr U, Dobe M, Meyer A, Hübner-Möhler B, Wamsler C, Blankenburg M (2012) Characteristics of highly impaired children with severe chronic pain: a 5-year retrospective study on 2249 pediatric pain patients. BMC Pediatr 12(1):54

Diagnostic Tools

9

Michael Dobe and Boris Zernikow

Contents

M. Dobe (✉)
German Paediatric Pain Centre (GPPC), Children's and Adolescents' Hospital,
Witten/Herdecke University, Dr.-Friedrich-Steiner Street 5, Datteln 45711, Germany
e-mail: m.dobe@kinderklinikdatteln.de

B. Zernikow
German Paediatric Pain Centre (GPPC),
Children's and Adolescents' Hospital, Witten/Herdecke University,
Dr.-Friedrich-Steiner Street 5, Datteln 45711, Germany

Chair Children's Pain Therapy and Paediatric Palliative Care,
Witten/Herdecke University, School of Medicine, Datteln 45711, Germany
e-mail: b.zernikow@deutsches-kinderschmerzzentrum.de

M. Dobe, B. Zernikow (eds.),
Practical Treatment Options for Chronic Pain in Children and Adolescents,
DOI 10.1007/978-3-642-37816-4_9, © Springer-Verlag Berlin Heidelberg 2013

The following pages present some diagnostic tools, the most important instructions for their use, and several worksheets used in our education.

The first six worksheets comprise two questionnaires on resources and stressful life events, a projective questionnaire, and three questionnaires just to become acquainted with the patient.

1. "Everything I judge as good" (A–Z)
2. "Everything I judge as bad" (A–Z)
3. "The 5 best events, the 5 worst events"
4. "Three things that should change soon…"
5. "'Wanted' poster"
6. "Complete the sentences"

The next 11 worksheets depict charts for psycho-education and instructions for certain therapeutic interventions.

7. "Distraction ABC"
8. "54321" technique for children and adolescents
9. Chart: attention to pain
10. Chart: distraction from pain
11. Chart: the vicious cycle of pain
12. "Describe your Safe Place"
13. Observation sheet for distraction strategies
14. Example Stress Day
15. List of pleasant activities
16. "That's me" poster
17. The three letters
18. Pain provocation

The last three worksheets refer to family interventions (Stress Test, parent's observation on the ward).

19. Observation sheet: Stress Test
20. Minutes – parent's observation on the ward: course of events
21. Minutes – parent's observation on the ward: reflection

9.1   Worksheet #1

"Everything I Judge as Good" (A–Z)

A	B
C	D
E	F
G	H
I	J
K	L
M	N
O	P
Q	R
S	T
U	V
W	X
Y	Z

9.2   Worksheet #2

"Everything I Judge as Bad" (A–Z)

A	B
C	D
E	F
G	H
I	J
K	L
M	N
O	P
Q	R
S	T
U	V
W	X
Y	Z

9.3   Worksheet #3

Which five events have been the best ones in your life so far?

Which five events have been the worst ones in your life so far?

9.4   Worksheet #4

Write down at least three things that should change soon.

Write down at least three things that shouldn't change at all.

Write down at least three things that should change soon but that take time to change.

9.5   Worksheet #5

"Wanted" Poster

Name:

Age:

Hobbies:

What I would like to learn:

What I can dispense with without difficulty:

What I wish for during my time on the ward:

Something weird I would like to do:

9.6 Worksheet #6

Name: Test supervisor: Date:

Please complete the following sentences:

Going to school is…

When I am grown up, I'd like to…

My father is…

The best I know…

I often dream about…

Having brothers and/or sisters…

The person making decisions within our family…

It is awful if…

The only thing I really fear…

I enjoy…

My mother is…

I'd like my father to…

In my opinion, my teacher…

My classmates…

The person preferred in our family…

My father is probably thinking that I…

I think my pain…

Name:	Test supervisor:	Date:

Please complete the following sentences:

If I don't obey…

If I could make decisions at home…

My mother is probably thinking that I…

What I don't like at all…

It is disgusting when…

What I like doing most is…

I get sad if…

The other boys/girls probably think I…

The worst thing I know…

I wish my mother…

If I could change myself…

If I had 100 euros then…

If three of my wishes came true:

   1st wish:

   2nd wish:

   3rd wish:

Which animal would you like to be?

Why?

Which animal would you not like to be?

Why?

What would you like to do by profession?

Why?

9.7 Worksheet #7

"Distraction ABC"

The distraction ABC is one of the most effective distraction techniques available for children with pain. It may be adapted to the abilities and preferences of every child and combined with nearly every other pain reduction technique. With increasing expertise, older children develop unique variants of this technique tailored to their specific skills and habits of distraction. Hence, teaching this method is complex and requires a very creative therapist. He/she should not focus too much on a fixed plan but should rather explore the individual abilities, resources, and spontaneous suggestions of the patient. The exploration of failures will offer valuable hints for the development of more individual and effective variants. As a rule of thumb, a distraction score of 7 and up (scale 0–10 (0, no distraction at all; 10, totally absorbed by the exercise, I don't take notice of my environment at all)) indicates that the exercise is perceived as helpful. A distraction score of 5–6 refers to a pain reduction of about 1 score (NRS, 0–10); a distraction score of 7–8 refers to a pain reduction of about 2 scores (NRS, 0–10); a distraction score of 9–10 refers to a pain reduction of about

3 scores (NRS, 0–10). By no means should one query the effect on pain directly, because this bears the risk of classical conditioning.

After the technique has been presented by the therapist, the child and therapist develop suitable variants. These are tested together once. The homework then is to perform and document the distraction ABC at least four times. For documentation, a sheet of paper with the columns (1) time, (2) type of ABC, and (3) distraction score (0–10) is used. If the exercise is complex enough, the technique may be suitable for controlling flashbacks, stopping thoughts, and reducing fear in children with high fear sensitivity.

Step 1

In the first and simplest step, the child is instructed to find any item matching a chosen topic for each letter of the alphabet from A to Z.

1. Topics may be specific such as animals, horse breeds, foods, things we like/dislike, swear words, or "things one is noticing or hearing."
2. The "Chaos ABC" is well suited to children in need of a fast distraction. For this exercise, the first association matching the respective letter is taken. In our experience, it is advisable to exclude the topic "animals," since the task is too easy otherwise. In a variant of the exercise, using an item more than once is not allowed, making the course of the exercise more demanding. Some children feel more distracted if the "Chaos ABC" is carried out repeatedly or with time pressure.
3. Performing the "Chaos ABC" in various languages (i.e., English, Spanish, French…) is another variant of the game.
4. Children like the variant in which each sentence or poem starts with the respective letter (variant: The sentences are not logically connected; the poem has/doesn't have meter).
5. The math whiz may like the variant looking for numbers in a logical sequence (e.g., $1,000 - 1^1$, -2^2, -3^3, and -4^4 up to say $-1,000$, then in reverse up to $+1,000$).

Step 2

In the second step, a sensory channel (visual, auditory, haptic, olfactory, gustatory) is added to verbalization. This will result in a higher degree of distraction in most children. This can only be done successfully if the child is able to sufficiently imagine that channel. A child with difficulties in figurative imagination should, for example, avoid the visual channel.

1. If the first exercises from step 1 fail to reach sufficient distraction (distraction score of 7 and up out of 10), the additional visualization (or imagination of animal noises) will increase the degree of distraction.
2. For step 2, some children like to "google in their head." This means to freely associate words and images to a given item starting with the respective letter (A–Z), similar to a search engine's list of hits. *For example*, given letter: D; associated word: dog. The child can now search for hits, verbal and figurative images (e.g., dog tag, dog breed; puppy; hot dog).
3. Another popular variant is the "jukebox." The child has to find a music title, artist, or album matching the given letter (A–Z). Then he/she has to play a 10-, 20-, or 30-s clip of the title song, another song of the artist, or of the album in his/her head.

4. Another task is to find sequences of a movie instead of music ("brain TV"). Younger children may alternatively watch the animals from animal ABC in their "brain TV" (freeze image or movie).

Step 3

In the third step, two or more sensory channels (visual, auditory, haptic, olfactory, gustatory) are added to verbalization. Techniques of step 3 are rarely applied right away. Usually they emerge while doing exercises from the previous steps, for instance if the degree of distraction is too low or if the children unleash their creativity.

1. The "jukebox" might be upgraded by superimposing the lyrics.
2. A bit more complex is the "music clip." In this exercise, the "jukebox" is combined with "brain TV" (such as Viva or MTV).
3. Two fun but very complex variants are "X-ray" and "camera." In "X-ray," the child watches a memory, a movie, a performance, or a current visual stimulus through an X-ray device (this can also be watched on mobile phones or smart phone). In "camera," everything that is happening (including the child performing the exercise) is seen through a camera's perspective. The resulting alienation or distancing can also be used to emotionally stabilize a traumatized child.
4. Although much less technical, the variant involving animals (visual imagination of the animal, hearing its sounds, stroking the animal, huddle against the animal) is very popular. This variant can only be practiced if the child has a good enough kinesthetic imagination.

Step 4

In step 4, the techniques proven helpful during steps 1–3 are combined with another technique (e.g., the Safe Place). That step is especially helpful for children with a comorbid trauma disorder who need both a higher degree of distraction and emotional stabilization and who have an excellent figurative imagination. The techniques of step 4 are very complex and require a lot of creativity and figurative imagination. The exercises need to be presented very clearly. The best way is to describe the examples from below as one *possible* way to perform this exercise. Most children will react spontaneously and unambiguously ("That sounds tiring," or "Great, I've already got an idea"). Different examples for this step are listed below.

1. Notice things you see, hear, or feel in your Safe Place (Sect. 6.4.2) starting with a given letter (A–Z).
2. Perform an ABC to a given theme in turn with the help of an "inner helper" (e.g., Pain Fighter) (Sect. 6.4.2). A more complex variant is to invite your "inner helper" to a nice place and search for items starting with the respective letter (A–Z) in turn.
3. Use the "screening technique" (Sect. 6.5.2) to look for funny/beautiful/relaxing movies/documentaries/etc. on "TV."

It is very rare that a child cannot perform the distraction ABC at all after a detailed description of the exercise and after having understood the vicious cycle of pain during education. Inadequate education excluded, this may indicate severe depressive symptomatology or a high degree of somatic fixation ($\rightarrow$ "If I am convinced that I am severely ill, I am not interested in techniques meant to reduce my symptoms, because this won't help me to get rid of my illness.").

9.8 Worksheet #8

"54321": Technique for Children and Adolescents

Instruction

Make yourself as comfortable as possible. Keep your eyes open for now. The only important thing is that you focus on what you are seeing, hearing, or feeling. Since we humans are lousy observers, this exercise may be more difficult for you than it sounds. However, it may also well happen that you succeed at once.

The Technique

Go over the things you notice right now in your head. It is also okay to just focus on your current perception.

5 times: **I am seeing**…! $\rightarrow$	5 times: **I am hearing**…! $\rightarrow$	5 times: **I am feeling**…! $\rightarrow$
4 times: **I am seeing**…! $\rightarrow$	4 times: **I am hearing**…! $\rightarrow$	4 times: **I am feeling**…! $\rightarrow$
3 times: **I am seeing**…! $\rightarrow$	3 times: **I am hearing**…! $\rightarrow$	3 times: **I am feeling**…! $\rightarrow$
2 times: **I am seeing**…! $\rightarrow$	2 times: **I am hearing**…! $\rightarrow$	2 times: **I am feeling**…! $\rightarrow$
1 time: **I am seeing**…! $\rightarrow$	1 time: **I am hearing**…! $\rightarrow$	1 time: **I am feeling**…!

1. It is all right to repeatedly name the same thing.
2. If a noise is distracting you while observing things you see, just switch your observations to the auditory channel.
3. Don't worry if the exercise gets out of sequence. This shows that you are doing a good job.
4. Speaking aloud and listening to one's own voice may help in performing the exercise.
5. The sequence of 54321 is nothing but a suggestion. Any combination is possible. For instance, you could focus on seeing, listening, and feeling in sequence.
6. Try different paces and stick to the one that suits you best.
7. For some children, it is easier to focus on more than one sensory channel at the same time. Others find it more pleasant to focus on just one channel.

(54321-technique, modified for use in children and adolescents (original in German language: Steffen Bambach (2003), http://www.traumatherapie.de/users/bambach/index.html)

9.9   Worksheet #9

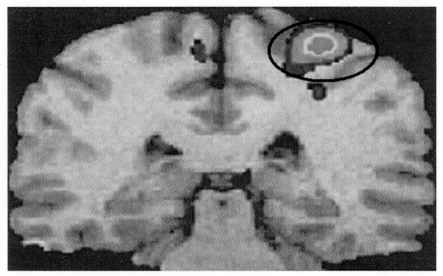

Attention to Pain

Taken from: Dobe M, Zernikow B (2013) "How to stop chronic pain in children: a practical guide." Carl-Auer-Verlag, Heidelberg. Printed with permission (Modified after Bushnell et al. 1999)

9.10   Worksheet #10

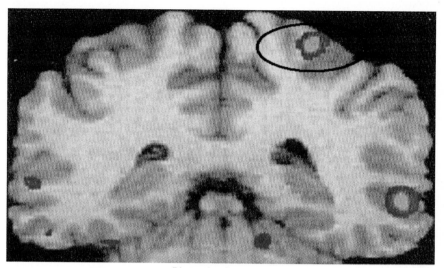

Distraction from Pain

Taken from: Dobe M, Zernikow B (2013) "How to stop chronic pain in children: a practical guide." Carl-Auer-Verlag, Heidelberg. Printed with permission (Modified after Bushnell et al. 1999)

9.11   Worksheet #11

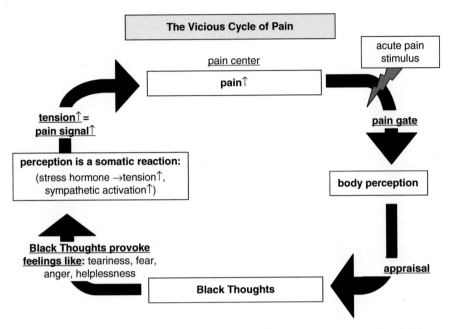

Modified from: Dobe M, Zernikow B (2013) "How to stop chronic pain in children: a practical guide." Carl-Auer-Verlag, Heidelberg. Printed with permission.

9.12   Worksheet #12

Describe Your Safe Place!

What can you see there?

What can you hear?

| Describe Your Safe Place! |
| What can you smell? |

| What can you do there? |

| What can you feel? |

| Which mood are you in? |

9.13   Worksheet #13

Observation Sheet for Distraction Strategies

When (time)?	Which technique?	Distraction score (0–10)?
For example, 8:45 am	ABC (double chaos)	6–7
For example, 10:10 am	ABC (jukebox)	8
For example, 1:45 pm	54321 (seeing, listening, feeling each quality once, fast, went over it in my head)	7

9.14   Worksheet #14

Tanja's Stress Day

In the following, we describe an example Stress Day on our ward (see Sect. 6.4.5.3). The Stress Day is discussed with the patient and his/her parents in advance. It is important that the child receives a detailed list of tasks for the day including a time schedule. In order to "stress" the child, a Stress Day comprises a high number of tasks.

Importantly, the child has the chance to take a break. He/she receives a certain number of "time-out cards" that allow a 10-min break at any chosen time, for instance, to practice a stress- or pain-reducing technique. Of course, the child is allowed to interrupt the Stress Day anytime. This is very important so that the child is always in control of the situation.

6.00	Get up, wash, and tidy up your room.
6.20	Wake up the other children.
6:45	Check if all other children are up.
6:47	Room check (all beds should be made).
6:48	Collect any pain questionnaires still missing from the other patients.
6:50	Set the table for both groups.
7:20	Rate your "Mood Barometer."
7:22	Call all patients for the morning round. Call the NET. Conduct the morning round. Distribute the notes with the scheduled appointments.
7:30	Breakfast (if any item is missing on the table, you have to get it).
8:00	Clean the table for both groups.
8:15	Set up a biography for 3 of your nurses (you may chose for whom).
9:00	See that all children pack their bathing suits.
9:10	Take all children to the swimming lesson.
10:15	See that each child hangs up and dries his/her bathing suit and bath towel.
10:20	Walk along the hall, singing a child's song aloud.
10:25	Tidy up your room and have it checked by a nurse.
10:30	Stand outside the nurse's room for at least 10 min and ask the nurses passing by various questions.
10:40	Look for the book "Wizard of Oz" on the book shelf, make a short summary, and present it to the nurses during a nurse meeting.
10:55	Count all lighthouses on the ward and give the number to the nurses.
11:05	Query 3 nurses or therapists on what they like about you.
11:15	Set the table: clear out the cart from the kitchen, and heat up the food in the microwave.
11:30	Lunch time (if any item is missing on the table, you have to get it).
11:50	Clean the table for both groups.
12:00	Rate your "Mood Barometer." Call all children for the group session.
12:10	Group therapy.
13:00	Prepare the seagull table for coffee time.
13:15	Break time spent in the patient's room. See that all children go to their room and engage in something quiet.
13:20	Write a French text (1 sheet) on "How to cope with chronic pain" and hand it to your nurse.
14.00	Rate your "Mood Barometer."
14.05	Biofeedback therapy.
14.30	Single therapeutic session.
15:15	Organize the joint afternoon for all children.
17:30	Set the table for both groups.
17.55	Rate your "Mood Barometer."

18:00	Dinner (if any item is missing on the table, you have to get it).
18:30	Clean the table for both groups.
18:40	Collect any pain questionnaires still missing from the other patients.
18:45	Prepare a plate of fruits and vegetables for the late-night snack.
18:55	Call all children for the evening round.
19:00	Conduct the evening and "beef" round.

Congratulations. You did it!

9.15   Worksheet #15

List of Pleasant Activities
- Sleeping
- Reading a book
- Listening to music
- Tabletop soccer
- Going for a 20-min run
- Polishing toenails
- Polishing fingernails
- Trying a new haircut or a new hairstyle
- Visiting the hairdresser
- Enjoying a face mask
- Body peeling with salt/oil/peeling
- Taking a bath
- Spending time at your PC/tablet
- Making a phone call
- Taking pictures
- Browsing through photographs
- Setting up a photo album
- Writing a letter
- Doing my make-up
- Buying something
- Going shopping
- Buying a newspaper/magazine/comic or reading a novel
- Watching TV
- Borrowing a DVD, watching a DVD
- Cooking or baking something tremendous
- PMR or autogenic training
- Listening to the radio
- Doing a crossword puzzle, sudoku, etc.
- Chatting
- Tinkering
- Painting using Window Color
- Playing soccer

- Playing basketball
- Kidding around
- Contacting friends using my smartphone
- Going for a walk
- Playing a board game
- Playing cards
- Making music
- Playing Nintendo, DS, PSP
- Lying in the sun/in bed/elsewhere, snuggling and dreaming
- Playing the piano
- Painting
- Going for a swim
- Collecting things outdoors (flowers, stones, sticks, chestnuts, etc.)
- Getting a massage
- Taking a really warm shower
- Writing a story
- Listening to a story being read out for me
- Meeting a friend
- Decorating my room
- Going for a stroll
- Visiting the playground
- Having tea and cookies
- Arranging photographs
- Playing with LEGO/Playmobil
- Swinging
- Picking flowers or buying flowers
- Paying someone a compliment
- Playing Sing Star
- Playing Wii console
- Riding my bicycle
- Setting up night lights and enjoying the beautiful atmosphere
- Knitting
- Tidying up the clothes closet and sorting out clothes
- Looking through the window and watching what is happening outside
- Singing
- Visiting someone
- Gardening
- Visiting an ice cream parlor and having an ice cream
- Planning my holidays
- Making oneself up and going out
- Arranging shelves and looking at all the things on them
- Kneading
- Enjoying a piece of chocolate
- Practicing a distraction technique
- Staying at a friend's house overnight

- Planning and preparing a party
- Boxing
- Relaxing
- Surfing the Internet

9.16 Worksheet #16

"That's me" Poster

Please set up a picture, a collage, or something similar, showing your:
- Characteristics
- Skills
- Previous successes
- Wishes/dreams
- Friends/family
- Other things important to you

   Feel free to choose any style or any type of artwork (painting, writing, photograph, symbols, etc.).

9.17 Worksheet #17

The Three Letters

Dear _____, I would like to give a brief introduction to a somewhat more extensive exercise. It will help you to better grasp your abilities and skills. It will also make clear in which aspects you could still need some support from us or someone else in order to reach your goals.

   The main exercise is to write 3 letters. As you can imagine, these letters are not letters as "usual" but letters in which you scrutinize and anticipate yourself and your life with much detail. I would also like to point out what kind of side effects writing these letters might have. Since you will look at all important aspects of your life with much more detail than usual, you will be able to see some issues much more clearly. Apart from the chance to reach your personal goals more precisely, this also means that you may see any obstacles on your way to reaching these goals much more clearly. This realization and clarity is *irreversible*. Is this a risk you are willing to accept? Or would you like to ponder it for a while? (In case of unambiguous acceptance, proceed with this introduction. Otherwise, support the child to find his/her answer, e.g., by using a list of pros and cons.) Well then, now I will explain the content of the three letters. Please feel free to interrupt me immediately in case of any question.

   Let's start with an essential point: The letters should cover *all* important areas of your life, e.g., apart from your pain, they should cover your family, friends, relationship, leisure time activities, school, future, and everything that is important to you. This means you will need at least 1 page to describe everything. Of course, some children manage to say everything in just half a page, but most children need more than one. Is that doable for you? Okay, here is another important point: Between letter 1 and letter 2, you may take a break of hours or even some days; that doesn't matter. But, having finished letter 2, you should directly proceed to letter 3 (of course, a few minutes' break is allowed). It is very important to write letter 3 immediately after letter 2. This means, for letter 2 and 3 together, you have to take at least 2 h in order to avoid getting pressed for time. Is that doable for you? When we get to the letter content, I will explain why that is so important. Okay, now I will explain the different letters' content in detail.

Letter 1. In this letter, you describe the ideal course of your life after this appointment (alternatively: inpatient therapy, outpatient psychotherapy…) for the next 2 years to come (alternatively: until your next birthday, your next but one birthday, your 18th birthday, any other special events in the future…). The most difficult thing is to write the letter from that date in the future using a first-person perspective and addressing it to yourself in the present (e.g., "Dear _____, 2 years have passed since you opted for the inpatient pain therapy. Since then…."). In order for this exercise to work, the letter should be as detailed as possible, describing the development of *all* relevant areas of your life (e.g., not only pain but also friends, relationship, school, family, leisure time activities). Moreover, you should describe which decisions, judgements, and behavior made your life go in that direction; only focus on those aspects that you performed on *your own* (so refrain from telling about winning the lottery or that suddenly everyone has been so nice, but instead describe exclusively *your own* changes and efforts). Do you understand the instructions? Or are there any questions left?

Letter 2. Letter 2, in a way, is the counterpart of letter 1. In this second letter, you report to yourself the worst possible course of your life from the future. The procedure is analogous to that from the first letter ("Dear _____, since your last stay on the ward, everything turned out for the worse. You decided to…"). You should describe as realistically as possible which of *your own* decisions, judgements, and behaviors contributed to that catastrophic development. The aim of the letter is to make you ponder what would be the worst imaginable course *for you* with respect to pain, family, friends, relationship, leisure time activities, etc. (for clarification: not the worst thinkable course but the worst course imaginable for *your* development). After having finished letter 2, don't forget to immediately proceed with letter 3. If you are under time pressure when starting with letter 2, it's better to not start with it until you are sure you will have enough time to also finish letter 3. Otherwise letter 2 will remain in your memory for too long, which will definitely be unpleasant. Is that doable for you? Are you sure you will be able to proceed with letter 3 immediately after having finished letter 2, no matter how you will be feeling then?

Letter 3. Most children think letter 3 is the most difficult one to write. It is not too difficult to imagine the best possible or the worst possible scenario, but it is a real challenge to imagine a realistic course (a probability of at least 50.1 % that something will happen) taking into account one's personality and perception of one's own abilities. And letter 3 aims exactly for that: to tie yourself down to a course as realistic as possible. The formal content and structure of letter 3 are no different to those of letter 1 and 2. The point is to tie yourself down with regard to each relevant aspect of your life between the extremes of letter 1 and letter 2 in order to describe a realistic course *from your point of view*.

9.18 Worksheet #18

Pain Provocation (Instruction)

"By now you know how to influence your pain a little bit. You also know you could increase your pain at will. In order to do so you have to focus on the current (or usually) most painful area of your body (remember the vicious cycle of pain). How long do you think it takes for the pain to increase if you are simultaneously thinking black thoughts associated with your pain? (Wait for the answer.) Some patients succeed at once; some need a few minutes. It is important for me that you know that with this exercise we will ONLY provoke pain that is stored in your cerebral pain memory. As we discussed previously, your brain has difficulties distinguishing between the different components of pain (pain due to tissue damage/inflammation; mood; attention; memory). Hence, the only thing you perceive during this exercise is a more or less slow increase of your pain.

At the beginning of the exercise, pain intensity should increase by just one score. Please focus on the area where your pain is (usually) worst, and think of black thoughts associated with the pain. As soon as the pain intensity has increased by one score, please say aloud 'STOP.' Please apply the distraction technique(s) that proved most helpful so far (e.g., distraction ABC, 54321 technique, colored thoughts, or Safe Place) *immediately* afterwards. As soon as pain intensity is back down to its starting point, repeat the exercise once in order to exclude any random effect and to gain more experience with the exercise. If you think you are not making any progress, please don't hesitate to ask me for support. Can I count on that? (Wait for the patient to confirm.) You still know the STOP signal? (Wait for the patient to confirm and demonstrate.) Can I definitely count on you using that STOP signal? (Wait for the patient to confirm.) Is everything 100 % clear? (Wait for the patient to confirm. If there is even the slightest hesitation, do query at once what remains unclear.) You tell me when you want to start."

9.19 Worksheet #19

Observation Sheet: Stress Test
Aims agreed on:
Child/adolescent: *Parents*:
If any therapeutic agreement cannot be realized (e.g., attending school at home), please inform the ward by phone as soon as possible.
For best cooperation, we ask you to answer the following questions:
What worked out best during the Stress Test?
Child/adolescent: *Parents*:

Observation Sheet: Stress Test

What turned out to be especially difficult?

Child/adolescent: *Parents*:

Aims for the next Stress Test:

Child/adolescent: *Parents*:

Wishes for us:

Current permanent medication:

Current medication on demand:

We wish you a pleasant Stress Test. – Your pain team

9.20 Worksheet #20

Parent's Observation on the Ward: Course of Events

Date/time (start/end):

Child's name:

Nurse's name:

Morning shift (MS):

Afternoon shift (AS):

Name of the guest (parent):

Aims of the observation on the ward:

•

•

•

•

•

Planned schedule for the day:

9.21 Worksheet #21

Parent's Observation on the Ward: Reflection

	Parents	Nurse (NET)
MS		
AS		

MS morning shift, *AS* afternoon shift

Reference

Bushnell MC, Duncan GH, Hofbauer RK, Ha B, Chen JI, Carrier B (1999) Pain perception: is there a role for primary somatosensory cortex? Proc Natl Acad Sci USA 96(14):7705–7709

Printed by Printforce, the Netherlands